Psychosocial Aspects of Cardiovascular Disease

Psychosocial Aspects of Cardiovascular Disease

The Life-Threatened Patient, the Family, and the Staff

Edited by:

James Reiffel
Robert DeBellis
Lester C. Mark
Austin H. Kutscher
Paul R. Patterson
and Bernard Schoenberg

with the editorial assistance of
Lillian G. Kutscher

Columbia University Press • New York • 1980

Library of Congress Cataloging in Publication Data

Main entry under title:

Psychosocial aspects of cardiovascular disease.

Includes Bibliographies and Index
    1. Cardiovascular system—Diseases—Psycho-
logical aspects.   2. Cardiovascular system—
Diseases—Social aspects.   3. Terminal care—
Psychological aspects.   4. Terminal care—Social
aspects.   I. Reiffel, James.   II. Kutscher,
Lillian G. [DNLM: 1. Attitude to death.
2. Cardiovascular diseases—Psychology.
3. Terminal care. WG100 P9735]
RC669.P79   616.1'001'9   79-27765
ISBN 0-231-04354-6

Columbia University Press
New York   Guildford, Surrey

✻ Acknowledgment

THE EDITORS WISH to acknowledge the support and encouragement of the Foundation of Thanatology in the preparation of this volume. All royalties from the sale of this book are assigned to the Foundation of Thanatology, a tax exempt, not for profit, public scientific and educational foundation.

Thanatology, a new subspecialty of medicine, is involved in scientific and humanistic inquiries and the application of the knowledge derived therefrom to the subjects of the psychological aspects of dying; reactions to loss, death, and grief; and recovery from bereavement.

The Foundation of Thanatology is dedicated to advancing the cause of enlightened health care for the terminally ill patient and his family. The Foundation's orientation is a positive one based on the philosophy of fostering a more mature acceptance and understanding of death and the problems of grief and the more effective and humane management and treatment of the dying patient and his bereaved family members.

Acknowledgment

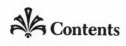 **Contents**

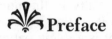 **Preface**

In conceiving this volume to introduce a thanatologic perspective on cardiovascular disease, the editors were aware that previous models proposed for the psychosocial care of life-threatened patients, the members of their families, their caregivers, and their survivors have focused on approaches designed for the cancer patient. Differentiations were not made to accommodate either individuals with other disease involvements or with the professionals who offered specialized care. Although it should be obvious that no universal design for care can be imposed on patients, their families, and their caregivers, popular attention has nevertheless been attracted to a cancer paradigm of discrete stages leading eventually to death—even though in the United States, the mortality rate for cardiovascular disease is approximately 66 percent as opposed to that of 16 percent for malignant disease.

The psychosocial differences between cardiovascular patients and cancer patients surface not only in relation to the impact of the symptomatology affecting these individuals but also in relation to the basic theoretical, practical, emotional, moral, and ethical issues inherent in each particular disease entity. The range in therapeutic modalities employed in the treatment of these two categories of pathology relate to each other in reverse order. For example, the primary approach to malignant disease is generally through surgery, followed thereafter by radiation therapy or chemotherapy, and, perhaps, at a time of the disease's recurrence, by whichever of these curative or palliative measures seem to be indicated. For cardiovascular disease, surgical procedures are generally measures of last resort. The patient stricken with hypertensive disease, congestive heart failure, a cardiac infarct, rheumatic heart disease, a cerebral or pulmonary embolus, or end-stage cardiovascular disease can often be treated with pharmacotherapeutic agents that control acute or chronic malfunctions or disabilities. Only when these fail to control symptoms in the specific systems affected are invasive therapeutic measures considered or performed.

Most of the literature describing the terminal trajectory of patients is specific to cancer, and theories of psychotherapeutic intervention emphasize the maintenance of quality in the numbered days of life that remain. Subtle though it is, the prevalent undercurrent connotes that the cancer patient is a dying patient whether or not he or she truly is. For the cardiovascular patient, as this book gives testimony, the goal is adaptation to life regardless of the deficit from the pre-disease physical state and performance levels. Utmost assurance is provided so that this patient does not become "crippled" by symptoms or diagnosis. Indeed, the "approach" is that the cardiovascular patient may well live as complete a life—and for a decent span of years—even though professional care and medications become a routine part of this life. While the atmosphere of the cardiac intensive care unit can be threatening, it is also reassuring; the attitudes of its staff are optimistic in terms of predicting long-range survival. Cardiologists themselves, to generalize, appear to have a more positive demeanor than do their professional counterparts in the field of oncology. Once having left the hospital to return home, the cardiac patient is rarely considered to be a dying patient.

Included among the authors of this book are cardiologists, cardiac surgeons, nurses, and patients themselves. It is the feeling of the editors that what may be interpreted as a form of denial in the way the contributors accept cardiovascular disease is more the glow of optimism which acknowledges the success of caregivers and patients in coping with the problems and issues of therapy. While the above cited mortality data cannot be faulted, their interpretation should take into account the fact that our population is living longer and that, inevitably, stages of system failures must be reached.

The issues addressed in this book should serve a wide audience, including not only the general physician, the cardiovascular specialist, the nurse, the social worker, and other professionals but also the patient and those members of the family who learn to live in an environment that, although not completely free from stress, does not always echo with the threat of disaster. Even when death occurs, grief can be tempered by those gratifications that have accrued when life goals have been fulfilled and when years of living in comfort have been given the patient stricken with cardiovascular disease.

The Editors

The editors acknowledge with much appreciation the wise counsel and guidance of many individuals who assisted in the planning of this book. In particular, they would like to give recognition to the contributions of Dr. Frederick O. Bowman, Jr., and the late Drs. Henry O. Heinemann and Nathan Lefkowitz.

Introduction: Principles of Thanatology

Arthur C. Carr

Preamble: Simply by being human, we are confronted with experiences related to death and dying. Consequently, a healthy view of life recognizes the finite nature of our lives and affirms death as an inevitable part of the living process.

Principle 1: A Healthy Outlook on Life Necessarily Comprehends Death

Preamble: Although forces in our culture seem to lead on the one hand to repression and denial, and on the other to exploitation and sensationalism, death and dying should ideally be accepted as inevitable aspects of reality that need not be imbued with anxiety and fear.

Principle 2: Death and Dying Are Not and Should Not Be Taboo Topics

Preamble: Since death and dying have traditionally been taboo topics in our culture, the logical means of combating the influences of repression, denial, exploitation, and sensationalism is through education. Education at all levels is indicated, beginning in kindergarten and continuing through courses for the mature adult and the aged. Training should be related, where appropriate, to all aspects and ramifications of death and dying, including loss and grief, care of the terminally ill, and recovery from bereavement—that is, to the discipline of *Thanatology*.

Principle 3: Education in Thanatology Is Necessary

Preamble: While the medical profession is usually most intimately involved with care of the dying patient, a continuous program of education in Thanatology requires a multidisciplinary approach that unites nursing, social work, philosophy, psychology, psychiatry, and religion, as well as other professional and lay groups. The development of adequate programs in the sensitive areas of Thanatology requires service, training, and research workers.

Principle 4: Education in Thanatology Requires a Multidisciplinary Approach

Preamble: Dying patients should neither be abandoned nor exploited. They are entitled to the same respectful care as those patients who are expected to fully recover. They should be given, where this is appropriate, information about their illness and treatment, and know that they have the right to refuse treatment. Confidentiality should always be respected. Care should be responsive and considerate and should always be given by qualified personnel.

Principle 5: Dying Patients Have Human Rights That Should Be Respected

Preamble: While the circumstances surrounding dying vary greatly, the care of dying patients should give emphasis to their psychosocial as well as to their physical needs. In usual circumstances, patients should be entitled to a relatively pain-free death, and with the maximum maintenance of control of self and self-esteem—in short, since death with dignity often seems hardly achievable, the goal to be sought should be death with as few indignities as possible.

Principle 6: An Ultimate Ideal in the Care of Dying Patients Should Be That of Death without Indignity

Preamble: Earlier formulations in Thanatology may have created the impression that terminally ill patients always know or always should be told they are dying. While patients differ greatly in their ability, need, or desire to acknowledge imminent death, the concept "death without indignity" subsumes the right of patients to express, or not to express, their fears, hopes, gratitudes, and dissatisfactions about their fate. Therefore, absence of shared communication about dying should maximally reflect the patient's choice, or circumstances, rather than the anxieties or impatience of caregivers and relatives.

Principle 7: Death without Indignity is Most Likely to Occur in an Atmosphere of Open Communication

Preamble: The capacity of one person to form an affiliation with another carries with it the potential for grief and mourning when that affiliation or relationship is broken. These reactions can be observed even in the very young child. Thus, there is nothing unusual or abnormal about grief and mourning among relatives after the death of a loved person.

Principle 8: Bereavement is a Normal Response to the Death of a Loved One

Preamble: Bereaved persons should not be exploited; nor should they have to experience undue loss to their own self-esteem. These goals are most likely to be achieved when the bereaved have had information concerning the illness and treatment of the patient, when the patient has experienced death without indignity, and when communication surrounding the patient's dying has been marked by clarity, candor, and compassion.

Principle 9: Bereaved Persons Have Rights That Should Be Respected

Preamble: Bereaved persons bring special physical and psychological needs to the health-care professional; these needs should not be ignored. Among the effects of bereavement are disruptions of normal bodily and sensory reactions, loss of appetite, tearfulness, insomnia, feelings of numbness, fatigue, irritability, and diminished sexual interest—all these occur and support the contention that a grieving person is in a physically vulnerable state that may include a susceptibility to other illnesses.

Principle 10: Although a Normal Response, Bereavement Has Physiological and Psychological Manifestations That Qualify It Symptomatically as a Temporary Illness

Preamble: The course of bereavement is usually predictable and is characterized, in time, by a returning of the person to a state of productivity and well-being, even if not totally unaffected by the nature and the extent of the loss. When, in addition to expected depression, the reaction includes undue loss of self-esteem, feelings of self-condemnation, suicidal thoughts, or grief that is inappropriate to the occasion, special professional assistance may be necessary.

Principle 11: Especially Severe Reactions to Bereavement May Require Special Professional Care

Preamble: The overwhelming context of Thanatology resides primarily in approaching what should be the ideal routine doctor–patient–family care relationships, such care forming the indispensable base upon which the core of care specific to Thanatology can and will easily be extended.

Principle 12: The Essence of Good Thanatologic Care Is Good Patient Care

Summary Preamble: Thanatology encompasses the broad areas of death and dying, loss and grief, and the accompanying issues and problems. It stresses the need for comprehending dying as part of a healthy outlook on living. It emphasizes the need for education and communication in these sensitive areas. It stresses the rights and needs of dying patients and their families to competent, considerate care responsive to their particular physical and psychosocial needs. It recognizes the necessity for new and better approaches to the care of the dying and the bereaved. It encourages inquiry into how attitudes and approaches to loss, grief, death, and dying can lead to fuller, happier living.

Summary Principle: Thanatology Is Both an Art and a Science. As an Art, It Emphasizes Humanistic Approaches to Death, Dying, and Bereavement. As a Science, It Stresses the Need for Education, Inquiry, Systematic Investigation, and Research in Approaching These Once Taboo Topics.

Part I
Psychosocial Aspects of Care

1
Care of the Patient with Coronary Heart Disease

H. D. Ruskin

THE MOST DRAMATIC clinical manifestation of coronary heart disease is the onset of acute myocardial infarction. On the assumption that the stricken individual survives long enough to reach a hospital, it is now customary for such patients to be treated in coronary care units suitably equipped and staffed. The psychological implications of a life-threatening illness which may occur with little or no warning have been clearly documented by Hackett and Cassem (1972) in their studies of coronary care patients and amplified more recently by Pranulis (1975). The nursing staff of these units should consist of highly trained individuals who are knowledgeable in the field of cardiology and alert to the psychological needs of their patients. It is not enough for professionals to be able to recognize and treat arrhythmias, they must also be able to cope with varying degrees of anxiety, denial, or depression.

The Coronary Care Unit and Its Staff

The nursing staff serves many additional functions, not the least of which is to form a positive and supportive relationship with the patient's family. One might expect that the patient's physician would provide such support, but the amount of time he can spend with each patient and his family is minimal, whereas the coronary-care staff is always available, has close contact with the patient at all times, and can do a great deal to bolster the family. An important staff function is teaching both patient and family what a heart attack really means. Patients and their families do not always understand what actually took place. Their ignorance may continue indefinitely, although the illness has probably changed their whole lives.

Working in community hospitals without a trained resident staff, coronary-care nurses have to assume great responsibility in the management of this unpredictable disease. Consequently, they are frequently more knowledgeable than many of the attending physicians. Some doctors are able to accept suggestions from skilled nurses, while others feel threatened, so that coronary-care personnel may have to exercise great tact in order that the patient's well-being remains paramount. Despite every effort, difficult situations do arise and the cardiologist in charge of the unit may have to intervene. Clearly, the nursing staff acts as a central pivot for patient, family, and physician. The importance of the nurse's role is frequently recognized by patients who continue to praise them long after discharge from hospital. Such praise is well deserved. My experience has been that almost all the coronary-care nurses that I have trained, and later worked with, turn out to be part of a rather special group, showing great pride in their role.

In coping with a patient's spouse and his or her reaction to the news of what must correctly be perceived as a major threat to life, the physician may be met with an entire range of reactions extending from disbelief to acute anxiety. Anger and hostility may often be directed at the physician and the staff. Occasionally there is a feeling of culpability. Other members of the family will add their reactions to the bad news and, at times, the management of a family will pose a harder task for the physician than caring for the patient. Not infrequently these difficulties are felt by the nursing staff too, as they attempt to establish a relationship with the family.

During the past few years it has become increasingly clear that early physical activity can be undertaken in uncomplicated cases of acute infarction. Under careful supervision, a graduated program is started in the coronary-care unit and continued until discharge from hospital. Included in these physical activities may be group meetings which are meant to be educational and psychotherapeutic. Such programs are aimed at shortening the convalescent period and allowing patients to experience a more rapid return of physical well-being. More rapid physical progress should, and probably does, have psychological benefits, although it does not seem to provide the whole answer to the prevention or amelioration of postinfarction emotional difficulties.

Leaving the security of the coronary-care unit is a cause for concern not only for the patient, but for family and staff as well. The use of an intermediate-care area, in which patients are monitored by telemetry, makes the transition to an open ward less abrupt and less threatening. The family has more opportunity to deal with its own anxieties, and the staff is aware that with each passing day, the danger to life recedes. Visits from members of the coronary-care staff have a most reassuring effect on patients as well as on the physician, who now knows that his patient is being watched by concerned individuals.

Posthospital Care

The patient is ready to be discharged from hospital following recovery from the acute phase of an infarct. The concept of what constitutes the acute phase is undergoing considerable change at present and the tendency is toward a shorter hospital stay (Hutter et al., 1973). It is customary to send the patient home with a set of instructions (which vary from the fairly specific to the very general). The spouse may or may not be present at this time, and he or she may or may not be encouraged to ask questions. Frequently, patients are instructed to see their physicians in the office several weeks later. They find themselves at home with very little to do but mark time. Many simple aspects of daily living now present problems for the patient, the spouse, and the family. The quality of the pre-illness interpersonal family relationships tends to become intensified, so that good feelings become even better while dislikes and disagreements are exacerbated. The patient who has little to do but worry about his future becomes depressed, those close to him often become engulfed in his feelings.

Although the need for the spouse's presence whenever the patient is seen and instructed by his physician is obvious, physicians must be reminded of it constantly (Klein et al., 1965). It is not unusual for the spouse to say during a follow-up visit, "I think I am going to have a heart attack," or "I should really be the patient."

Postcoronary Emotional Status

The incidence of anxiety and depression six to twelve months after an infarct has been shown to be extremely high (Wishine et al., 1971), and these findings are substantiated by our own study (Ruskin et al., 1970). One cannot escape the conclusion pointed out by Nagel et al. (1971) that the fault lies with the physician who fails to supply adequate information about the patient's health, detailed instructions regarding changes in life style, advice about such vital matters as sexual activity and a return to work. While sexual difficulties and fears are being discussed more readily and with greater confidence on the part of the physician, mainly because of Hellerstein and Friedman's (1970) work, the average clinician is poorly equipped to offer more than general advice concerning occupational rehabilitation. This uncertainty often leads to overprotection of the patient and the creation of yet another "cardiac cripple."

Personal experience with private patients, followed for varying periods up to 20 years after myocardial infarction, leads me to feel that it takes at least two years for a patient and his family, who have reasonable emotional stability, to adjust to this illness. During these two years one finds anxiety, depression, or denial in the majority of cases. The family has to live and deal with these states from day to day. The physician has to face it infrequently by comparison, and to deal with it mainly when he sees the patient. His skill in handling the situation may make a vast difference to the patient, and, therefore, to the family. It is a recognized fact that the physicians' role in determining the success of rehabilitation is enormous (Gulledge, 1975). Denial, which was a protective way of coping with the acute phase of the illness, instead of continuing in an intellectualized manner may become a hazard. There is now a need for the patient to test himself continually so that he often undertakes unwise and even dangerous tasks and activities. The spouse and the family are forced to exert constant vigilance in order to prevent possible trouble. This policing role justifiably increases their anxiety or despair. The physician may see the need for skilled psychotherapy, which may well include the spouse, in order to limit the patient's activities or to ease the spouse's anxieties.

Postcoronary Care and Rehabilitation

The physician can now back up his educated guesses with such modalities as submaximal stress tests and 24-hour electrocardiographic monitoring. Information obtained in these ways will often provide patients and their doctors with an objective measurement of the kind of physical activity and emotional stress which is reasonably safe. Physicians are often surprised at the latitude which they may now permit a given patient in his daily living and working.

An area where the physician may function poorly is in making use of community resources. He often is not aware of the availability of rehabilitation facilities, be they social, physical, psychological, or vocational. Economic pressures may become crippling and force patients into unwise decisions. A knowledge of appropriate agencies capable of providing temporary help may relieve both patient and family of this type of anxiety.

Avoiding Sudden Death

Sudden death is so defined when it occurs within an hour of the onset of symptoms. Approximately 50 percent of sudden deaths occur outside the hospital and involve individuals who appear to be in good health as well as those known to have coronary heart disease. The public is being educated to seek help rapidly at the nearest hospital, yet there are studies which indicate that delays for a variety of reasons are all too frequent. It is of considerable interest that the victim's spouse is usually an influence in reducing any delay in obtaining help, whereas physicians not infrequently put off prompt hospitalization. In an effort to bring skilled help to stricken individuals, Pantridge and Geddes (1967) working in Belfast pioneered the concept of rescue units which are now available to some American communities. Regrettably, since time is of the essence, even rescue teams cannot salvage all the hearts that are too good to die.

Mouth-to-mouth breathing and external cardiac massage are life-saving measures which can be taught to the general public. It has been reported that 25 percent of the adult population of Seattle has received such instruction. It would seem that such instruction in this type of first aid should become routine for all high school students; it should occur in a setting where it can be taught accurately and repeated at intervals. Places where groups of people congregate to work or to be entertained should have a cadre of trained individuals available. Simple thumping of the chest following sudden collapse may be all that is needed to resuscitate an individual with ventricular fibrillation.

The ability to act in the face of an emergency transforms helpless spectators, often family members, into active participants in what may turn out to be a life-saving process. Not only is such a role of great psychological value to the family of the stricken one, but also it is emotionally reassuring to the patients with coronary heart disease to know that their families can act in an emergency.

Sudden death may occur during hospitalization, but the incidence decreases rapidly with each passing day and hour. In the hospital, cardiac arrest is managed by a trained and equipped team. It has been my experience that coronary-care nurses, in particular, have come to feel that every arrest due to coronary disease should be treated successfully; when they fail, they tend to become unduly upset even though they have carried out their duties in a highly efficient manner. Perhaps what appears to be an unrealistic overreaction is related to the generally optimistic and constructive attitude nurtured in coronary-care units, as well as to the high standards which these same nurses place upon themselves.

Sudden death may involve anyone, but the incidence is clearly higher among individuals with known coronary disease. Much clinical research is now involved with attempts to identify those who are at high risk and to determine how best they may be protected (Prineas and Blackburn, 1975). It is well known that intense emotional experiences in addition to many other factors may be associated with sudden collapse and so, once more, the spouse and family may become involved in the patient's well-being. That is not to say that such an event is another individual's fault; it may well reside within the patient's own personality. Fear of such a catastrophic event may alter many important interpersonal relationships.

The possibility of sudden death is rarely broached by patients or their families. While it is statistically frequent, very few patients being cared for by an individual physician meet this fate, so that he too has no desire to discuss this negative subject.

The Physician's Role

No less important than sudden death (for which one cannot really prepare) is the need to help those patients who die less dramatically. It becomes the ultimate test of nursing to look after such patients and to make their emotional and physical comfort the only thing that matters. The physician, however, exerts a marked influence on how patients are managed during a terminal coronary illness. The controversial area in which therapeutic efforts have to be weighed against patient comfort when the outcome is really not in doubt has received a great deal of public attention recently.

The management of a patient with acute myocardial infarction and his subsequent course reveals a great deal about the patient's physician. An overcautious attitude on the part of the physician may be visible early and will be followed by a serious delay in full rehabilitation. Failure to clarify the illness to patient and family occurs too frequently. Instructions upon discharge from hospital may consist of a prescription and an admonition to take it easy at home for the next month or more. Further advice can only be elicited by means of questions from the patient or from members of the family, who sometimes find it difficult to ask for information. As has already been stressed, it is essential for the spouse to be present when any instructions are given, especially in relation to the period of convalescence at home. This part of the recovery process constitutes the weakest link in the medical management of individuals who are now permanent patients and who, therefore, require ongoing guidance.

The majority of patients seen in the cardiac work evaluation unit with which I have been associated had only a fragmentary understanding of the illness that had befallen them and of its implications for the future. Many of them had been kept away from their jobs for periods of six months to a year, and some were told by their physicians that they would never work again. A startling observation was the general ignorance concerning the correct use of nitroglycerin.

A recent study (Mayou et al., 1976) substantiates the impression that communication between physician and patient is inade-

quate, vague, and conflicting and that the degree of understanding of medical advice is low. It is frequently pointed out that
physicians are too busy to devote enough time for proper discussion, particularly of an illness that has such profound effects on
every aspect of living. It should also be remembered that physicians have not been adequately trained to listen to what their patients are saying, and as a general rule they do not encourage
questions.

Can it also mean that the reluctance on the part of many
physicians to depart from what is now felt to be outmoded management of uncomplicated myocardial infarction is a reflection of
the fear engendered in these physicians by the disease itself? The
incidence of coronary heart disease is very high among physicians
themselves, and one gains the impression that some doctors feel
uncomfortable when dealing with patients who suffer from it. In
general, patients with heart disease are referred to internists or
cardiologists much more frequently than is any other single
group. The attitude of physicians toward the management of patients with coronary heart disease needs to be examined in depth,
particularly outside the supportive environment of the hospital.

The Spouse's Role

The importance of the spouse's role in the rehabilitation process
has already been alluded to several times in this presentation.
Gulledge (1975) has reviewed some of the literature concerned
with the subject, including the reaction of the spouse to the patient's illness.

Because of the recognition of the importance of the spouse, a
study was undertaken, using the MMPI, which was administered
at the same time to 128 male patients with proven myocardial infarction and to their wives (Ruskin et al., 1970). Some 83 percent
of the patients showed statistically significant depression as measured by the MMPI scale. In two-thirds of the cases, this finding
was present six months or longer after the myocardial infarction
had occurred. The mean scores of the group were significantly
elevated in the scales relating to the neurotic triad—
hypochondriasis, depression, and hysteria. By contrast, the
spouses had mean scores in all the scales which were within normal limits. Further study of the same data (Stein et al., forthcoming) indicates that the spouse's emotional makeup and life style

play a greater role in the patient's postinfarction vocational adjustment than any personality attributes of the patient himself. In other words, the more stable the wife, the more likely is the patient's vocational adjustment to be successful. Further study of an expanded group of these patients (Bailey et al., unpublished data) produced the same basic findings and suggests that disturbed thinking on the wife's part probably interferes with the patient's ability to concentrate at work, and emotionally unstable wives produced enough effect on their husbands to keep them from working effectively. Approximately 50 percent of the wives in this group were working at the time of study. Role reversal, often dictated by economic necessity, may provide special problems in psychological adjustment. Since the spouse's contribution may make the difference between success or failure in the patient's rehabilitative process, it would seem worthwhile to determine her strengths and weaknesses, so that she may be helped to play a more positive role.

Although we are not presently dealing with matters related to causation of coronary heart disease, it is interesting to note that a study from Finland (Rahe et al., 1973) suggests that the recent life changes may have significance as a possible risk factor. At the head of the list of personal and social life-change events during the six months prior to a myocardial infarction are death of spouse and divorce. The role of the spouse can be seen to emerge before the onset of myocardial infarction and to take on increasing importance during and after the acute illness.

The Team's Role

The large majority of people who recover from a myocardial infarct return to gainful employment. However, there is a sizable number of patients who either have problems related to work or who simply stop working permanently. Cardiac work evaluation units, consisting of physicians, psychiatrists or psychologists, vocational experts, and social workers have played a pioneering role in demonstrating that a professional team can help most of these individuals to return to work, provided it is work suitable to their physical and emotional needs. The unit with which I have been associated for the past 15 years has dealt with more than 900 patients during this time, most of whom have coronary heart disease. These patients were selected largely because of occupational difficulties. It became obvious early in our experience that psychological factors were far more frequent than were any physical handicaps. Consequently, the unit's orientation has been directed toward attempting to advise patients and their spouses in dealing with these psychological barriers to satisfactory adjustment.

For more than 10 years, as knowledge concerning work physiology has grown, great emphasis has been placed on physical rehabilitation, and most cardiac work-evaluation units have become incorporated into newly established physical-stress testing and rehabilitation facilities. This trend is understandable, but it does not solve the problems associated with psychological rehabilitation. If anything, it has placed the accent where it was already known to be—that is, the heart heals long before the psyche.

The failure of physicians to provide guidance necessary for rehabilitation has led to the formation of hospital groups and heart clubs. The concept is a good one, since it allows patients and their spouses to exchange experiences and air common problems. It permits them to realize very rapidly that they are in no way unique. Use can be made of coronary-care nurses, dieticians, psychologists, social workers, vocational counselors, and physicians. Patients and their spouses can begin to attend meetings before discharge from hospital and continue during the period of convalescence at home, a time when all available support is sorely needed. It should be emphasized that groups or clubs require skilled leadership and professional guidance, without which they can rapidly deteriorate into gripe sessions. The ultimate value of groups and clubs is as yet unproven.

Summary

Advances in cardiology have been truly astounding and have outdistanced those in any other field of medicine. There is good reason for optimism in the management of patients with coronary heart disease. In addition to a reduction in mortality resulting from more effective management of the acute infarct, bypass surgery undoubtedly alters the quality of life for the majority of carefully selected patients who undergo this procedure. There are preliminary indications that it may increase longevity in certain subgroups (Logue et al., 1976).

Early physical rehabilitation for myocardial infarction has been thoroughly tested and its benefits are encouraging to patients, family, and staff. It is now time to focus attention on primary psychological rehabilitation in its broadest sense, because it is in this area that the greatest damage is produced by this chronic disease. It has been estimated that four million Americans suffer from coronary heart disease and it is clearly impossible to provide expert help on so large a scale. A partial solution may lie in more intensive public education so that knowledge will lessen the fear of heart disease and its long-term consequences. A better understanding of stress and how to make it less destructive (Selye, 1974), as well as modification of behavior based on personality characteristics (Friedman and Roseman, 1974) may help in the prevention of coronary heart disease as well as increase longevity and improve the quality of life once it has manifested itself.

References

Bailey, M. A., H. D. Ruskin, and L. L. Stein et al. Unpublished data.

Friedman, M. and R. H. Rosenman. 1974. *Type A Behavior and Your Heart.* Greenwich, Conn.: Fawcett.

Gulledge, A. D. 1975. "The Psychological Aftermath of a Myocardial Infarction." In Gentry and Williams, eds., *Psychological Aspects of Myocardial Infarction and Coronary Care,* pp. 107–23. St. Louis: C. V. Mosby.

Hackett, T. P. and N. H. Cassem. 1972. "Psychological Effects of Acute Coronary Care." In Meltzer and Dunning, *Textbook of Coronary Care,* pp. 443–52. Philadelphia: Charles Press.

Hellerstein, H. K. and E. H. Friedman. 1970. "Sexual Activity and the Postcoronary Patient," *Archives of Internal Medicine,* 125:987.

Hutter, A. M., Jr., V. W. Sidel, K. I. Shine, and R. W. DeSanctis. 1973. "Early Hospital Discharge After Myocardial Infarction," *New England Journal of Medicine,* 288:1141.

Klein, R. F. et al. 1965. "The Physician and Post-Myocardial Invalidism," *Journal of the American Medical Association,* 194:143.

Logue, R. B., S. B. King, and J. S. Douglas. 1976. "A Practical Approach to Coronary Artery Disease, with Special Reference to Coronary Bypass Surgery," *Current Problems in Cardiology,* vol. 1, no. 2. Chicago: Yearbook Medical Publishers.

Mayou, R., B. Williamson, and A. Foster. 1976. "Attitudes and Advice After Myocardial Infarction," *British Medical Journal,* 1:1577.

Nagel, R., R. Gangola, and I. Picton-Robinson. 1971. "Factors Influencing Return to Work After Myocardial Infarction," *Lancet,* 2:454.

Pantridge, J. F. and J. S. Geddes. 1967. "A Mobile Intensive-Care Unit in the Management of Myocardial Infarction," *Lancet,* 2:271.

Pranulis, M. F. 1975. "Coping with an Acute Myocardial Infarction." In Gentry and Williams, eds., *Psychological Aspects of Myocardial Infarction and Coronary Care,* pp. 65–75. St. Louis: C. V. Mosby.

Prineas, R. J. and H. Blackburn. 1975. "Sudden Coronary Death Outside Hospital," *Circulation* Supplement no. 3, vol. 52.

Rahe, R. H., L. Bennett, and M. Romo et al. 1973. "Subjects' Recent Life Changes and Coronary Heart Disease in Finland," *American Journal of Psychiatry*, 130:1222.

Ruskin, H. D., L. L. Stein, I. M. Shelsky, et al. 1970. "MMPI: Comparison between Patients with Coronary Heart Disease and their Spouses together with Other Demographic Data," *Scandinavia Journal of Rehabilitation Medicine*, 2:99.

Selye, H. 1974. *Stress without Distress.* Philadelphia: L. B. Lippincott.

Stein, L. L., M. A. Baily, and H. D. Ruskin. *Rehabilitation of the Postcoronary Patient: Role of the Spouse.* Forthcoming.

Wishine, H. A., T. P. Hackett and N. H. Cassem. 1971. "Psychological Hazards of Convalescence following Myocardial Infarction," *Journal of the American Medical Association*, 215:1292.

❧ 2
Care of the Severely Ill Cardiovascular Patient

Irving S. Wright

DURING MY PROFESSIONAL life, I have been privileged to observe and participate in the remarkable evolution of the care of severely ill cardiovascular patients. As a student and resident, I witnessed countless patients as they died, quickly or slowly. The weapons were few and frequently ill-used—digitalis, morphine, and low salt diets. Oxygen was used sparingly and diuretics were being investigated. There were no methods of controlling shock, or arrhythmias, or preventing thromboembolism—the problems we consider of greatest importance in precipitating death today. Even then, drawing conclusions regarding death, prolongation of life, or temporary improvement was hazardous for the physician. A few patients regarded as beyond help surprised the experts by struggling back to a remarkable degree of activity, sometimes living for months or years.

Today, despite our vastly improved armamentarium, accurate prognosis is even less secure. We generally know when the patient is seriously ill but are too frequently embarrassed by a sudden death which occurs within a few hours or days after an examination which failed to reveal any ominous abnormalities.

When he is ill, we can evaluate a patient's status, but for some years I have refrained from making a definitive statement to the family as to an immediate outcome or long-term outlook, indicating instead that we have and will use all available weapons to restore the patient to acceptable life so long as there is any chance whatever—examples of hopeless situations being a total neurological death secondary to a stroke, totally intractable failure, or really severe shock (the causes of 85 to 90 percent of all deaths). Even with severe shock, the use of an intra-aortic balloon as an accessory heart pump may occasionally sustain life long enough to permit the heart to regain its capacity for life. Recently, a physician who seemed in hopeless shock in the hospital coronary-care unit was restored to a life-sustaining level by the use of the aortic balloon. Arrhythmias were controlled with Lidocaine and Propanalol and his O_2 deficit met constantly. He then survived multiple large pulmonary emboli which were arrested with Heparin and Coumadin. He has returned to good health and is ready to resume practice—we hope on a moderate scale instead of the 15-hour, seven day a week program of the past. This is not a unique case, but it does indicate the long distance we have traveled in a few decades. We are, however, still confronted with the fact that although we have great resources in our hospitals for the care of these patients, 60 percent of those who die from acute myocardial infarctions do so before they reach the hospital. Therefore, our new advances must, in large measure, be in this area. How do we accomplish this?

The public must be educated to recognize the warning signs of heart disease. These include difficulty in breathing (dyspnea), tightness or pain in the retrosternal area, locally or extending across the anterior chest, into the arms, neck or jaw, swollen ankles, faintness, blackouts, and unexplained sweats or weakness. These symptoms may not be due to heart disease but a physician, not the patient, must evaluate them. Physicians are now becoming much more sensitive to these warning signs, and there has been a great change within the past decade. If the physician knows the patient, he will be much more able to evaluate the patient's telephone call and hence to instruct him whether to go by ambulance or car directly to the emergency unit in the hospital, remain at home until he sees him, or come to the physician's office. This points to the need for patients to have a primary physician, either a well-trained family physician or an internist, and to see him for regular checkups, at least once a year, but with increasing frequency if he is known to have cardiovascular disease. The majority of patients who develop "heart attacks" of whatever nature have warning signs—sometimes for months or years—and good medical advice can often forestall or postpone serious attacks, the outcome of which may be questionable at the time of the attack. Therefore, the patient with a known heart condition must keep in close communication with his physician. The physician must encourage this and should instruct the patient and his family regarding what steps are to be taken if his condition suddenly becomes worse and he cannot immediately reach his physician. This type of specific instruction is too often neglected by either the physician or his patient, yet it may mean the difference between life and death. Lives can be lost because the patient does not understand his symptoms or he acts out what is now termed the "denial syndrome" until it is too late. In the past, physicians often belittled the telephoned complaints, but my experience suggests that this is now rare. The name of the game is "Immediate Action and Play it Safe." Textbooks on the treatment of heart disease abound. Consideration will be given to the broad concepts involved in modern care. The primary step is the correct diagnosis—for example, valvular heart disease vs. atherosclerotic heart disease, and evaluation of the immediate state and the rate of progress—for example, gradual failure due to valvular or myocardial disease vs. progressive angina vs. sudden ischemia associated with a myocardial infarction. Clearly, the methods of attack are quite different and must be individualized in each case. We do have new weapons to stay or improve these complex conditions. A few examples will be discussed, but detailed discussion of all possible problems would be too voluminous for this report.

Hypertension is responsible for increased strain on the heart and ultimate failure in thousands of cases a year. It is estimated that 22 million persons in the United States have hypertension, but fewer than one-half know it, fewer than one-half of these are receiving any treatment, and fewer than one-half of these are adequately treated! The vast majority of sufferers from hypertension are not seriously ill in any one year, but this affliction is a cause of thousands of strokes secondary to cerebral vascular disease, as well as many thousands of heart attacks. It can now be treated with a marked reduction in pressure levels in the majority of patients, and the evidence is strong that this will reduce the incidence of catastrophic and terminal complications. There are numerous effective medications, including reserpine, the chlorthiazides, methyldopa, as well as mild tranquilizers. Singly or in combination, they should be tried until a formula which is both effective and tolerated by the patient is found. Most of these patients require long-term or lifelong therapy.

For many patients *arrhythmias* are annoying. Quinidine sulphate, digitalis preparations, or propanolol hydrochloride will control many of the premature contractions or paroxysmal tachycardias, but "blackouts" secondary to prolonged asystole or Stokes-Adams syndromes may produce serious injuries due to falls or death. The development of artificial pacemakers represents one of the great new advances in medicine and today nearly one hundred thousand patients are alive and active thanks to these implanted devices. In the past, pacemakers have had a lifespan of about 18 months, after which they required replacement, with the unpleasantness of minor surgery. Several thousand patients have lived to have one or more replacements (some of our patients are now living with their fifth pacemaker) and the likelihood of their survival prior to this era would have been close to nil. Recently lithium and atomic pacemakers have been developed, which will, it is hoped, provide longer life between replacements. Most of these patients, who previously would have been considered as seriously or fatally ill, are now leading active and quite normal lives. Very recently monitors have been developed which make it possible for the patients to check the function of their pacemakers by telephone with a central control unit, even though they are many miles away.

The majority of patients with *rheumatic heart disease,* usually contracted in the first 30 years of life, were in the past faced with a life of progressive invalidism as the valves, most commonly the mitral or aortic valves, progressively stenosed, until not enough blood was able to reach the vascular tree and sustain life throughout the body. I have watched helplessly as many of these patients died. The first successful mitral commissurotomy was reported by Henry A. Soutar, a London surgeon, in 1926, but it was many years before this was an accepted procedure. Indeed, his own reputation suffered for his having dared to operate on the human heart. Years later, after World War II, American surgeons began to use this technique. Then Soutar was knighted and honored in other countries. This pioneering step led the way to a wide variety of valvular surgery and ultimately innumerable prosthetic valves were developed in an effort to find a material and valvular mechanism which would continue to function uncomplicated by wear, leakage, and thrombosis. Successful surgery is based on careful selection of suitable cases. Prior to this type of surgery, cardiac catheterization, cardiac angiography, and (in some cases) echocardiography are essential. These patients, formerly so desperately ill, can today usually be offered markedly improved outlooks with valve prostheses when combined with long-term anticoagulant therapy.

Myocardial infarction, usually the result of atherosclerotic coronary disease, remains the most dreaded of the serious heart syndromes and the one which has received the most concentrated attention during the past decade. The introduction of coronary care units and intensive care units has changed the entire approach toward the patient stricken with a myocardial infarction once he reaches the hospital. More recently, this type of intensive care has been extended to the time when the patient is first picked up by an ambulance with a highly trained team, modern equipment, and radio telephonic communication with experts in a center who can direct his care while he is being brought in. Physicians and laypersons alike are familiar with these new developments. The means for controlling arrhythmias, thromboembolic complications, failure, and (in many but not all cases) shock and cardiac arrest, are now widely available in hospitals throughout the country. However, the quality of this care is not uniform, because of the lack of the most highly trained personnel or optimal equipment. The trend is toward marked improvement throughout the United States.

Patients who develop progressive *angina pectoris* due to ischemia of the myocardium secondary to stenosis of the coronary arteries were usually confronted with steadily increasing disability, ultimate myocardial infarction, and frequently death. Today we have a new approach which is helpful for many of these patients. Careful coronary cine angiographic studies will depict the state of the coronary circulation, how badly it is affected by atherosclerosis, how many points of severe stenosis there are and whether the condition is one that can justifiably be approached with modern surgery. The approach of choice today is usually a bypass procedure from the aorta to the effected artery beyond the site of stenosis or occlusion, using a segment of the patient's saphenous vein. In some cases a mammary artery bypass is used. This may be performed by bypassing from one to four arterial stenoses. In carefully selected cases, the results are usually helpful and frequently remarkable, with the patient freed from his angina. The preliminary angiographic studies show that some patients are not suitable for this approach. The myocardium may be too badly damaged, or there is inadequate runoff due to too great damage to the coronary artery wall for a graft to be attached. On the other hand, in some, more advanced surgery may include excision of a ventricular aneurysm at the same procedure as the bypass operation with excellent results. This type of surgery is still relatively new even though an estimated 50,000 cases have been done. The ultimate evaluation of its indications and the determination of prolongation of life are not complete. Many of the bypasses occlude within 3 to 12 months and atherosclerosis continues to involve other coronary arteries. This step represents progress but not complete control of the disease. The control of atherosclerosis involves heredity, smoking, lipid metabolism, hypertension, diabetes, and overeating of cholesterol and saturated fats. But this is another chapter—one of prevention.

Heart transplants and artificial hearts will not be included in this discussion since their general usefulness is far from established at this time. Belief in their future value is presently based on faith rather than results.

A few days after acute infarction or failure, or after serious cardiac surgery, the patient is moved out of the intensive care area—usually to a general medical service. This occurs frequently after five to seven days but unfortunately many complications occur during the following week or two. They include recurrent myocardial infarction, serious arrhythmias, pulmonary emboli, thromboembolic strokes, peripheral arterial occlusions and thrombophlebitis. These complications can be reduced greatly by anticoagulant therapy and early ambulation if this is possible. Because of these complications, such patients should ideally remain in areas adjacent to the intensive care units, where careful observation and appropriate monitoring can be continued with emergency care immediately available. In older hospitals, this may not be possible but no new hospitals should be constructed without consideration of this type of plan. As the patient improves he can be moved to a continuation-care unit. There he can convalesce under observation without the need for the highly intensive and expensive resources required during the acute stages of his illness.

Toward the terminal stages of heart disease with an irreversible downhill course, the decision as to whether the patient can be cared for at home or in a nursing home must be faced. Keeping the patient at home involves plans for 24-hour coverage by family, nurses, or other auxilliary personnel. It may go on for very long periods and be exhausting in terms of both physical and financial resources. The alternates now available are not very satisfactory. If the patient is affluent or well insured, a high-quality nursing home may be the only solution. If the resources are limited, the local social service, by whatever name, can usually be helpful—especially with elderly patients covered by Medicare or Medicaid. Unfortunately, this service is still uneven in this country, but it is usually to be found if the physician and the family are persistent.

Need for the compassionate physician. With all of these highly technical advances, the patient's chance of survival following extremely serious cardiovascular crises has improved. However, in many services the emphasis on emergent procedures is so strong that the emotional reactions of the patients are not handled ideally. There is an understandable conflict here between what has to be done as a lifesaving measure at the moment—for example, external cardiac massage, mouth-to-mouth breathing, and D.C. shock for conversion to normal rhythm—and being thoughtful and compassionate, taking the time to explain to the patient and his family what is happening and why. Granted, that at the moment of crisis there is little time for explanations to the patient, but someone must try to clarify the picture to the family and, if the patient does survive the crisis, to reassure and calm him. The average CCU is a frightening experience to a patient. He may see other patients being resuscitated—not a pleasant sight—and being taken out dead. He pictures himself in that spot. He is receiving I.V. fluids and O_2 by tube with frequent throat suction. He is catheterized and has many wires attached to the monitors. He may also be given DC shocks several times to restore his rhythm. While all of this is going on, he is surrounded by strangers. Rarely is there a face he has ever seen before. Above all he is examined, probed, tested, and discussed so many times in each 24 hours that he gets little normal rest. This aspect of Coronary-Care Units is unfortunate, and in some progressive hospitals steps are being taken to minimize the psychic trauma which by itself can adversely effect the blood pressure, and cardiac rate and rhythm.

It is well established that severe emotional stress can precipitate myocardial infarctions and strokes in patients who already have atherothrombosis in key arteries, even though the patient may have been asymptomatic or had only minor warning symp-

toms before. It appears clear that the stress involved in the realization by the patient of his serious immediate state, his dubious
long-term outlook with all of the implications involved, and the
frightening experiences of many C.C. units, can produce aggrava-
tion of the patient's already hazardous state—even to the point of
jeopardizing his life. Many physicians are fully aware of this paradoxical therapeutic dilemma, but my experience has led me to
believe that in some services the feelings of the patient have a
fairly low priority and that the concentration is too purely technical, that the team is acting primarily as a group of technicians,
not of physicians. While the technical aspects are vital, so, often,
are the humanistic aspects of the care of the patients. Here the
primary physician, whom the patient has known before, can play
a major role, even if he leaves the technical aspects to the CCU
team. He should be welcomed by the unit team and he can play
an important role in advising and reassuring the patient and his
family that everything is being done for the patient during his
critical period and his fight to return to health. There is, at this
time, a need for the entire staff responsible for the technical
aspects of the care of the seriously ill cardiac patients to bear in
mind the emotional stress which is inevitable in such situations,
and to give the patients and their families the psychological support essential to help them to face their problem in the most constructive way possible. This may be as important in obtaining a
good therapeutic result as some of the more dramatic steps they
are taking.

❧ 3
Approaches to the Seriously Ill Cardiac Patient

Marvin Moser

A PATIENT WITH heart disease confronts death differently from the patient with a terminal illness resulting from a malignancy or kidney failure. The cardiac patient is unique in that he often finds himself in a position where death is a strong possibility but not a certainty. His situation is also different because he is frequently more aware of what is happening to him than the patient who is suffering from a terminal malignancy, uremia, a stroke, or the patient who is dying from severe injuries. In these other situations, large amounts of narcotics or analgesics may be given because of pain or, in the case of kidney failure, for example, the patient may remain semiconscious for days or weeks, unaware of his surroundings or the implications of actions around him.

The physician's approach to the cardiac patient and his own attitude about life and death also determine the patient's feelings about the future, perhaps to a greater degree than most of us will admit. I should like to discuss the problems of the cardiac patient when faced with the possibility of death, physicians' and relatives' attitudes, and his own perception of what has occurred.

The Role of the Physician and the Hospital

A patient who has had severe chest pain is rushed into the emergency room or coronary-care unit fearful that he has had a heart attack. The fears are reinforced when pain recurs, an electrocardiogram is taken, and members of his family or his friends show concern. Although almost everyone has known someone who died of a coronary or has visited someone on a coronary-care unit, the surroundings usually are not familiar to the patient. His first contacts are with concerned nurses, orderlies, or a new doctor—a stranger covering the emergency room or "on call" in the coronary-care unit. The physician with whom he has had a long-term relationship may not be available or, as frequently occurs in the large medical center, may refer the case to a specialist. The anxiety of unfamiliar surroundings, the problem of being labeled a "case," the unfamiliar faces and voices, and the sense that everyone is rushing around trying to save his life compound the original fear.

The moment a patient enters the hospital as a "heart case," he is in a setting of gadgetry which, unless explained, is another source of anxiety. In the emergency room, he is hooked up to monitoring equipment, then wheeled to the coronary unit, where he is wired for the sound of his heartbeat, frequently audible to the patient. Nurses are moving quickly. If he is unlucky enough to be in a hospital that still has an open coronary-care unit where beds are contiguous and separated only by a screen or curtain, the patient is exposed to the problems of other patients. In many large teaching hospitals, for example, there are still open coronary-care units where beds are in one large room. When the chief of cardiology makes rounds with four or five residents, several interns, and an array of medical students, the patient is exposed to all of the talk and discussion of his potentially serious condition. Diseases may be discussed about which the patient has little understanding; someone might discuss the implications of heart block and sudden death in full view and earshot of the patient. In such units it is extremely difficult for the patient to obtain privacy or quiet rest without being heavily sedated.

Add to the above two other common problems: a monitoring system with an audible beeping sound that signals heart-rate changes and the middle-of-the-night emergency. Changes in the noises of the heart beeper can be the result of a malfunctioning electrode or a loose connection. When the patient moves in bed and pulls the electrode away from his chest wall, an alarm may sound, with frightening results to the patient. There are other problems, too: at any time, another patient may experience cardiac arrest; at any time, an acutely ill patient may arrive. Suddenly, 15 or 20 people are scurrying around, alarms are sounded, the terms "shock him again," "defibrillate him" are used; the anesthesiologist is called, noises of punching on the chest are heard, and then, if the patient expires, the room is silent, leaving all the other patients in the coronary care unit aware of what has happened and naturally quite upset.

These are some of the anxiety-producing episodes that a patient experiences in a coronary-care unit. They are aware that they have a possibly death-dealing illness; they are aware that death is all around them. What effect does it have on them, and can the physician and other personnel modify these effects? What do these anxiety-ridden episodes do to the patient?

First, there are physiological considerations. It is well known that we excrete a great deal more adrenalin during periods of anxiety than we do during periods of calm. The normal heart can handle this very well; heart rate speeds up, the amount of blood pumped out is increased, the work of the heart and the oxygen demand on it are increased. The patient with a coronary occlusion, or even an episode of so-called coronary insufficiency, is more vulnerable to the added work and oxygen demand on the heart. The anxiety and increased adrenalin may be just enough to cause heart failure or a serious rhythm change. From a simple physiological point of view, preventing anxiety is extremely important.

Second, there are psychological considerations. How do patients respond to the bigness, the inhumanity of the gadgetry, the fear of sudden catastrophe, the viewing of catastrophe all about them? There are some patients who feel secure when they are hooked up to monitoring equipment. They feel protected by the atmosphere of the coronary-care unit and are not disturbed by the specialist who treats a patient as a "case" without knowing much about him—or about his reactions to pain or illness. They feel secure that they are in the hands of an expert. Several follow-up studies have been done on patients who have survived either cardiac arrest, when technically they died and were resuscitated by defibrillation and cardiac resuscitation, or the experience of the coronary-care unit itself. These studies have demonstrated that, because of this fear of catastrophe, for months and years many patients wake up with anxiety dreams, are afraid to be left alone for long periods of time, and are unable to function in their daily jobs.

Patients who have been put into single rooms with a degree of soundproofing and have not viewed the serious events described above generally do much better. Women tolerate the procedures that are performed and the gadgetry more easily than men do. It should be remembered that the vast majority of these patients are alert and feel well after the first few minutes or hours of the "attack" that signaled the life-threatening coronary event.

Are the patients who seem to ignore the "coronary-care experience" just being brave; are they denying their fears and their illness? Interviews with patients who have experienced a massive coronary occlusion or who have been resuscitated and who know that they were "saved from death," clearly establish that denial is a factor, often an important one, in their survival as effective individuals. Denial is a defense many of us employ in similar situations. It is relatively easy to disbelieve the seriousness of an illness, especially when we feel well. This is in contrast to the patient with a terminal malignancy or kidney failure—tired, weak and sleepy, his senses dulled by narcotic drugs. Here, reality frequently overcomes the defense of denial. The coronary patient is often alert when last rites are administered and, depending upon the manner in which the priest handles this delicate situation, a great deal of harm can be done and a good prognosis changed by physiological reaction to fear.

Can the personnel of a modern hospital utilize the latest equipment and handle the cardiac emergency efficiency without sacrificing the dignity or privacy of the patient? Can they handle the fear of a frequently catastrophic illness and alleviate anxiety without sacrificing the advantages of modern technology? Planners must keep these factors in mind when designing special-care units; nothing is lost to care by using soundproofing liberally and installing opaque walls where monitoring equipment is following the patient and direct visualization is not always necessary. Nurses and aides, medical students, and house staff must be trained to be patient, move quickly but quietly, and not talk too much or too loudly.

Approach to the Patient

The physician's role is extremely important in the patient's perception of his illness and his view of chances for survival. A patient's feeling about death depends largely upon the way he has lived his life. Has he been fearful of crossing the street; has he been an eager, active person; does he view things optimistically or pessimistically? Even a positive outlook can be shaken by a gloomy prediction from a physician; a naturally pessimistic outlook can be converted into a long-term neurosis by a "cold turkey" approach during the first few frightening days following a coronary occlusion.

My own experience leads me to a firm conclusion that no one should be told that death is inevitable, especially a cardiac patient. In dealing with a patient who has had an acute coronary occlusion, nothing is gained by saying, "You have had a massive heart attack," or "You are in danger of dying," or "Your condition is terribly serious,"—and much can be lost. I firmly disagree with those who believe that the patient must face facts, but each physician has his own way of approaching this and his reasons for doing so. My feeling is that this approach accomplishes nothing; that only if the patient were to do something that interferes with his recovery, need the physician use strong, frightening terms to gain compliance to a treatment program. In my experience, this is rarely necessary. The anxieties produced, with their secondary effects upon the heart and need for oxygen, frequently make matters worse and affect long-term recovery.

It is a simple matter to tell a patient that he has had some spasm of the coronary arteries or perhaps a closure of a small blood vessel which has injured a small portion of the heart, but that, barring something very unusual and unforeseen, he will do very well, and recovery will be excellent. This is an honest approach, an optimistic one, and can be followed in the vast majority of cases. The extent of his illness, if he is seriously ill, need not be conveyed, except in very special circumstances. If the patient totally ignores the physician's advice later on and engages in activities that might be dangerous to him, there is time then to talk about "heart damage." Generally, this is not necessary; in fact, we often have had to convince patients to go about their normal activities, to exercise more than they had been exercising before, to live a vigorous, healthy, and productive life and not to be too protective of themselves after a "heart attack."

Approach to the Family

The manner in which the physician approaches the family has a great deal to do with the patient's perception of his illness. Physicians often make the drama worse by using the words "critical" or "very serious" or by delving too deeply into explanations of complications. Frequently, because of legal implications, a patient's family, or the patient himself, is told of the worst possible complications that can result from a procedure before it is done or of the miraculous results after it is performed. A physician treating a cardiac patient has several options. He can begin his journey toward becoming a hero by his initial approach to the patient's family, with such comment as, "Your spouse has had a serious heart attack and is in critical condition—we'll do everything to help him [her] survive." The image of death begins to loom larger in the eyes of the family. More anxiety is built up, perhaps guilt about what they may or may not have been doing just prior to the onset of symptoms; guilt about an argument they may have precipitated; guilt about intercourse that may have precipitated the coronary attack.

The family cannot help but transmit gloom to the patient by facial expressions, by oversolicitousness when they visit, or by staying around for hour after hour grimly viewing the bed and this "dying man." What does the physician gain by this approach? He has protected himself. If the patient dies within a few days, "Doctor Smith warned us; he told us my spouse was quite ill." If the patient lives, the physician is a hero: "He's pulled my husband through a terrible illness—we are indebted to him forever." Perhaps this is an overstatement of a point, but it does occur.

What has been lost? Anxiety and fear of catastrophe or death have been implanted in the minds of both the family and patient for the rest of the patient's life unless there is a great deal more discussion of the patient's illness and subsequent recovery. Usually this is not done. The spouse becomes overprotective, always remembering the seriousness of those first few days; the patient may develop a true cardiac neurosis.

The other approach, which we have found to be useful, but which may not be appropriate in all cases, omits phrases such as "massive heart attack," "your spouse is dying," or "critical condition." I believe that the same message may be conveyed and overanxiety prevented if the episode is minimized. Obviously, if a patient is in shock or has a serious rhythm change, the situation changes, but the majority of cases do not present these complications. A family should be told that a heart attack has occurred, that a vessel has closed, that heart attacks can be quite minor, and that "your relative will do very well"—a positive, optimistic statement. The risk to the physician of minimizing, or seeming to minimize, the coronary attack is that if something does happen during the next few days, he is blamed: "Didn't he realize how seriously ill my spouse was?" The odds are with the cardiologist, because over 80 percent of patients who are admitted to coronary-care units survive with the kind of care that is now available. If the patient recovers, "Well, it was a routine coronary so the doctor didn't have to do much anyway." (Not much of a hero for a job well done.) In the long run, the family and the patient are healthier and less frightened. Coronary heart disease is unpredictable, and we have all seen patients who were given a poor prognosis but lived for many years as productive, active people.

Resuscitation—How Much and How Long?

The treatment of cardiac arrest, with either a fibrillating heart or a heart with no beat at all. is effective in many instances. Heart massage, breathing for the patient, and using an electric shock to get the heart beating normally have saved many lives. Some people who recover remember feelings of death or dreams and are aware for years that they died and were brought back to life. Eventually, they recover from these feelings and most adjust fairly well. There are cases, however, when physicians refuse to accept the fact that some people cannot be resuscitated and continue heroic measures long after they are indicated. An 85-year-old patient, who has suffered a coronary occlusion, who has a huge heart which is beating inefficiently, who suffers four or five episodes of cardiac arrest, and is resuscitated each time but who suffers increasingly severe brain damage, is an example of a patient who might be best treated by fewer heroic acts. Obviously, this is a difficult decision to make, but it is one that physicians are facing more and more. We are able to keep someone's heart beating or keep him breathing for days or weeks. Technically, the patient is alive. The definitions of death are a great deal more important today than they were 10 or 15 years ago, before we had the mechanical means either to resuscitate patients or to keep them alive indefinitely, even with severe brain damage.

There is a point when one must say to oneself, "The patient is technically alive but will never function as a feeling, thinking individual; he will become an economic as well as an emotional and psychologic burden." At that point (and it is a difficult one to determine) resuscitative measures should probably be stopped. If an electroencephalogram shows that brain-wave activity has ceased, the decision is easier.

Valvular surgery, or the use of arteries or veins to increase the circulation of the heart itself (the "coronary bypass operation") has been performed on thousands of patients. Results are frequently quite gratifying. Patients are asked to face the risk of death during and after surgery. The role of the physician and his approach to the patient are extremely important in preparing these patients for surgery. Some of them are seriously ill, some might not live too long without surgery; but far too often the patient is told, "If you don't have this operation, you will be dead in a week, or two, or six months." Many patients, with all three of their major coronary arteries partially or almost completely closed, with a heart functioning only on so-called "collateral circulation" and rejected for surgery as "too great a risk" lead productive lives for many years; no one can predict their longevity. We must be careful not to frighten lest we create severely anxious patients whose last years are spent waiting for the prediction to come true.

I think that both surgeons and cardiologists, in approaching the patient who is to undergo cardiac surgery, must say, "Yes, there is a risk to this procedure, but we believe that it is a reasonable one and that surgery will be helpful." I do not believe that a pessimistic approach is generally helpful. There are some cases, obviously, where risks are enormous and the patient's family must be made aware of them.

The group of patients with chronic heart failure from advanced arteriosclerotic heart disease, and the elderly patient whose heart is so badly damaged from progressive coronary artery disease that it can no longer function, require a somewhat different approach. Despite medication, the patient is continually short of breath, loses weight because of poor appetite, is unable to walk effectively, and slowly goes downhill. The patient is older, is usually more tolerant of the idea of potential death and can often face it. Even here, the physician's role should be that of encouragement, since we have all seen patients of 75 or 80 go well beyond the number of years predicted. These people usually lead reasonably satisfactory lives and are different from the patient with a terminal malignancy who might be in severe pain.

There are other patients, somewhat younger, who have inflammatory disease of the heart muscle, which also causes heart failure and death. Despite their certain prognosis, an optimistic point of view has proved to be much better than informing the patient that death is inevitable.

I believe that the patient with heart disease, in most instances, faces the prospect of death as a possibility but not as a certainty and should be handled in an optimistic way. No one is capable of predicting duration of life in most patients with heart disease. A note of optimism, a vote for humane care, and the isolation of the patient from contiguous, catastrophic situations, from too much discussion, from too much gloom, and from too much instrumentation, will allow the patient with an acute, threatening heart attack to become a much healthier person after his recovery.

I do not believe that overemphasis of the possibility of death is useful in dealing with the patient's family, since this is transmitted to the patient, resulting in physiological changes as well as emotional stress. There are some categories where death eventually appears inevitable, such as infectious diseases of the heart muscle, or the older patient with chronic heart failure; but here too, since no one can predict the time, an optimistic approach seems to work a great deal better than pessimism or being too realistic.

Most patients will deny their illness. This is perhaps true in heart disease (coronary artery disease) more than in other illnesses. The male of 40 does not want to lose his manhood or to cease being the breadwinner, the father of his kids, or the companion of his wife. He will seek to deny it at every turn. He will only hear what he wants to hear. Nine out of ten times, these patients deny the fear of death when interviewed. This denial is protective and useful, and I do not believe that any effort should be made to break down this response or label it "unhealthy, bizarre, or unrealistic." I think we should accept this as protective and, in the long run, useful and helpful to the patient. We should remain optimistic, so that our patients do not become invalids or cardiac neurotics.

4
Psychological Intervention During Transfer from the Cardiac Intensive Care Unit

Lillie Shortridge

EARLY IN THE morning of Mr. Timothy Davis's sixth day in the coronary-care unit, his physician reported to him, "You're getting along really well. You'll be transferred to the ward today." Mr. Davis responded, "I'm glad you think I'm doing better. When do I get moved?" His doctor replied, "The nurse will take you over there sometime today. You're going to be fine."

Later that morning one of the nurses told Mr. Davis that he was being transferred to the ward. She organized his belongings and assisted in moving him to the new unit, a four-bed ward near the nursing station. The other patients in the room were stable, but required various interventions, such as intravenous fluids or oxygen; and there was one with a Foley catheter, which made them appear quite ill.

Mr. Davis, 44 years old and married, had three children, two sons, 13 and 8, and a daughter, 10. He owned a real estate business and employed three men. His wife was not working at the time, but had taught science in high school before they had children.

This was Mr. Davis's first admission to a hospital and the first indication of coronary problems. He experienced no complications immediately following the myocardial infarction. During his stay in the unit he was quite talkative, asked questions, laughed frequently, and made such comments as, "I'm too strong to let a little thing like this get me down," and "I needed a little rest anyway." During the transfer from the unit, however, he asked the nurse, "Do you really think I am well enough to leave this unit?" The nurse assured him that he was improving quite rapidly and would be out of the hospital soon.

That night Mr. Davis was unable to sleep; he called the nurse frequently to check his intravenous. He complained of the noise in the hall and asked to be put in a room where patients were not so ill. He asked for an extra blanket, as his hands and feet were cold although the palms of his hands were sweaty. He also said that he thought that "they should still be checking my heartbeat." His blood pressure, pulse, and respiration rate were markedly increased. However, his pulse remained regular.

The next day, he complained about the food, medications, visiting hours, and the aide who bathed him. The following night, he complained of severe chest pain and was extremely restless, agitated, and diaphoretic. He was transferred back to the coronary-care unit when electrocardiogram changes consistent with infarction became apparent.

Mr. Davis's experience is typical of situations that indicate the deleterious effects of a new environment on unprepared patients. In a study by Klein and others (1968) it was found that patients had a high occurrence of severe psychological reactions and increased urinary catecholamines after being transferred from the CCU. Related factors contributing to these changes were identified by these investigators as abruptness of the transfer from the unit; private room to ward seen as a demotion; critically ill patients in the new room; decreased numbers of physicians and staff; fewer medications; increased physical activity; and possible changes in diet.

Garrity and Klein (1975) have reviewed the literature of studies considering the role of glucocorticoids in heart diseases. The overproduction of glucocorticoids in response to stress can lead to myocardial electrolyte imbalance or increased sensitivity of heart muscle to the effects of catecholamines. In their own study of patients' adjustment to myocardial infarction, they found that there was a decreased mortality rate within six months for those adjusting to the attack. This finding indicates the importance of psychological factors in coronary disease.

Engel (1976) discusses several studies in an editorial on psychological factors related to sudden death, showing that arrhythmias and sudden death have been induced in animals by electrical stimulation of the brain and by subjection of the animals to situations in which they cannot control the noxious stimulus. These adverse effects do not occur if the animal is given control of the stimulus. In humans, feelings of helplessness, disappointment, dissatisfaction, depression, and uncertainty are associated with occurrence of arrhythmia and sudden death.

In a review of the literature from 1970 through early 1975 on psychological and social-risk factors for coronary disease, Jenkins (1976) presented several studies of psychosocial variables associated with coronary disease. Suffice it to say, for the purposes of this paper, that many psychosocial factors were identified as increasing the risk of developing angina pectoris and myocardial infarction. These factors—including sociological indexes, social mobility, status incongruity, anxiety, neuroticism, other reactive characteristics, life dissatisfactions, interpersonal problems, stress and life change, and coronary-prone behavior pattern—must be given careful consideration in efforts to reduce the incidence of heart disease or resulting complications.

In our example, Mr. Davis may have had several psychosocial risk factors operative in his life. However, the focus of this paper is to discuss the importance of *psychological interventions* during the transfer from the Coronary-Care Unit. Mr. Davis was progressing well in the unit, moving from the initial anxiety denial to admitting on the day of transfer that he was ill in his question, "Do you really think I am *well enough* to leave this unit?" Just as his defenses were beginning to be used less and he became more aware of possible changes in his life because of the infarction, the transfer occurred. It took place without his having had time to deal with the thoughts of a new environment, discuss feelings about the change with family and staff, ask questions, meet the staff on the other unit, or mobilize strong defense mechanisms.

What psychological interventions have been shown to be effective in the prevention of the acute anxiety and its potential complications that may be experienced in a new environment? The primary focus should be a full assessment of the patient's pyschological responses to the myocardial infarction. Efforts to determine psychosocial factors that may have contributed to his attack should be made. From this assessment, potential areas of concern, as well as usual coping behavior pattern, may be identified for the patient and family. This information will serve as a guide in supporting the patient throughout his hospitalization and after discharge. The patient should be prepared early to expect a transfer from the unit to an intermediary unit or ward as soon as his condition no longer necessitates close observation (Andreoli et al., 1971; Granger, 1974; Robinson, 1976). He should be made aware of the fact that when his condition warranted his transfer, he would be moved. Klein et al. (1968) found that assignment of a nurse to the patient during the stay in the unit and a physician during the entire hospitalization assisted in reducing complications from the transfer. Any measures that can facilitate the patient's expression of feelings about the unit and ward should be taken. Does he see the unit as a protective, comfortable, safe environment, and the ward as noisy, unprotected, and understaffed? Andreoli et al. (1971) and Grace et al. (1972) recommend the use of a "weaning" or intermediary unit as being highly desirable in helping the patient and family accept the transfer. Monitoring by telemetry can provide additional support for the patient in both the intermediary unit and ward. If no monitoring is to be done after transfer, Scalzi (1973) recommends disconnecting the monitor a few hours before the transfer.

Scalzi also suggests that the ward nurse visit the patient in the unit before the transfer to discuss differences in routines and to answer his questions. If possible, the family should be included at the time of this meeting. The transfer should be emphasized as a positive step in the recovery process. Any negative feelings that the patient has should be discussed.

At the time of the transfer, the presence of a relative can provide additional support. The patient should be introduced to the new staff and told that the plan for his care will be shared with the ward staff. Introductions to the other patients in the room should be made. If possible, these patients should be nonacute. Several experts have suggested that the patient should be visited by nurses from the coronary-care unit (Andreoli et al., 1971; Robinson, 1976). Klein et al. (1968) found that having a nurse spend an hour each day with the patient, talking with him and providing care, was an effective measure. Teaching the family and patient and helping them to adjust to the changes become a part of the nurse's caregiving responsibilities.

Other measures that can be used to decrease anxiety on transfer to the ward are explanations of hospital routine, call lights, location of things in the room, and visiting hours. The patient should be encouraged to verbalize feelings and concerns, with the nurse staying with him during extremely anxious periods. Defense mechanisms should be recognized and supported until the patient is able to deal with the threatening situation. Allowing the patient and family to be involved in the decision-making increases their knowledge and control of events. Participation in as many activities as possible should be encouraged (Andreoli et al., 1971; Bragg, 1975; Foster and Andreoli, 1970; Grace et al., 1972; Robinson, 1976). Cassem and Hackett (1973) found that a consistent exercise program begun on the third day of hospitalization and continued through the rehabilitation period had psychological benefits for the patient. The program provides the patient with something to do and confirms to him that he is alive (Bragg, 1975). Andreoli et al. (1971) suggest that discussion of discharge plan should be done during preparation for the transfer and until discharge to assist patient and family to focus on the eventual outcome.

During the transfer and for a period of time after the move, the patient should be assessed for adverse psychological reactions as well as physiological complications. The patient may again experience anxiety, denial, anger, hostility, depression, and other responses in the process of accepting the changed environment.

As noted in Mr. Davis's case, psychological reactions to the transfer can be deleterious. Application of the interventions described in this paper has been shown to decrease the complications that result from a transfer. These psychological interventions are required for both the patient and family to make the transfer less threatening, support them during the adjustment, and provide for the patient's continued recovery.

References

Andreoli, K. C., et al. 1971. Comprehensive Cardiac Care. St. Louis: C. V. Mosby.

Bragg, T. L. 1975. "Psychological Responses to Myocardial Infarction," Nursing Forum, 14:383–95.

Cassem, N. H. and T. P. Hackett. 1973. "Psychological Rehabilitation of Myocardial Infarction Patients in the Acute Phase," Heart and Lung (May-June), 2:382–87.

Engel, G. L. 1976. "Psychologic Factors in Instantaneous Cardiac Death," The New England Journal of Medicine (May 18), 294(12):664–65.

Foster, S. and K. G. Andreoli. 1970. "Behavior Following Myocardial Infarction," *American Journal of Nursing* (November), 70:2344–48.

Garrity, T. F. and R. F. Klein. 1975. "Emotional Response and Clinical Severity as Early Determinants of Six Month Mortality After Myocardial Infarction," *Heart and Lung* (September-October), 4(5):730–37.

Gentry, W. D. and T. Harvey. 1975. "Emotional and Behavioral Reaction to Acute Myocardial Infarction," *Heart and Lung* (September-October), 4(5):738–45.

Grace, W. J. et al. 1972. "Intermediate Care After Myocardial Infarction," *Heart and Lung* (November-December), 1(6):818–20.

Granger, J. W. 1974. "Full Recovery From Myocardial Infarction: Psychological Factors," *Heart and Lung* (July-August), 3(4):600–10.

Klein, R. F., et al. 1968. "Transfer from Coronary Care Unit," *Archives of Internal Medicine* (August), 122:102–8.

Jenkins, C. D. 1976. "Recent Evidence Supporting Psychologic and Social Risk Factors for Coronary Disease (Parts One and Two)," *New England Journal of Medicine* (April 29, May 6), 18:294; 19:987–94, 1033–38.

Robinson, L. 1976. *Psychological Aspects of the Care of Hospitalized Patients.* Philadelphia: F. A. Davis.

Scalzi, C. C. 1973. "Nursing Management of Behavioral Responses Following an Acute Myocardial Infarction," *Heart and Lung* (January-February), 2:1:62–69.

Additional Bibliography

"Anxiety Recognition and Intervention: Programmed Instruction." 1965. *American Journal of Nursing* (September), 64(4):124–52.

Elms, R. and R. C. Leonard. 1968. "Effects of Nursing Approaches During Admission," *Nursing Research* (Winter), 25(1):39–48.

Meyers, M. E. 1964. "Effect of Types of Communication on Patients' Reactions to Stress," *Nursing Research* (Spring), 13:126–31.

Poslusny, E. 1975. "Anxiety: Patient Behavior and Nursing Intervention." Unpublished lecture content handout. New York: School of Nursing, Columbia University, September.

Shortridge, L. 1976. "Client Care Plan for New Environment." Unpublished class handout. New York: School of Nursing, Columbia University, Fall.

"Understanding Defense Mechanisms: Programmed Instruction." 1972. *American Journal of Nursing* (September), 72:1–24.

Wishnie, H. A. et al. 1971. "Psychologic Hazards of Convalescence Following Myocardial Infarction," *Journal of the American Medical Association,* 215:1292ff.

5
The Psychosocial Needs of the Cardiovascular Patient

Steven A. Moss

WHILE WESTERN JUDEO-CHRISTIAN tradition has taught that we are children of God and little lower than the angels, it has also presented the teaching that "for dust thou art, and unto dust shalt thou return." It has been, I believe, the attractiveness of the former, with its promise of immortality, that has blinded us to the reality of the latter, which guarantees our finite nature and the ultimate fact of death. Our blindness to our finitude has caused us to go on a course that is destroying our environment and ourselves. The food we eat, the air we breathe, the stressful life we lead—all demonstrate this guise of immortality we live under. Even the speeds at which we drive our cars, or our disregard of the cautions of doctors, and of the surgeon-general, point to the fact that most of us believe we shall live forever.

How very often I hear the comment from a person who is sick, "I thought this happened to someone else, not me!" Such a comment implies an assumed invulnerability on the part of the sick person, the feeling that he or she could not get sick. Implied also is the wishful assumption that he or she could not die.

For those who live with these assumptions of invulnerability and immortality when a disease occurs that attacks these assumptions, the result is devastating. Whether it is cancer or cardiovascular disease or some other life-threatening ailment, the general attack on the physical and psychosocial system is the same. The result is one of shock, confusion, groping for proper defense mechanisms, as the reality of sickness and death hits that person who for possibly a lifetime has said, "I never get sick," or "I can't die." Now the possibility presents itself that he *can* die. And it is this realization of vulnerability which hits the cardiovascular patient as a "ton of bricks." The symptoms are not, generally speaking, so insidious or unnoticeable, as those of various malignancies. (Unnoticeable that is, if the victim wants them to be so.) And how often he does want them to be unnoticeable, as he continues that "invulnerable" hectic pace which probably helped bring on the disease in the first place. The following vignette from Louis S. Levine's book *Heart Attack!* is most instructive in showing the victim's denial reaction to the very noticeable warning signs of the worsening cardiovascular disease.

> Hurrying from the restaurant, I walked to my automobile, parked at the top of a hill. About midway, my breathing became heavy and labored; but I knew that the client would be waiting at my office and I struggled on. Then it happened. As I continued, an invisible weight seemed to press against my chest just to the right of center. The pressure, almost centrally located at first, started to spread across both sides of my chest; I began gasping for air. My breathing became so labored that with each step I took I experienced a crushing and constricting sensation in my chest and lungs as though I were being squeezed in a vise. The struggle to breathe, combined with the struggling pressure across my entire chest and the accompanying pain in my lungs and throat, forced me to stop instantly. I felt as if I could not take another step without losing consciousness. For less than one minute, I stood absolutely still. All signs of pressure, pain and breathlessness disappeared completely.
>
> Not quite sure what had happened, I continued to walk to the car. There was no trace of the frightening phenomenon. In spite of the fact that my bodily functions had all returned to normal, I got into the car shaken and cursed quietly to myself. This was a new experience. As I sat behind the steering wheel, reflecting, before starting the motor, I cursed my secretary for making the appointment that had upset my entire day's schedule, the client for not accepting a later date, the accident, which had made me late, and the slow service at the restaurant, which had forced me to hurry with my meal. . . . I refused to visit a physician. . . . But I attributed all that to middle age and mental strain, whether real or imaginary. (1976, pp. 23–24).

What is so instructive with this quotation is that after the attack, Levine continues on his pre-attack pace. Is this not a manifestation of some kind of death wish? Surely, it is an example of denial, and how this mechanism can dangerously affect one's health. And, of course, as he is unaccepting of this attack on his physical vulnerability at the first sign of disease, recovery later on becomes equally as difficult, at least until acceptance does come about.

I am obviously basing the above comments on the presumption that personality and way of life are primary causes of cardiovascular disease, or at least strong influences on it. Dr. Paul Dudley White observed that the majority of young male coronary patients in his series of studies were mesomorphs (in Kastenbaum and Aisenberg, 1972, p. 299). The mesomorphs' traits "include assertiveness, desire and aptitude for vigorous physical activity, and a tendency to dominate others. This constellation is coupled with the relative absence of sensitivity to one's own inner feelings" (ibid., p. 399). This is obviously the "what make's Sammy run" personality, a personality conducive to causing and instigating cardiovascular disease. And it is just this type of personality which will find it difficult to cope with a new outlook on life, necessary for recovery and for a minimizing of the recurrence of attack.

As this type of personality denied the facts of disease, as he denied his physical vulnerability, this same denial process can go on during the recuperation period. Denial, repression, rationalization can take over as the patient assumes various activities, and certainly "normal" daily activities. He can also become so immobilized by fear, as his realization of vulnerability and the shattering of his image of immortality come to light, that these also can contribute to further disease and difficulties for recovery. It is my belief that these processes, whichever they be or in whatever combination they are formed, begin to take shape once the confirmation of disease takes place, be it by physical pain itself, or the doctor's diagnosis and prognosis. In other words, the processes of coping and accepting, or the mechanisms of denial and repression, begin in the hospital or doctor's office. These fears, expectations, acceptance of limitations are aspects of the psychosocial person which must be dealt with immediately and not once the patient is discharged. Those lonely isolated hours in the cardiac-care unit give much time for thought. And if the thoughts are not communicated or worked through, the question must be raised as to their eventual effect on the patient's recovery.

The cardiac-care unit monitors the inner physical workings of the patient, but what or who monitors the psychosocial workings of the person? While in the hospital, cardiac patients are given verbal instructions, as well as booklets—on diet, exercise, work load, the mechanisms of the heart, and of what happened to the organ. But does anyone discuss with him his fears of future attack, death, coping with the instructed limitations on what was before a "normal" active way of life, and the accepting of a new philosophy toward stress, scheduling, and life itself. A weakness in loving, caring, support, open communication, appropriate respect for the patient as person by the hospital team and by the family can affect a patient's isolation and difficulties in coping with his future life under disease, in and out of the hospital. As with the cancer patient, the following is also important for cardiovascular patients.

> Unprepared to meet the constant questions of the dying patient, they tend either to avoid him or to adopt an unfamiliar manner. The distance between them and the dying can quickly become enormous. Deception cannot flourish where openness and honesty have been the rule. One of the saddest dramas enacted is the silent conspiracy between a doctor and relatives to keep the patient happily uninformed, when, all the while, the patient has been playing his assigned role and protecting the feelings of the other actors. (Reeves, 1973)

Such closed communications and cut off relationships can have the same effect on the cardiovascular patient as on the terminal cancer patient. And it is my belief that as so much work has been done in the area of more open communication with the terminal cancer patient, so too it should be carried over into relationships with the cardiovascular patient. Such work must begin in the hospital, to assure the patient the optimum chances for recovery and living his life to the fullest, learning to cope and accept in the face of various degrees of physical and psychosocial limitations. Specialized teams of nurses, doctors, psychiatrists, social workers, clergymen should be trained in this very important task. It is time for all hospitals and their cardiac staffs to treat not only diseased hearts and vascular systems, but also diseased human beings, their ways of life, their attitudes toward living. When they do so, they will aid the cardiovascular patient in getting back to living life with an attitude conducive to optimum enjoyment, within the limitations of his own body and life. Levine wrote:

> I have often thought about those dark days when I teetered between life and death. I have contemplated what I could have done to prevent that heart attack . . . being aware of this problem would have made me conscious of my own stressful personality and emotional make-up. I might have striven to be less tense, less of a perfectionist.

If these precautions did not prevent the heart attack, they might have delayed it until a much later time, when the chances of survival would have been vastly improved because my collaterals would have been more developed.

If the heart attack was predestined, I realize now that I required assistance from sources other than my own strength to survive. I know now that I had to rely on values that have been cherished by the human race for so many centuries—the love of a wife and children, and faith in God. (1976, p. 12.)

References

Levine, L. S. 1976. *Heart Attack!* New York: Harper & Row.
Kastenbaum, R. and R. Aisenberg. 1972. *The Psychology of Death.* New York: Springer.
Reeves, R. B., Jr. et al. 1973. *Pastoral Care of the Dying and Bereaved: Selected Readings.* New York: Health Sciences Publishing Company.

Part II

Personality Patterns and Coronary Heart Disease

☙ 6
Introduction to Part II:
The Cardiovascular Patient

Arnold A. Hutschnecker

IF LIFE, IN the words of Herbert Spencer, is a continual adjustment of internal relations to external relations, we find the cardiovascular patient engaged in a relentless struggle of inner hostile-aggressive feelings against the external psychosocial demands of his group and his own set of values. This type of patient is conditioned to meet the challenges of life by fight rather than flight and by a relentless need to excel in order for the world to consider him worthy of love. Early experiences of rejection cause him to compensate for his feelings of vulnerability or insignificance by setting extraordinary goals for himself, and by pursuing difficult tasks to attain the recognition he craves. Striving for positions of power, status, and money, he does not allow himself to relax nor is he overly concerned about intrinsic values that would help him to mature and to relate affectionately with another human being.

In his studies of hypertension, at the Chicago Institute for Psychoanalysis, Franz Alexander, found that most of these patients "as children are prone to attacks of rage and to be aggressive. Then, at some point, a change of attitude takes place . . . unable to assert himself, the aggressive child then becomes overly compliant."

Compliance in the hostile-aggressive person, who eventually

becomes a cardiovascular patient, is the mask that covers the fire that burns within. Pride and ambition stir and he can never allow himself to appear weak. He is like the captain on the bridge who never sleeps. Or, the politician whose deeds must stand out and at all times attest to his brilliance, his magnificence, and his human concern for others.

Different from the mentally depressed and suicidal individual, the cardiovascular patient is psychodynamically a person who chooses to die with his boots on. It is not society that makes continual demands on this patient. It is his interpretation of what he believes society demands of him that feeds his inner aggressive drives. It is his autoplastic disease picture—the picture he has of himself in relation to his illness—that causes the difficulties such a patient creates for other people, primarily his family, friends, and physicians.

The psychosocial aspects of the life-threatened cardiovascular patient then must be considered in the light of his specific psychodynamic functioning and his established reaction pattern. His inner will and emphasis on the heroic, namely to die at the peak of power rather than to go on with a prospect of vegetating, are decisive factors in the outcome of the illness. These are patients who will say "Doc . . . give it to me straight" and, as a rule, will not settle for a promise to be taken care of. Life's ultimate meaning for them is achievement, for on their achievement depends their feeling of worthiness to be loved. Whenever there is a break in this hope, the life-threatened cardiovascular patient will tend to turn his aggression against himself and must then be considered a potential suicide.

7
Psychosocial Aspects of Cardiovascular Disease

Raymond Harris

PHYSICIANS HAVE LONG known empirically that psychosocial stresses and strains can affect the cardiovascular system and, in some patients, induce cardiac arrhythmias, angina pectoris, and even death (Levine, 1963; Wolf, 1969; Engel, 1971). John Hunter, an outstanding eighteenth-century surgeon, accurately predicted the manner of his own demise when he said, "My life is at the mercy of any scoundrel who chooses to put me in a passion." But, as scientific medicine developed in the late nineteenth century, such ready acceptance of clinical experience declined. The new scientific approach downgraded empiricism and insisted a cause of death had to be established at autopsy and in the laboratory rather than by clinical experience or observation. More recently, the development of new techniques has renewed interest in psychosocial stresses and has stimulated new research into the pathogenesis of cardiovascular diseases, particularly hypertension, cardiac arrhythmias, and ischemic heart disease, that indicate emotional states may affect hormonal and neuronal functioning and produce cellular changes in the body which can alter behavior.

The American Heart Association, estimating that during 1976 about 1,060,900 persons died of heart attacks or related heart ailments in the United States, strongly maintains that attention to the risk factors that produce heart disease can decrease the risk of developing such disease. Psychosocial stress is certainly one of the most important risk factors which contribute to cardiovascular disease. If the incidence of heart disease is to be lowered, people must learn how to handle and cope with the psychological and physical stresses that modern society inevitably exerts.

What Is Stress?

According to Selye (1976), stress occurs when stimulation raises the activity of an organism more rapidly than its adaptation response can lower it. A "stressor" is a change in the internal or external environment of such magnitude that it requires from the organism more than the usual adaptation and defense reactions to maintain its life or homeostasis. It differs from a stimulus, which means any change in the environment. A stress, because of its intensity, is therefore more than a stimulus and the difference between a stimulus and a stressor is often quantitative rather than qualitative. It also depends on the sensitivity of the organism at a certain moment. Stresses (like stimuli) may be physical, chemical, viral, bacteriological, biological, or interpersonal.

It is essential to distinguish between a stressor as a causative agent and stress (the nonspecific response). Dr. Selye defines biological stress as a nonspecific response of the body to any demand made upon it. It is a specific complex of physiological responses to nonspecific changes in the environment. Stress is characterized by increased catecholamine or corticoid secretion, thymus atrophy, or gastrointestinal ulcers. Stress which accompanies all normal biological reactions is not necessarily harmful. In the form of nonspecific therapy such as exercise, cold, heat, electroshock, it can even effect curative responses.

When a psychosocial response occurs as a response to memories or signals no longer corresponding to reality, or when it continues to appear because the organism cannot adapt, the machinery of the body is being misused. This physiological pattern of response is harmful and strain ensues.

Much stress results from the inevitable conflict between man's genetically determined, fixed-action pattern and the demands of his modern psychosocial environment. Unlike our less-cultured caveman ancestors, we no longer strike or flee from someone whom we dislike intensely. Although our whole circulation and metabolism may become mobilized in preparation for fight or flight, we "grin and bear it" on the surface; inside, we seethe, boil, and build up stress. These reactions can become harmful and produce disease if they are mobilized repeatedly during the course of a day, without being adequately discharged by exercise, relaxation, or other appropriate techniques.

Psychosocial stresses, representing the general malaise of a modern society and reflected in unavoidable feelings of tension, anxiety, and alienation, are often as devasting as the more obvious and measurable physiological stresses. They exert their effects on the body through various mechanisms, depending upon the person's personality, disposition, coping and habituation, appraisal of threat to safety, frustration, challenge, and gratification. They arise from the societal interrelationships experienced in familial relationships, social relationships, work and work-related problems, such as promotions, success, retirement, and other social pressures associated with aging and the cultural attitudes of society. The individual psychosocial stressors—such as threats to security, self-esteem, way of life, or safety—contribute enormously to stress and strain. The uncertainty in cultural changes—the products of today's constantly changing technological society—is sometimes more than most individuals can safely bear. These pressures, together with the uncertainty of employment, rising inflation, death and living, and other societal factors, produce stress and eventual exhaustion, leading to capitulation of the patient and to the development of some form of heart disease, such as hypertension, cardiac arrhythmias, ischemic heart disease, or other stress-induced illnesses.

Short-term reactions to these psychological stressors may include damaged performance, emotional changes, and reversible behavioral signs and disturbances; long-term reactions may produce neurosis, disturbed social adjustment, and stress-related disease, including cardiovascular illness and gastrointestinal and other disorders.

In our well-to-do type of Western culture, the main social stressors include emotional deprivation, lack of group support, and loneliness in the midst of the crowd, coupled with material affluence. In the poorer sociological stratum, these same factors, coupled with material deprivation and overcrowding, compound these difficulties. The problems of aging, retirement, and inflation also constitute significant social stressors for most people.

Psychosocial Stress and Clinical Heart Disease

Although it has been widely accepted that obesity, hypertension, diabetes, overconsumption of animal fat, cigarette smoking, and too little exercise enhance the likelihood of coronary atherosclerosis, myocardial infarction, and sudden death, there is also growing evidence that a pattern of behavior (Type A), characterized by tireless striving and doing things the hard way without commensurate satisfaction, may also be implicated (Friedman and Rosenman, 1974).

Engel (1971) noted that life settings for sudden death fall into eight categories which involve events impossible for the victims to ignore or overlook and to which they respond by becoming overwhelmingly excited, giving up, or both. This noxious combination provokes basic neurovegetative reactions involving both the flight/fight response and preservation/withdrawal systems which may be conducive to lethal cardiac events, particularly in individuals with preexisting cardiovascular disease. Other investigators reported that an increased rating in a scale of major life changes, such as death of a spouse, divorce, loss of a child, and so forth predicts persons who will develop myocardial infarction or die from a coronary accident with as much accuracy as the more traditional physical risk factors of high blood pressure and high serum cholesterol. Such studies imply that life-change variables may precipitate cardiac illness and death and suggest that if persons had not been exposed to these major psychological stresses, they may not have developed myocardial infarction or have died when they did.

Wolf (1969) and others (Friedman and Rosenman, 1974) have emphasized the importance of psychosocial factors in the causation of myocardial infarction and sudden death. They believe an increased risk of myocardial infarction is present in persons with certain personality and behavioral characteristics classified as Type A. Persons striving and struggling to succeed and not enjoying success when it comes are more susceptible to serious heart disease. They follow a life-style characterized as the Sisyphus pattern, in which myocardial infarction occurs when their life patterns are overtaxed or decompensated. This situation is often associated with depressive manifestations. Dr. Wolf found that 28 patients dying within the seven-year period of his study had deaths associated with a severely stressful episode. His patients displayed greater psychological disturbances and reacted to stresses in life with depression—not that they had more stresses, but that they handled them badly and reacted poorly to them.

Research and Psychosocial Aspect of Heart Disease

Roadblocks to ascertaining the precise influence of stress and higher nervous system activity on cardiac rhythm and function have included the very complex nature of the psychological variables, the difficulty in defining and quantifying emotional responses, and the susceptibility of the heart itself to arrhythmias. Nevertheless, progress is being made in developing appropriate research designs which permit the application of psychological stimuli and stresses to the body and measuring their effects upon the cardiovascular system and the brain.

Sound experimental data demonstrate that psychologic stress can actually alter the ventricular threshold of cardiac vulnerability and provoke major arrhythmias in animals with experimentally produced coronary occlusion. For example, Corbalan et al. (1974) found that the production of psychological stress during myocardial infarction in the conscious dog provides a good experimental model for the systemic investigation of the roles of psychological factors in the development of cardiac arrhythmias. They noted that before coronary arterial obstruction, psychological stress lowered the vulnerable-period threshhold for repetitive ventricular responses by 82 percent; after myocardial infarction, presentation of stressful stimuli provoked diverse ventricular arrhythmias, including ventricular tachycardia and early extrasystoles with T-wave interruption.

Other experiments have linked psychological and neural activity with the production of ventricular fibrillation or other life-threatening cardiac arrhythmias even in the absence of organic heart disease. Lown et al. (1976) demonstrated that neurophysiologic activity can change electrical properties of the myocardium and precipitate fibrillation in the absence of demonstrable cardiac disease. There is also evidence that hypothalamic stimulation can provoke ventricular fibrillation in animals with coronary arterial-occlusive disease, and even in normal animals, midbrain stimulation can substantially reduce the ventricular fibrillation threshold.

A major difficulty has been to devise experiments showing how psychosocial stresses affect the human heart. Now it has been demonstrated that stress interviews can induce significant

ST-T depressions in the electrocardiogram confirming that emotional stress affects the heart, especially in patients with angina (Schiffer et al. 1976).

These experiments and other data suggest that in the intact individual, the central nervous system exerts a continuous regulatory tone and possesses the capacity for making powerful adjustments. Autonomic and neuroglandular mechanisms are activated through neurons in the hypothalamus that respond in turn to impulses resulting from integrative processes in the cerebral hemispheres. The latter interprets events and experiences, and consciously or unconsciously relates them to attitudes, conditioning, and other characteristics peculiar to the individual. The capability to make major modifications in cardiac function may be found in the limbic system, an association area that handles input signals from visceral and somatic sensory nerves, as well as from the parts of the brain that interpret experiences.

The Detection of a History of Psychosocial Stress

A good psychosocial history is the first step in detecting the presence of psychosocial stress. It should be suspected in any patient with a history of, for example, death of a spouse or family member, divorce, separation, jail term, severe injury or illness, marriage, pregnancy, loss of a job, change in financial status, foreclosure of mortgage, change in residence, vacations, minor law violations, or retirement. Each of these stressors may produce some type of stress; their total effect depends upon the tolerance of the individual.

Symptoms of stress include complaints of tense muscles; sore neck, shoulders and back; insomnia; undue fatigue not brought on by extreme physical exertion; boredom, depression, listlessness, dullness and lack of interest; drinking too much, eating too much or too little; gastrointestinal complaints such as diarrhea, cramps, gas, constipation, palpitations, heart skip, and chest pain; phobias or fear of enclosed places, heights; facial tics, restlessness, itching, and undue worry.

A Tape-Recording Technique

I recently began using a tape-recording technique that has brought to the surface many interesting psychosocial problems in older cardiovascular patients. Although some patients have been treated over long periods of time, many of these problems did not emerge until I began tape recording. The success naturally depends upon the skill, experience, interests, and available time of the interviewer and the cooperation of the patient. Patients often provided highly significant information when asked simple nondirective questions. During such questioning, the nonverbal responses of the patient were often more revealing than their answers.

The technique itself is simple. After the patient sits down, I turn on a small standard tape recorder that is already on my desk in front of the patient and say, "I would like to tape record our conversation so that I can get a good history for your record and to help you better. Is it all right with you to tape our discussion?" Almost invariably, the patient assents. I do not attempt a complete life-cycle review of the patient at any one visit. Usually, I continue these discussions during several office visits to save time. The information often pinpoints some of the psychologic factors behind the patient's illness and complaints and helps me to better understand what is bothering him and to determine how to treat him. The tapes are transcribed, and the transcriptions filed in the patient's chart for further review.

The psychosocial interview technique provides the astute physician or therapist with additional background information that illuminates how and why his patient's cardiovascular condition developed and what happened to the patient on his way to old age and cardiovascular disease. Many patients seem to have dammed up within them psychic pressures, built up by the stresses and maladaptation to them over the years, which this technique decompresses. An observation was made to me that this technique "undressed the patient mentally and left him stark naked." This was an intriguing observation. For a good physical examination, we undress the patient physically; is there any reason not to undress him mentally to obtain information about his mental and emotional state? Of course, the interviewer using this technique must be familiar with the inherent dangers of allowing the patient to undress himself mentally too rapidly lest it promote an emotional crisis. I have been careful to end the interview or to change the subject by inserting an appropriately different question if I notice the patient is becoming too agitated, upset, or disturbed by my questions or his responses.

Occasionally, a patient refuses to have the discussion taped.

When this occurs, I turn the recorder off and ask the patient why he does not want the conversation recorded. The answers often prove equally informative and helpful in assaying the situation and shed light on the patient's personality and condition. Some patients object to being recorded if a medical-legal examination is being done. Others eventually permit themselves to be recorded, and as a matter of fact, look forward to being taped when they come in again. One such hypertensive patient, who declined at first to be taped, explained later that he thought I wanted to record our conversation to protect myself against malpractice! This idea had not occurred to me, but it is a practical defense against the rising cost of malpractice. This 68-year-old patient with a 20-year history of hypertension provided a fascinating life-cycle history on his next visit. Although for almost 20 years I had treated him medically for his hypertension, the taped interview provided the first inkling of the background problems that underlay his hypertension and his life. For example, even at 68 years of age, he was still disturbed by the intermarriage of his Jewish father and Catholic mother. He was brought up with no religious education and found it difficult to find his identity as a result of the intermarriage of his parents and, subsequently, of his own intermarriage and that of his son who later became psychotic. As I listened silently without prodding or attempting depth analysis, this man related his story without prompting. His nonverbal responses were dramatic; at times, his face became florid, his hands hyperactive, and his blood pressure rose and fell as I took it, despite the fact that he was on medication.

Stress in the Coronary Care Unit

There is evidence that patients with acute myocardial infarctions in coronary-care units are under severe stress and may require psychiatric consultation (Gentry and Williams, 1975). Hackett and Cassem (1975) note the three most common reasons for psychiatric consultation in the coronary-care unit are anxiety, depression, and management problems. Anxiety occurs early in the coronary-care-unit patient, usually on the first or second day; depression peaks on the third day, and management problems of a bimodal distribution with a higher peak coming on the second day and a lower peak emerging on the fourth day. There is usually no relationship between anxiety and the seriousness of the illness or the patient's socioeconomic background. Anxiety usually stems from either the prospect of sudden death or the appearance of death's heralds—breathlessness, severe chest pain, or other complications.

It is important to recognize that emotional states can occur quite independently of pathophysiological processes. The patient may well be emotionally disturbed, but this may have nothing to do with the disease process itself.

The taping technique and/or psychiatric consultations enable the physician to focus on the patient's life functioning and to decide whether to recommend psychotherapy or to offer supportive therapy in his own office. Very often the patient with a psychosomatic disorder who cannot externalize his inner feelings may actually be better off coming to his physician's office for reassuring conversations instead of being referred for psychiatric care. It is the patient who is verbal and intelligent enough to explore his own feelings who is likely to have the degree of insight needed to benefit from such short-term psychotherapy.

How Patients Regard Their Illness and Themselves

In studying psychosocial stresses, it is important to know how patients with life-threatening cardiovascular disease regard their illness. To find out, we conducted a study of attitudes toward living and death in 100 elderly patients with known cardiovascular disease (Ninivaggi and Harris, 1976). We found that subjects regarded their illness as a significant impediment to carrying on a fully active and meaningful existence. Concern about imminent death and the search for increased responsibilities and relatedness were the two most important recurrent themes that came out in these interviews.

Like the tape recordings mentioned earlier, these interviews themselves appeared therapeutic and afforded patients the opportunity to engage in a meaningful interpersonal activity that reaffirmed their worth and ability to contribute toward both personal and social understanding and betterment.

Most of these patients understood their "heart trouble" to mean a functional impairment or the experience of physical symptoms. They spoke with feeling of the impact on them of significant limitation of physical activities. Of the 100 patients, 21 percent were overtly depressed, and the remaining 79 percent optimistic.

Almost all related positively toward their physician and described his role as significantly related to their well-being. Their goals in life included health, travel and vacation, remaining independent, and not becoming helpless. Concern for others, especially spouse and children, and their wish to stay alive were considered the most important tasks in life at this time. Three-fourths of the patients felt satisfied or helped by discussing their illness during the course of the interview.

The most outstanding features of this survey were consistent with the theme that meaningful human existence is a function of interpersonal relatedness and that the threat of its loss constitutes a primary concern of those who face imminent death from a potentially lethal disease such as cardiovascular disease. This quality of being related in a responsible and caring way to others appears to impart meaning and a sense of personal satisfaction to life. It would appear from this study that interpersonal relatedness is a basic motivating force in formulating attitudes toward living and death in the elderly.

Summary

Clinical and basic investigations into the psychosocial factors of cardiovascular disease demonstrate the importance of such psychosocial factors in producing stress situations that may lead to strain-induced illnesses, such as hypertension, cardiac arrhythmias, and death from cardiovascular disease. For the physician, patient, and family, and others concerned with treating patients with life-threatening cardiovascular conditions, it is important to obtain and understand the individual psychosocial factors behind the conscious and unconscious attitudes, façade, and life experiences of the patient, which build up physiological and psychological stresses. Attention to their mechanisms and their influence upon the patient offers hope in preventing further serious cardiovascular illness.

The research techniques for investigating these factors require a combined basic sciences and behavioral-sciences approach. Such coordinated studies can unravel the still-hidden connections between psychic, social, and cultural stresses, which eventually lead, in some way, to cardiovascular illness. As has been pointed out, there are too many clinical observations relating emotional and psychic stresses to the development of cardiovascular disease and death for such relationships to be coincidental rather than causal.

The taped life-cycle review, as described above, is a useful clinical technique for eliciting important psychosocial history and, at the same time, providing therapeutically helpful information to the life-threatened cardiovascular patient, his family, and the medical and health-care staff.

Better understanding of the potentially lethal life situations and identification of individuals at risk may lead to the development of practical prophylactic measures. In time, we may yet have a better explanation than divine edict for the death of Ananias who fell down dead when he was charged by Peter, as the Bible tells us, "You have not lied to man, but to God" (Engel, 1971).

References

Corbalan, R., R. Verrier, and B. Lown. 1974. "Psychological Stress and Ventricular Arrhythmias during Myocardial Infarction in the Conscious Dog," *American Journal of Cardiology*, 34:692–96.

Engel, G. L. 1971. "Sudden and Rapid Death during Psychological Stress," *Annals of Internal Medicine*, 74:771–82.

Friedman, M. and R. H. Rosenman. 1974. *Type A Behavior and Your Heart*. New York: Knopf.

Gentry, W. D. and R. B. Williams, Jr., eds. 1975. *Psychological Aspects of Myocardial Infarction and Coronary Care*. St. Louis: C. V. Mosby.

Hackett, T. P. and N. H. Cassem. 1975. *Coronary Care. Patient Psychology*. Booklet, American Heart Association.

Levine, S. A. 1963. "Benign Atrial Fibrillation of Forty Years' Duration with Sudden Death from Emotion," *Annals of Internal Medicine*, 58:681–84.

Lown, B., J. V. Temte, P. Reich et al. 1976. "Basis for Recurring Ventricular Fibrillation in the Absence of Coronary Heart Disease and Its Management," *New England Journal of Medicine*, 294:623–29.

Ninivaggi, F. J. and R. Harris. 1976. "Attitudes Toward Living and Death; in Chronic Cardiovascular Disease," *New York State Medical Journal*, 76:1493–96.

Schiffer, F., L. H. Hartley, C. L. Schulman, and W. H. Abelmann. 1976. "The Quiz Electrocardiogram: A New Diagnostic and Research Technique for Evaluating the Relation Between Emotional Stress and Ischemic Heart Disease," *American Journal of Cardiology*, 37:41–47.

Selye, H. 1976. *The Stress of Life*, rev. ed. New York: McGraw-Hill.

Wolf, S. 1969. "Psychosocial Forces in Myocardial Infarction and Sudden Death." (Suppl. 4) *Circulation*, 40:74.

❀8
Sudden, Unexpected Death in Patients with Healed Myocardial Infarction

Stewart G. Wolf, Jr.

WHEN DEATH OCCURS following myocardial infarction, the heart itself is usually not severely damaged. It stops beating, therefore, not because of weakness or incapacity of the myocardium but because of a disturbance in the mechanism that regulates the rhythm of the heartbeat and, hence, the effectiveness of its pumping action. Death then results from inadequate profusion of the brain.

It is paradoxical that a heart, only slightly damaged or not damaged at all, should suddenly stop, since it has a very effective intrinsic mechanism to maintain its beat. Even when cut out of an animal's body and perfused in vitro the heart will continue to beat for a long period of time. Indeed, Kountz (1934, 1932), years ago revived the heartbeat of dead Egyptians and with appropriate perfusion observed them to continue beating for hours. When, therefore, the heart of an intact person perfused with adequately oxygenated blood stops suddenly, the explanation may lie outside the heart itself.

Neural Control of the Heartbeat

Leriche, Hermann, and Fontaine, in 1931, implicated the nervous system when they demonstrated in animals that excision of the upper thoracic sympathetic ganglia greatly reduced the likelihood of extrasystoles and ventricular fibrillation immediately following sudden occlusion of a coronary artery. The findings were extended in the studies of Manning, McEachern and Hall (1939), and of de Takats, Beck and Fenn (1939), who demonstrated reflex coronary constriction after pulmonary embolization. The Canadian group and later LeRoy and Snider (1941) described a generalized vasoconstriction in the heart of dogs immediately following experimental occlusion of one coronary artery. They observed that "the uninfarcted part of the myocardium gradually becomes as dark as the infarct just before ventricular fibrillation commences." Seventy-five percent of the animals in which a coronary artery had been ligated died in this fashion. In as many as two-thirds of such animals, however, both groups of authors were able to prevent ventricular fibrillation and death when they effected partial deafferentation of the heart by sympathectomy, by performing the procedure under deep anesthesia, or by pretreatment with atropine or atropine plus theophylline derivatives. More recently, Porter and French (1960) demonstrated an important central element in the reflex, namely an increased excitability in the reticular activating system, which can be induced by hypoxia, hypoglycemia, hypercapnia, and also by light anesthesia. Other workers have adduced intriguing evidence that instability in the cardiac regulatory mechanisms resulting in fatal arrhythmia may be triggered by emotionally stressful experiences.

Forebrain Mechanisms

It is likely that modifications in cardiac function attributable to psychosocial forces involve connections in the limbic system, an association area that handles input signals from visceral and somatic sensory nerves, as well as from the parts of the brain that interpret experience. The limbic system, beginning in the septum between the two cerebral hemispheres and arching laterally along the lower border of the temporal lobe to include the hippocampus, fornix, amygdala, and gray matter that surrounds the aqueduct of Sylvius, interacts with the frontal lobes above and the hypothalamus below, where synapses provide connections to the nuclei of autonomic effectors in the medulla. The cerebellum is also capable of modulating the rate and rhythm of the heart as it is the performance of skeletal muscle structures. Atrial and ventricular arrhythmias, including ventricular tachycardia, have been induced in cats and monkeys by stimulation in the various sites described above (Proceedings, Brain Research Symposium, 1972). Such serious arrhythmias have also been induced in human subjects by the technique of the stress interview (Wolf et al., 1955).

Myocardial Infarction

In Western industrialized societies, myocardial infarction is the most frequent cause of sudden death. A wealth of published anecdote and the personal experience of hosts of physicians attest to the importance of psychological factors in the precipitation of myocardial infarction—intense disappointment, frustration, failure after vast effort, and bereavement. With respect to the latter, epidemiological studies have shown myocardial infarction and sudden death to be significantly increased among the recently bereaved (Parkes, 1967; Rees and Lutkins, 1967).

Increased risk of myocardial infarction has also been identified with certain personality and behavioral characteristics. From published descriptions of many clinicians (Osler, 1910; Dunbar, 1943; Arlow, 1945; Weiss et al., 1957; Wardwell et al., 1963; Cleveland et al., 1962; Russek, 1959; Cathey et al., 1962) going back more than 60 years, a characterization of the coronary-prone person has emerged for which we have suggested the term "Sisyphus reaction" (Wolf, 1969).* The pattern is that of an "effort oriented" person who strives against odds, but with very little sense of accomplishment or satisfaction, a person driving and struggling to succeed and not enjoying success (Arlow, 1945; Ostfeld et al., 1974; Dunbar, 1943; Weiss et al., 1957; Russek, 1959; Friedman and Rosenman, 1959; Wardwell et al., 1963; Cleveland and Johnson, 1962; Cathey et al., 1962; Groen, 1965). Although several psychological tests in wide general use have failed to delineate a personality or behavioral type characteristic of ischemic heart disease (Mordkoff and Parsons, 1968), questionnaires fo-

* Sisyphus, King of Corinth, banished to Hades, was required to push a huge stone up the side of a hill. Each time he was near the top, it would roll down again, requiring him continually to labor without success.

cused at attitudes toward work and satisfaction have confirmed the clinical judgment referred to above (Theorell and Rahe, 1972). So also have careful observations on identical twins, one of whom developed manifestations of ischemic heart disease (Liljefors, 1970; Liljefors and Rahe, 1970). Moreover, extensive studies by Friedman and Rosenman (1959) have afforded strong support for a closely related formulation designated as behavior pattern A. Myocardial infarction or sudden death seems to occur when the coping pattern is overtaxed or decompensated with accompanying evidences of depression and "emotional drain" (Dreyfus, 1959; Bruhn et al., 1968).

Sociological studies in widely scattered cultural groups have yielded remarkably similar interpretations (Syme and Reeder, 1967; Smith, 1967). Myocardial infarction has increased in prevalence among societies where incongruity has developed between the culture of the group and the demands and expectations of the prevailing social situation. The resemblance to the "struggling" model described by those who have approached the problem from the standpoint of personality or behavior is apparent.

Since autonomic mechanisms appear to provide the major final common pathway for the effects of psychosocial forces on the heart and other viscera, our work has focused on the possible relevance of autonomic behavior to the process of myocardial infarction. Autonomic and neuroglandular mechanisms are activated through neurons in the hypothalamus that respond in turn to impulses resulting from integrative processes in the cerebral hemispheres. The latter interpret events and experiences and, consciously or unconsciously, relating them to attitudes, conditioning and other characteristics peculiar to the individual.

Attempts to relate psychosocial data to disease states are difficult to validate because they are based on circumstances that are not strictly replicable; there is no available measure of the emotional significance of an event; and the intervening visceral regulatory circuits and mechanisms are poorly understood. Another problem, that of post hoc observer bias, can be partly circumvented by recourse to prediction of outcome in a prospective study, thus allowing for more rigorous testing of hypotheses. Accordingly, the prognostic significance of a global personality assessment, the Sisyphus pattern, was tested in a 10-year prospective study. There were 124 subjects, 62 having suffered a well-documented myocardial infarction two months or more in the past and an equal number of healthy controls, individually

matched for age, sex, race, height, weight, educational background and type of job.

Predictions were made of the likelihood of myocardial infarction or sudden death on the basis of the Sisyphus pattern, extreme type A behavior, and depression in the total group of patients and controls. Raters were kept as blind as possible with
respect to diagnosis.

The results indicate a close correlation between the Sisyphus
pattern and extreme type A behavior (Friedman and Rosenman
1959). Furthermore, both were significantly more frequent
among patients than controls and both were predictive of poor
prognosis in those who had suffered a myocardial infarction in the
past. Autopsies in nearly 80 percent of those who died revealed a
fresh myocardial infarct in less than half of them. The remaining
hearts showed only the old scar of the original insult.

We found the Sisyphus behavior with depressive manifestations in 11 among 33 of the patient group who died during the
period of study. The electrocardiograms of 10 of the 11 displayed
prolonged QT, more than 10 percent PVCs or both. Among 29
patients who survived the period of study, 7 had been found to
display the psychosocial characteristics described. Three of these
had prolonged QT intervals, more than 10 percent PVCs, or both,
but 4 had neither. Only 3 of the 62 controls had been tagged with
the psychosocial criteria. One of them had more than 10 percent
PVCs.

The findings suggest that the psychosocial manifestations described are reflected in electrocardiographic abnormalities, especially PVCs and long QT intervals, both of which correlated
highly with the risk of sudden, unexpected death.

As social deprivation (including bereavement and other contributors to emotional drain) may predispose to sudden, unexpected death, other social forces (notably family cohesiveness and
community support) may actually counteract or stave off psychosocial forces that precipitate fatal cardiac arrhythmia. Such was
our experience in the Italian-American town of Roseto, Pennsylvania. Although the conventional coronary risk factors (diet high
in saturated fats, cigarette smoking, lack of exercise, and elevated
serum cholesterol concentration) were at least as prevalent in
Roseto as elsewhere in the region, the death rate from myocardial
infarction in Roseto was found to be less than half that of four surrounding towns. The outstanding features of the community of
Roseto were its close family and community ties, the respected

status of the elderly, and the stable, unambiguous man–woman relationship in which the man is automatically conceded the number one position.

Sula Benet, a Professor of Anthropology at Hunter College, New York, tells of the remarkable health and longevity of the Abkhasians of Georgia in the USSR. She emphasizes similar peculiarities of that culture, "the high degree of integration in their lives, the sense of group identity that gives each individual an unshaken feeling of personal security and continuity and permits the Abkhasians as a people to adapt themselves—yet preserve themselves—to the changing conditions imposed by the larger society in which they live," (Benet, 1968). The resemblance to the prevailing philosophy of Roseto is evident.

Also in common with Roseto, and in contrast to most American communities, the place of the elderly in the community of Abkhasians is very special. Dr. Benet writes that as "a life-loving, optimistic people, [they are] unlike so many very old 'dependent' people in the U.S. who feel they are a burden to themselves and their families—they enjoy the prospect of continued life. . . . In a culture which so highly values continuity in its traditions, the old are indispensable in their transmission. The elders preside at important ceremonial occasions, they mediate disputes and their knowledge of farming is sought. They feel needed because . . . they are." The similarity to the situation of the elderly in Roseto is striking.

Death as Adaptation

If there is an adaptive significance in a mechanism that results in cardiac death, one must consider that death at times is the ultimate solution to a pressing problem. Thus, in the midst of intolerable suffering from an incurable disease or life situation, death may best serve the needs of the individual. Physicians as well as most laymen find it difficult to acknowledge such a possibility, and naturally cling to the conviction that their ultimate responsibility is to postpone death. Certain poets and writers have been more perceptive. Referring to sudden death, Robert Browning, in his poem "Prospice" had this to say: ". . . in a minute pay glad life's arrears of pain, darkness and cold." Earlier, Shelley wrote in "Queen Mab": "How wonderful is Death, Death and his brother Sleep." Two hundred years earlier, Shakespeare had Roderigo in

Othello (I,iii) say: "It is silliness to live when to live is torment, and then have we a prescription to die when death is our physician." And in *King Henry VI* (Part I, II,v) the Earl of March said: "just death, kind umpire of men's miseries." Two thousand years before that, in the golden age of Greece, Aeschylus perhaps best characterized the adaptive value of death: ". . . of cureless ills thou art the one Physician." (Fragment 250). A few years ago, Zvi Oster told of his experience in Israel with a patient whom he had resuscitated following a cardiac arrest. On regaining consciousness the man was bitter and dejected. "For two years I have been trying to summon courage to kill myself," he said, "and now when I die legitimately you have to bring me back to life" (Oster).

Conclusion

The evidence reviewed supports the thesis that fatal cardiac arrhythmias, with or without associated myocardial infarction, may often be attributable to autonomic discharges in response to either afferent information from below, or to impulses resulting from integrative processes in the brain involved in adaptation to life experience, or both. It is tempting to speculate that the oft proposed relationship of self-esteem, self-confidence, and optimism to health has a sound scientific basis. In any case, it seems appropriate to supplement our consideration of social stresses with attention to forces that counteract stress and sustain the person. Among these may be numbered strong and confident religious beliefs, family solidarity and all manner of love relationships, as well as the satisfactions of achievement, a sense of purpose in activities, and in a host of uniquely human experiences. Especially striking is the low prevalence of death from myocardial infarction in Japan, a highly competitive industrial nation but one marked by extraordinary lifelong support for the individual from family and even from employer.

References

Arlow, J. A. 1945. "Identification Mechanisms in Coronary Occlusion," *Psychosomatic Medicine*, 7:195.

Benet, S. 1965. *Abkhasians: The Long Living People of the Caucasus*. New York: Holt, Rinehart and Winston.

Bruhn, J. G., K. McCrady, and A. L. DuPlessis. 1968. "Evidence of 'Emotional Drain' Preceding Death from Myocardial Infarction," *Psychiatry Digest*, 29:34.

Cathey, C., H. B. Jones, and J. Naughton. 1962. "Relation of Life Stress to the Concentration of Serum Lipids in Patients with Coronary Artery Disease," *American Journal of Medical Science*, 244:421.

Cleveland, S. E. and D. L. Johnson. 1962. "Personality Patterns in Young Males with Coronary Heart Disease," *Psychosomatic Medicine*, 24:600.

De Takats, G., W. C. Beck, and G. Fenn. 1939. "Pulmonary Embolism. An Experimental and Clinical Study," *Surgery*, 6:339.

Dreyfus, F. 1959. "Role of Emotional Stress Preceding Coronary Occlusion," *American Journal of Cardiology*, 3:590.

Dunbar, F. 1943. *Psychosomatic Diagnosis.* New York: Hoeber.

Friedman, M. and R. Rosenman. 1959. "Association of Specific Overt Behavior Pattern with Blood and Cardiovascular Findings," *Journal of the American Medical Association*, 169:1286.

Groen, J., ed. 1965. *Het Acute Myocardinfarct, een Psychosomatische Studie.* Haarlen: De Erven F. Bohn N.V.

Kountz, W. B. 1932. "Studies on the Coronary Arteries of the Human Heart," *Journal of Pharmacology and Experimental Therapeutics*, 45:65.

Kountz, W. B., E. F. Pearson, and K. F. Koenig. 1934. "Observations on the Effect of Vagus and Sympathetic Stimulation on the Coronary Flow of the Revived Human Heart," *Journal of Clinical Investigations*, 13:1065.

Leriche, R. L., L. Herrmann, and R. Fontaine. 1931. "Ligature de la Coronaire Gauche et Fonction Chez L'animal Intact," *Compt. Rend. Soc. de Biol.*, 107:545.

LeRoy, G. V. and S. S. Snider: 1941. "The Sudden Death of Patients with Few Symptoms of Heart Disease," *Journal of the American Medical Association*, 117:2019.

Liljefors, I. 1970. "Coronary Heart Disease in Male Twins: Heredity and Environmental Factors in Concordant and Discordant Pairs," *Acta Medica Scandinavica*, 188 (Suppl. 511).

Liljefors, I. and R. H. Rahe. 1970. "An Identical Twin Study of Psychosocial Factors in Coronary Heart Disease in Sweden," *Psychosomatic Medicine*, 32:523.

Manning, G. W., C. G. McEachern, and G. E. Hall. 1939. "Reflex Coronary Artery Spasm Following Sudden Occlusion of Coronary Branches," *Archives of Internal Medicine*, 64:661.

Mordkoff, A. and O. A. Parsons. 1968. "The Coronary Personality: A Critique." *International Journal of Psychiatry*, 5:413.

Osler, W. 1910. "The Lumelian Lectures on Angina Pectoris," *Lancet*, 1:696–700, 839–844 and 974–977.

Oster, Z. Personal communication.

Ostfeld, A. M., B. Z. Lebovitz, R. B. Shekelle, and O. Paul. 1974. "Prospective Study of the Relationship between Personality and Coronary Heart Disease," *Journal of Chronic Diseases*, 17:265.

Parkes, C. M. 1967. "Bereavement," *British Medical Journal*, 3:232.

Porter, R. W. and J. D. French. 1960. "The Physiologic Basis of Cardiac Arrest during Anesthesia," *American Journal of Surgery*, 100:354.

Proceedings, Brain Research Symposium. 1972. "Limbic System Influence on Autonomic Function." Toronto, Canada, March, 1969.

Rees, W. D. and S. G. Lutkins. 1967. "Mortality of Bereavement," *British Medical Journal*, 4:13.

Russek, H. J. 1959. "Role of Heredity, Diet and Emotional Stress in Coronary Heart Disease," *Journal of the American Medical Association*, 171:503.

Smith, T. 1967. "Review of Empirical Findings," *Milbank Memorial Fund Quarterly*, 45(2), part 2:23.

Syme, S. L. and L. G. Reeder, eds. 1967. "Social Stress and Cardiovascular Disease," *Milbank Memorial Fund Quarterly*, 45 (2): part 2.

Theorell, T. and R. H. Rahe. 1972. "Behavior and Life Satisfactions Characteristic of Swedish Subjects with Myocardial Infarction," *Journal of Chronic Diseases*, 25:139.

Wardwell, W. I., C. B. Bahnson, and H. S. Caron. 1963. "Social and Psychological Factors in Coronary Heart Disease," *Journal of Health and Human Behavior*, 4:154.

Weiss, E., B. Dlin, H. R. Rollin, H. K. Fisher, and C. R. Bepler. 1957. "Emotional Factors in Coronary Occlusion," *Archives of Internal Medicine*, 99:628.

Wolf, S. 1969. "Psychosocial Forces in Myocardial Infarction and Sudden Death," (Suppl. 4) *Circulation*, 40:74.

Wolf, S., P. V. Cardon, Jr., E. M. Shepard, and H. G. Wolff. 1955. *Life Stress and Essential Hypertension*. A Study of Circulatory Adjustments in Man. Baltimore, Md.: Williams and Wilkins.

9

The Role of Type A Behavior Pattern in Coronary Heart Disease

Ray H. Rosenman

CLINICAL CORONARY HEART disease (CHD) is not a new disease, but its significant incidence did not begin until the second or third decades of the twentieth century, after which it occurred at a rapidly increasing rate in middle-aged males of Western countries. It has been shown that this rapid increase (to near-epidemic proportions) cannot be ascribed to a larger population of older men at risk, to improved diagnosis, or to some rather sudden and esoteric change of genetic factors.

The coronary epidemic has accompanied modern civilization, implying that the environment plays a major role. During the past two decades, the environmental role has been widely considered to be an excessive intake of saturated fats in the diet, combined with a lack of adequate physical activity, while individual specificity has been assigned to risk factors for CHD of which serum cholesterol, blood pressure, and cigarette smoking have been considered the most important. The attention given to these factors has led to the expectation that an altered diet, increased physical activity, and the elimination of the three risk factors would also eliminate the associated disease, even though much of the associations have been based on statistical correlations which cannot be equated with cause and effect relationships. Unfortunately, there is as yet little evidence that such an approach alone will significantly reduce the rate of CHD and, as several recent journal editorials have pointed out, the evidence that alterations of diet, exercise, or the risk factors will reduce the CHD rate is indeed minuscule in proportion to the remarkable aura of faith that surrounds such treatment.

Comparisons of large population groups with very different habitual diets have shown a direct, if not linear, relationship between mean serum cholesterol and mean dietary consumption of fats, particularly saturated fats. Moreover, changes of fat intakes have been found to lower serum cholesterol levels. This has given rise to the widespread belief that the association of diet with CHD incidence is mediated through serum cholesterol, with the implication that the individual serum cholesterol level is regulated primarily by the diet. However, the decrease of mean serum cholesterol in populations fed experimental diets reduced in saturated and enhanced in polyunsaturated fats is relatively small, and is in part, ascribable to statistical regression about the mean. In clinical practice the physician has often found that the effect of such dietary manipulations on the serum cholesterol level is small and in its long range effect often disappointing.

This is not surprising, since relevant studies of the relationship of the diet to the serum cholesterol of individuals have failed to find that the wide variance of cholesterols in any given population group can be explained by diet. Thus, in such studies there has not been found to be any correlation of serum lipids with the quantity or quality of foodstuffs, the proportion of nutrients, the intake of fats or cholesterol, the percentage of calories derived from total fats or their different sources, their degree of saturation or their ratio of saturated to polyunsaturated fatty acid. Thus, in any community susceptible to CHD there has not been found to be any correlation between serum cholesterol and the habitual diet. This does not appear to be because of any dietary threshold above which no simple effect of the diet is exerted on the cholesterol level. Lifelong community dietary habits may shift the distribution of serum cholesterol upward, but it has become clear that nondietary factors are responsible for the wide range of cholesterols observed in any given community. A role of genetic factors in the different physiological handling of both nutrient and endogenous input of lipid into the serum also has not been found to be responsible for the wide variance of serum cholesterol in the vast majority of individuals.

The mechanism underlying this wide variance remains unclear. Although cholesterol absorption is linearly related to the amount in the diet, the rate and amount of its absorption do not differ in subjects with normal and elevated serum cholesterol. On the other hand, the rate of cholesterol removal from the blood is impaired in hypercholesteremic subjects and it is now clear that the serum cholesterol level is regulated primarily by its rate of egress from the plasma rather than by its rate of input either from endogenous or dietary sources. Ingestion of unsaturated fats may reduce serum cholesterol to some degree, but this may be due only to a redistribution of cholesterol between serum and tissues and without any effect of unsaturated fats on the synthesis, excretion, or degradation of cholesterol.

The diet may play a significant role in the pathogenesis of coronary artery disease by some mechanism other than by regulation of serum lipids. In this event, several possible relationships should be found between the diet and the incidence of CHD. In the first place, a relationship should be found between the habitual diets of individuals and their subsequent incidence of CHD. Such a relationship, however, has not been found in prospective epidemiological studies of populations in Framingham, Chicago, San Francisco, and elsewhere, despite the fact that subjects exhibiting higher serum cholesterols in each of these prospective studies suffered a significantly higher rate of CHD. Even when the subjects in these studies with the highest and lowest intakes of saturated fats were contrasted there was no evidence of any relationship between diet and the subsequent occurrence of CHD.

In the second place, an association between diet and CHD incidence should be found in studies of large population groups. International comparisons have shown a general relationship between dietary fat intake and CHD incidence in such assessments, but closer scrutiny shows that even these are from linear relationships. There also are many discrepancies. For example, the frequency of coronary mortality rates is better than average in English and American farming communities subject to prolonged exposure to diets dominated by dairy produce and animal fats. A number of primitive groups have been identified who habitually ingest diets high in saturated fats and nevertheless exhibit enviably low serum cholesterols and freedom from CHD. The comparison of brothers who remained in Ireland with those who migrated to Boston found that the migrants had higher serum cholesterols and higher rates of CHD although they took in fewer calories and ate less animal fats, cholesterol, and carbohydrates. Comparisons between the east and west regions of Finland showed higher CHD rates in the east, which were not ascribable to differences of diet, including intake of animal fats. Clearly the relationship between dietary fat and CHD is not a simple matter of one cause and one effect.

In the third place, an association between diet and CHD incidence might be indicated by parallel increases in both. However, an altered diet was found not to account for the increased rate of CHD in Yemenites after migration to Israel, and for only a small proportion of the increased rate of CHD observed in postwar Japan. Little change has occurred during the past 200 years in the intake of animal fats in England and Wales, with a large population eating as much or more animal fats at the turn of the century as in the 1950s. In the United States, changes in dietary fat have not been very great over the past six decades with a slight increase of fat intake that, however, is due to an increased consumption of unsaturated fats. During the postwar 1940s the proportion of dietary fats provided by animal sources decreased, while that from vegetable sources increased significantly, owing to increased use of margarines, shortening, and salad and cooking oils. Studies of dietary changes have led experts to the conclusion that it is hazardous to lay primary blame for the twentieth-century epidemic of CHD on the diet.

In the fourth place, an association between diet and CHD incidence might be indicated by an effect of altered diet on CHD incidence. There have been a number of trials in which population groups have ingested diets reduced in saturated and increased in polyunsaturated fats. The results are not very striking, and the evidence that the CHD incidence has been reduced significantly by modifications of dietary fat intake is suggestive but hardly convincing to date. In spite of the above there is still good reason to believe that cardiovascular health will be promoted by a diet of appropriate total calories that is restricted in cholesterol, saturated fat and simple carbohydrate, even in normolipemic subjects. However, it would appear foolhardy at this juncture to believe that CHD has been shown to be prevented by diet modification.

Physical activity also has received much attention as a culpable factor in the twentieth-century increase of CHD. However, there is no evidence to indicate that our nineteenth-century ancestors remained largely free of CHD because of greater physical activity in riding horseback or in carriages, playing croquet, or strolling on dirt and cobblestone streets. Epidemiological studies have sometimes found a trend that less physically active subjects have higher rates of CHD. Physical conditioning improves cardiac performance, but there is little evidence that purposeful conditioning protects the coronary arteries, alters the coronary or collateral circulation, or, indeed, that it reduces either primary or secondary rates of CHD. International comparisons have shown striking differences in CHD rates of middle-age males in Finland, Italy, and Greece—all of which have low frequency of sedentary males, the lowest being in Finland, which has the highest rate of CHD. Like the diet, there is insignificant evidence to suspect inadequate physical activity as the sine qua non of the coronary epidemic.

During the past two decades, CHD has emerged as having a multifactoral etiology. It is, therefore, appropriate to look at the multivariate relationship of the classical risk factors to the CHD incidence. When the multiple logistic model is used to assess the data from the major prospective studies, it found that well over half of the CHD incidence occurring in each of these studies remains numerically unexplained when account is taken of age, blood pressure, serum cholesterol, cigarette smoking, and obesity. A recent comparison of comparable middle-aged male populations in Framingham, Honolulu, and Puerto Rico found that the CHD rate in Honolulu was not significantly related to serum cholesterol levels or that of Puerto Rico to cigarette smoking. At the same level of the traditional risk factors, the chance of a myocardial infarction or fatal coronary event was significantly greater in Framingham than in Honolulu or Puerto Rico. Another such comparison of male populations in Framingham and Yugoslavia found that at the same levels of the traditional risk factors, the incidence of CHD in Framingham was three times higher than in Yugoslavia, and in the latter population the incidence of CHD was almost twice as high in urban as in rural men. The study of Japanese men in Japan, Hawaii, and San Francisco also has found that the significantly higher rate of CHD in the westernized Japanese in San Francisco, compared to Japan, could not be ascribed to differences of either diet or the traditional risk factors.

It now appears to be clear that the Western epidemic of CHD cannot be ascribed per se to the diet, inadequate physical activity, or the traditional risk factors. It is just as clear that additional factors must play a major role. The evidence now strongly indicates that these are associated with the socioeconomic and psychosocial stress of modern Western civilization, as was intuitively suspected by Osler at the turn of the century. It is therefore not surprising that clinical CHD does not occur in the majority of individuals with the classical risk factors, that many victims of CHD do not exhibit high levels of such factors, and that rates of CHD remain low in many populations in which such factors are prevalent, even when habitual diets are high in fats. Conversely, it is just as clear that the incidence of CHD in the Western world is significantly related to the diet, less so to physical activity, and strongly to the classical risk factors. The point is not to denigrate the importance of these factors in the pathogenesis of CHD, but rather to emphasize that even when taken together these "multifactors" are far from providing a total explanation of the total effect.

Jenkins recently noted that there is now "a broad array of research studies that point out with ever-increasing certainty— that certain psychologic, social, and behavioral conditions do put persons at significantly higher risks of clinically manifest coronary disease." It is not possible to cite very many studies dealing with various aspects of this relationship, and they are reviewed elsewhere. Consideration has been given to the role of personality, emotions, stress, life changes, socioeconomic status, education, occupation, work load, religion, ethnic background, region of nativity, marital status, social mobility, graphic mobility, and status incongruity. Emotional factors which have been considered include anxiety, neurosis, depression, life dissatisfactions and rates of changes, stress and distress, coping mechanisms, and social supports. However, too many studies have been retrospective or contemporaneous, with imprecise measurements that lack scientific conviction.

Perhaps the greatest agreement concerns the personality traits of the coronary-prone subject. There is remarkable consistency in finding such characteristics as orderliness, self-discipline, devotion to work, inability to relax, aggressiveness, competitiveness, hostility, compulsive activity, and striving for achievement. However, personality characteristics interplay with the environmental milieu, with the exhibition of various patterns of overt behavior. My associates and I have found that a majority of coronary-prone individuals exhibit a pattern of overt behavior that we have defined as Type A. Type A's exhibit an action-emotion complex in response to their chronic and excessive struggle to achieve more and more, and to obtain more and more from their own environment in too short a period of time and against the opposing efforts of other persons or things in this same environment. This struggle may consist of attempts to do or to achieve more and more in less and less time, or of a chronic conflict with others, and this may be by preference or by necessity. However, Type A's never despair of losing this struggle, but strive to overcome challenges, in contrast with anxious persons who prefer to retreat in similar competitive and hostile situations. Type A's usually exhibit enhanced traits of aggressiveness, ambitiousness, and competitive drive. They are work-oriented and preoccupied with deadlines, and exhibit chronic impatience and time urgency, haste, restlessness, hyperalertness, tenseness of facial muscles, and explosive speech. Moreover, their personality and behavioral traits are present simultaneously. Subjects with the converse Type B behavior pattern are mainly free of such enhanced personality traits, feel no pressing conflict either with time or other persons, and are generally free of a chronic sense of time urgency. The Type A behavior pattern thus is an overt behavioral syndrome by which such individuals confront and cope with life situations. It must be distinguished from the vague concept of stress, strain, and distress as well as from simple neurosis associated with fears, anxieties, worry, and so on.

In our early studies, we observed a significant association of Type A behavior with increased prevalence of CHD in both sexes. However, the test of prediction is the most valid way of determining antecedent-consequent relationships, impelling us to do a prospective study in which the Type A behavior pattern was included in a rigorously designed investigation of all risk factors having relevance to CHD incidence. The Western Collaborative Group Study (WCGS) is a prospective study of 3,154 initially well men who were followed annually for a mean 8.5 years, during which 257 subjects developed clinical CHD. The participants were employed in 10 California companies and were aged 39 to 59 years at intake. The traditional risk factors and many other variables were determined. The behavior pattern was obtained by our structured psychological interview.

The WCGS data confirmed the relationship of the traditional risk factors to the incidence of CHD, including age, serum cholesterol, blood pressure, and cigarette smoking. The CHD risk was predicted using the additive multiple logistic model and was found to be significantly influenced by the behavior pattern. A twofold higher risk of CHD was found for Type A's compared to Type B's and this prevailed after adjustment for interactions with all other risk factors.

The relationship of Type A behavior pattern to CHD has also been studied by other investigators, who have confirmed a significant relationship of the rate of CHD either to Type A behavior per se or to its major facets. We also have observed a significant relationship of Type A behavior to the risk of sudden death and of recurring coronary events in subjects with prior clinical CHD.

Type A behavior is significantly related not only to the CHD incidence but also to the degree of basic coronary atherosclerosis. We observed this in subjects who died during the course of the WCGS, and several groups have confirmed this finding in patients undergoing coronary angiography, and in whom a significantly greater degree of basic coronary atherosclerosis was found in Type A subjects of both sexes compared to their respective Type B counterparts.

We do not clearly understand the relationship of any of the major risk factors to coronary artery disease and the same is true of Type A behavior pattern. Type A's compared to Type B's exhibit higher serum cholesterol and triglyceride levels, slightly higher prevalence of hypertension, and are more often the heavier cigarette smokers. However, the association of Type A behavior with increased prevalence and incidence of CHD is numerically independent of interactions with the other risk factors. Type A behavior is associated with significant neuro-hormonal differences compared to Type B behavior, including differences in growth hormone and in the hypothalamic-pituitary-adrenal axis. Stimuli arising in the central nervous system affect lipid metabolism in animals and neurogenic factors are significantly involved in the regulation of serum lipid levels.

Type A behavior is in part a response style to maintain control over the environment and therefore leads to chronic performance at or near maximum capacity, with hyper-reactiveness to actual or perceived threats. It is thus not surprising that it is associated with increased sympathetic nervous system discharge, which may be important in atherogenesis. In one prospective study, the cold pressor test, which reflects hyper-reactiveness of the sympathetic nervous system, had major predictive power for the incidence of CHD. In a primitive society, stress reactions prepare the body for violent action, and, once this is over, the body returns to normal homeostatis. The crises of Western civilization are different and the stress is often long-lasting and free-floating and often cannot be ended by some catharsis of physical action. The body of Western man thus is constantly poised for fight or flight, without the civilized possibility of either aggressive fighting or fleeing.

It has become clear to the discerning observer that the twentieth-century coronary epidemic of Western civilization has not occurred in a simplistic causal relationship with excessive saturated fat intake, along with inadequate physical activity, in which the victims always have elevated serum lipids, high blood pressure, obesity, parents with CHD, are cigarette smokers, or, for that matter, exhibit Type A behavior. However, Type A persons are at higher risk for CHD, and particularly if they exhibit other risk factors. By the same token, the prevention of CHD also is far from simplistic. Although we must use faith as our guideline rather than hard fact at this juncture, there seems little doubt but that the total elimination of risk factors should be our goal and at the earliest possible age. General health hazards such as excessive cigarette smoking and obesity should be corrected. Hypertension can almost always be controlled. It is more difficult to eliminate hypercholesterolemia, but dietary modifications should be attempted along with appropriate medication. Since habitual Western diet often is excessive in calories, carbohydrates, and total fats and is even poor in proper nutrition, there is good reason to correct this. However, there is every reason to believe that the primary and secondary prevention of CHD will require a holistic approach in which adequate attention is given to modification of the coronary-prone Type A behavior pattern.

References

Brand, R. J., R. H. Rosenman, R. I. Sholtz, and M. Friedman. 1976. "Multivariate Prediction of Coronary Heart Disease in the Western Collaborative Group Study Compared to the Findings of the Framingham Study," *Circulation*, 53:348.

Friedman, M. and R. H. Rosenman. 1959. "Association of a Specific Overt Behavior Pattern with Increases in Blood Cholesterol, Blood Clotting Time, Incidence of Arcus Senilis and Clinical Coronary Artery Disease," *Journal of the American Medical Association*, 169:1286.

Friedman, M., S. O. Byers, J. Diamant, and R. H. Rosenman. 1975. "The Plasma Norepinephrine Response of Coronary-Prone Subjects (Type A) to a Specific Challenge," *Metabolism*, 24:205.

Friedman, M., S. O. Byers, and R. H. Rosenman. 1967. "Factors Controlling Serum Lipids and Lipoproteins and Their Significance in the Etiology of Arteriosclerosis." In H. T. Blumenthal, ed., *Cowdry's Arteriosclerosis* (2d ed.). Springfield, Illinois: C. C. Thomas.

Friedman, M., S. St. George, S. O. Byers, and R. H. Rosenman. 1960. "Excretion of Catecholamines, 17-Ketosteroids, 17-Hydroxycorticoids and 5-Hydroxyindoles in Men exhibiting a Particular Behavior Pattern (A) Associated with High Incidence of Clinical Coronary Artery Disease," *Journal of Clinical Investigations*, 39:758.

Friedman, M., R. H. Rosenman, and V. Carroll. 1958. "Changes in the Serum Cholesterol and Blood Clotting Time in Men Subjected to Cyclic Variation of Occupational Stress," *Circulation*, 17:852.

Friedman, M., R. H. Rosenman, R. Straus, M. Wurm, and R. Kositchek, 1968. "The Relationship of Behavior Pattern A to the State of the Coronary Vasculature: A Study of 51 Autopsied Subjects," *American Journal of Medicine*, 44:525.

Jenkins, C. D., C. G. Hames, S. J. Zyzanski, R. H. Rosenman, and M. Friedman. 1969. "Psychological Traits and Serum Lipids. I. Findings from the California Psychological Inventory," *Psychosomatic Medicine*, 31:115.

Jenkins, C. D., S. J. Zyzanski, and R. H. Rosenman. 1976. "Risk of New Myocardial Infarction in Middle-Aged Men with Manifest Coronary Heart Disease," *Circulation*, 53:342.

Rosenman, R. H., and M. Friedman. 1961. "Association of a Specific Overt Behavior Pattern in Females with Blood and Cardiovascular Findings," *Circulation*, 24:1173.

Rosenman, R. H. and M. Friedman. 1963. "Behavior Patterns, Blood Lipids, and Coronary Heart Disease," *Journal of the American Medical Association*, 184:934.

Roseman, R. H. and M. Friedman. 1974. "Neurogenic Factors in Pathogenesis of Coronary Heart Disease," *Medical Clinics of North American*, 59:269.

Rosenman, R. H., R. J. Brand, and R. I. Sholtz. "Diet and the Regulation of Serum Lipids in the Western Collaborative Group." Unpublished manuscript.

Rosenman, R. H., R. J. Brand, and R. I. Sholtz. "Associations of Diet and the Incidence of Coronary Heart Disease in the Western Collaborative Group Study." Unpublished manuscript.

Rosenman, R. H., R. J. Brand, R. I. Sholtz, and M. Friedman. 1976. "Multivariate Prediction of Coronary Heart Disease During 8.5. Year Follow-up in the Western Collaborative Group Study," *American Journal of Cardiology*, 37:903.

Rosenman, R. H., M. Friedman, C. D. Jenkins, C. D. Straus, F. Wurm, and R. Kositchek. 1966. "The Prediction of Immunity to Coronary Heart Disease," *Journal of the American Medical Association*, 198:1159.

Rosenman, R. H., M. Friedman, R. Straus, M. Wurm, R. Kositchek, W. Hahn, and N. T. Werthessen. 1964. "A Predictive Study of Coronary Heart Disease," *Journal of the American Medical Association*, 189:15.

Rosenman, R. H., C. D. Jenkins, R. J. Brand, M. Friedman, R. Straus, and M. Wurm. 1975. "Coronary Heart Disease in the Western Collaborative Group Study: A Final Follow-Up Experience of 8.5 Years," *Journal of the American Medical Association*, 233:872.

❧ 10
Thoughts on the Current Status of Investigations of Personality Patterns and Coronary Heart Disease

James A. Blumenthal

MOST PHYSICIANS TODAY would agree that people suffering from hypertension, diabetes, obesity, and hypercholesterolemia, or who have a parental history of heart disease, or who smoke excessively are, relatively speaking, coronary-prone. Indeed, epidemiologic research has identified a number of risk factors as being related to coronary heart disease (CHD) including diet, smoking habits, physical exercise, serum cholesterol, and blood pressure (Epstein, 1965). It has become apparent, however, that these factors alone or in combination do not account for even half of the number of reported CHD cases. In an effort to discover other possible agents, researchers turned their attention to a consideration of personality patterns. That psychological variables may represent a new and significant risk factor has now been documented in over 200 publications. Obviously, it is beyond the scope of this paper to review the numerous studies that have investigated the relationship between psychological variables and CHD. For a comprehensive review of such literature, the interested reader is referred to several publications (Jenkins, 1971; 1976;

Caffrey, 1967). The purpose of this paper will be to focus on the major methodological and conceptual issues confronting researchers in this area: the problem of measurement of coronary-prone behavior, and the need for a theoretical integration of the coronary-prone literature.

Definition and Assessment of the Coronary-Prone Personality

The ambiguity of the term "coronary-prone personality" in itself poses a serious stumbling block in understanding the relationship of psychological variables and CHD. One particular problem that has emerged in evaluating the coronary prone individual is the question of "level of personality." For example, psychodynamic proponents view the behavior of a person to be the overt manifestation of internal, often unconscious, processes which are the critical determinants of behavior. Others view all behavior as a function of the laws of learning (for example, the individual's reinforcement history) with the significance of behavior to be understood by the way it operates on the environment. Consequently, investigators refer to an individual as being coronary-prone because of overt patterns of behavior, latent behavioral predispositions, or unconscious motivational states.

What kinds of data lead us to conclude that someone is coronary-prone? The early researchers relied on global clinical impressions. For example, Osler (1910) noted, "It is not the delicate neurotic person who is prone to angina but the robust, the vigorous in mind and body, the keen and ambitious man." In 1943, Dunbar reported a detailed study of 22 hospitalized patients with CHD. Her description of personality features included "compulsive striving, hard work, and self-discipline and a great need to get to the top." Arlow (1945; 1952) added the idea that although the CHD individual is driven to success, full satisfaction is rarely achieved. The Menningers (1936) also relied on the case-study method and emphasized strong unconscious aggression and hostility as central to the dynamics of the coronary-prone individual. While these reports received considerable attention, they were criticized because of small, select samples, inadequate controls, and a lack of standardized measurements.

In an effort to objectify their observations, researchers employed standardized psychological procedures. Initially, projective tests were utilized. For example, Kemple (1945) used the

Rorschach on CHD patients and found that "they manifest a persistent pattern of aggressiveness and drive which distinguishes them from patients in other groups." Cleveland and Johnson (1962) combined the TAT and Rorschach to identify characterologic personality features of CHD patients including high degrees of tension, activity and hostility. Still, these conclusions were based on subjective interpretations of responses and more objective measures were sought.

Investigators turned to a variety of paper-and-pencil questionnaires, self-report inventories, and rating scales. The Minnesota Multiphasic Personality Investory (MMPI) and Cattell 16 Personality Factor Questionnaire (16PF) have been two of the most popular instruments. In general, those studies utilizing the MMPI find CHD patients score higher on the "neurotic triad" (hypochondriasis, depression, hysteria) prior to the onset of disease relative to normal controls, especially for patients with angina pectoris. The subsequent occurrence of clinically manifest disease (i.e., myocardial infarction) further elevates the MMPI profile and results in the apparent deterioration of ego functions. Patients who developed a myocardial infarction scored higher on scales R (repression) and A (anxiety) and lower on scales K ("defensiveness"), H (hostility), and Es (ego strength) (Jenkins, 1971; 1976). One criticism of the MMPI is that the test is essentially a measure of the pathological features of personality. Some investigators chose the 16PF as a possible solution to this problem, only to discover that data were often inconsistent and contradictory. In spite of highly variable data, however, CHD patients generally appeared to be more unstable (low C), particularly patients with angina pectoris. Coronary patients also appeared to be more conforming (low E) and serious (low F), yet more self-sufficient (high Q2). They also appeared to be more shy (low H) and more apprehensive (high O) than normal controls (Jenkins, 1971; 1976). It should be noted that studies based on these multidimensional scales can be criticized because of their failure to consider profile or configural interpretations of data in addition to mere single score comparisons between CHD subjects and controls.

Perhaps the most integrated description of the role of psychological factors in the development of CHD has come from the work of Rosenman and Friedman of the Harold Brunn Institute, Mt. Zion Hospital and Medical Center, San Francisco. They defined the coronary-prone behavior pattern as "a characteristic action-emotion complex which is exhibited by those individuals who are engaged in a relatively chronic struggle to obtain an unlimited number of poorly defined things from their environment in the shortest period of time and if necessary, against the opposing efforts of other things or persons in this same environment" (Friedman, 1969, p. 84). This pattern, referred to as *Type A*, is characterized by extremes of competitiveness, ambition, impatience, time urgency, and aggressiveness. The converse *Type B* pattern is defined as a relative absence of these traits.

In a series of retrospective and prospective studies, the Type A pattern has been associated with significantly higher incidence and prevalence of CHD than the non-coronary-prone Type B pattern. Repeated followup over a 10-year period found Type A men to have roughly twice the rate of new CHD compared to their Type B counterparts (Rosenman et al., 1964; Rosenman et al., 1966; Rosenman et al., 1970; Rosenman et al., 1975). Other studies indicate that Pattern A is not only related to the clinical manifestations of CHD but that it is also associated with the disease process itself (Friedman et al., 1968; Jenkins et al., 1974; Blumenthal et al., 1975). In addition to CHD, Type A behavior has been found to be associated with elevated serum cholesterol (Friedman et al., 1958; Rosenman and Friedman, 1959; Friedman and Rosenman, 1959; Rosenman and Friedman, 1963) and triglycerides (Rosenman and Friedman, 1963; Friedman, Rosenman and Byers, 1964), a decrease in clotting time (Rosenman and Friedman, 1959; Friedman and Rosenman, 1959), an increase in the incidence of arcus senilis (Rosenman and Friedman, 1959; Friedman and Rosenman, 1959) and elevated levels of norepinephrine during the working day (Friedman et al., 1960).

Classification of the subjects as being Type A or Type B is customarily based on one of two procedures: first, a standardized semistructured interview that considers both speech stylistics and content of answers to the interview questions; and second, a paper-and-pencil questionnaire called the Jenkins Activity Survey (JAS). The interview consists of a series of standard questions designed to elicit Type A behavior (Rosenman et al., 1964). It utilizes four basic sources of information: (1) presence of characteristic speech and motor signs; (2) degree of ambition and drive; (3) degree of past and present competitive and aggressive strivings; and (4) degree and intensity of time urgency. Detailed descriptions of the development, validity, and reliability of the JAS have been published (Jenkins et al., 1967; Jenkins et al., 1971; Zyzanski and Jenkins, 1970). Essentially, the JAS was designed to objectively measure the coronary-prone type behavior pattern. However, the JAS has only modest validity and is unable to predict individual cases or even to discriminate between small groups of CHD cases and noncases (Jenkins et al., 1971).

One frequent criticism of the Type A-B classification is the imprecise method by which the pattern is assessed. Coronary-prone behavior represents a complex entity and more exact diagnostic criteria are needed. Although Friedman and Rosenman (1974) state that the coronary-prone behavior pattern "cannot be described in quantitatively acceptable terms," psychometric instruments designed to assess a variety of Type A characteristics would invariably facilitate the identification of coronary-prone individuals and add greater precision to the classification procedure. Clinical literature has in fact demonstrated the improved diagnostic accuracy by a combination of clinical and statistical procedures (Meehl, 1954; Meehl, 1956). Further research could facilitate the development of more suitable assessment tools. Such assessment must recognize the complexity of personality and behavior and the importance of the context in which behavior occurs. The use of multiple measures that assess personality and behavior at different levels (e.g., manifest-latent, conscious-unconscious) may further help to clarify the association of psychologic factors and CHD.

A Conceptual Model of Coronary-Prone Patterns and CHD

While much attention has been focused on the methodological problems with the coronary-prone–Type A variable, there has been relatively little effort aimed at providing a theoretical framework for interpreting the steadily accumulating data in the field. For example, one source of ambiguity in the Type A–Type B dimension lies in the concept of *type*. The notion of a neat dichotomy with Type A on the one side and Type B on the other is certainly an appealing one but most agree that this view is overly simplistic. Investigators today generally believe that there is a behavioral continuum with Type A on the one end and Type B on the other. Still there remains a good deal of heterogeneity within each subgroup, even with respect to the attributes connoted by the criteria defining the classification. A Type A individual need not have all the characteristics to be classified as coronary-prone and it is possible that particular variables may be more predictive of CHD than others. Several studies have begun to investigate the relative contributions of various subcomponents of the Type A pattern (Herndon et al., 1976), but findings are inconclusive at this time.

Rosenman and Friedman have contributed a great deal to understanding the role that behavior may play in the development of CHD. However, their investigations emphasize a description of overt behaviors and make no attempt to provide a framework for understanding the dynamics of the behavior. For example, Rosenman and Friedman repeatedly stress that the Type A pattern is not a personality trait nor a stress reaction but rather the overt behavior that emerges when a person, *predisposed* by his *character structure*, is confronted by a particular behavior-eliciting situation. Unfortunately there has been little effort to specify the nature of this character structure. One may assume that this predisposition is likely to be a relatively stable characteristic reminiscent of the concept of *acquired behavioral disposition* (Campbell, 1963). Such dispositions are believed to be functions of past learning experiences that increase the probability that an individual will view and respond to the world in a particular way.

In an effort to formulate a theoretical basis for the Type A-B dimension, a group of researchers at the University of Texas has conducted an extensive research program identifying certain situations eliciting the Type A pattern (Herndon et al., 1976; Krantz et al., 1974; Glass et al., 1974; Burnam et al., 1976; Carver and Glass, 1976). They view Type A as a coping style aimed at maintaining control over potentially uncontrollable events. An alternate formulation which I propose is that this behavioral style reflects a particular level of personality development and organization. The cardinal feature of the coronary-prone individual is that he is much *less able to tolerate psychic tension* than the Type B non-coronary-prone individual and that he engages in behaviors aimed primarily at tension reduction. From a psychodynamic viewpoint, this individual is narcissistic, counter-dependent and impulsive. The Type A individual does have a strong need to be in control and his behavior is designed to gain mastery over potentially uncontrolled situations. However, the underlying mechanism is that the situation presents an implicit threat *that the ego may not be able to secure gratification*. The behavioral repertoire of the coronary-prone individual is essentially *active, purposeful,* and *goal-directed*. The coronary-prone person is extremely manipulative, maneuvering people to the fulfillment of his demands. When his demands are frustrated, he may become hostile, irritable, anxious, or depressed. Such characteristics are likely to be common in the coronary-prone individual because his needs are so great that it is unlikely he would be satisfied and content for an extended period of time.

What might maintain such behavior? One common denominator may be that the coronary-prone individual engages in a high frequency of behaviors that are designed to secure reinforcement—either by gaining material goods, achieving ego gratifications such as attention and recognition, or by reducing anxieties.

How does this pattern develop? It is this author's conviction that interpersonal experiences represent the dominant force in the development of personality. Naturally, constitutional factors are inevitably codeterminants and interact with personality and environmental forces. The possibility that the coronary-prone individual, or the cluster of traits implied by that term, has a partially genetic basis has recently been investigated (Mathews and Krantz, 1976; Rosenman et al., 1976). Results have been generally negative, although the research can be criticized on such grounds as nonrepresentative sampling procedures, inadequate criteria for zygosity determination, and questionable behavior classification. I propose that the coronary-prone personality is acquired through learning, specifically by the identification of the child with certain significant others (primarily parents). Empirical evidence is necessary to support this hypothesis and a number of studies are presently being conducted to investigate the psychological processes by which the pattern may develop. Some data have suggested that the Type A Pattern is observable at age 5, and several studies have noted similarities in parent-child behavior types (Mathews and Krantz, 1976; Bortner et al., 1970).

A model for the interaction of the psychological variables and the traditional risk factors is present in figure 10.1.

Genetic Factors represent the inherited biophysical predispositions of the individual. These factors are likely to exert a direct influence on the biological risk factors or interact with the environment. While the role of genetics may be important, I believe that CHD is not transmitted genetically as such, but as a biologic predisposition that probably requires the operation of environmental influences. The *Biological Risk Factors* have been well documented and include such factors as serum cholesterol, blood pressure, family history of CHD, and advancing age. The

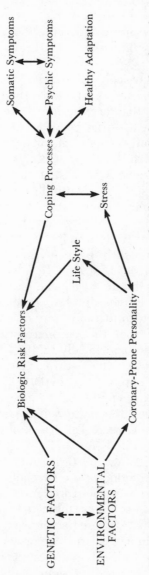

Figure 10.1 Development of Coronary Heart Disease: Proposed pathways by which various biophysical and psychosocial components interact in the pathogenesis and expression of CHD

Environmental Factors refer to the developmental and socio-psychological experiences of the individual that shape his personality. As previously described, there has been relatively little effort to identify the precursors of the coronary-prone personality, but indications are that the personality develops as a result of environmental forces. *Life Style* refers to certain behavioral, social, and demographic factors that are associated with CHD and may be considered independent of the coronary-prone personality. Diet, smoking habits, occupation, marital status, and social status may be considered to be some relevant variables and may operate via the biological Risk Factors or by other physiologic mechanisms. *Stress* denotes the external forces (i.e., environmental conditions; Type A-behavior-eliciting situations) that confront an individual. These may include ego-threatening situations, life changes, and uncontrollable events. How any particular situation affects a person depends upon his subjective appraisal of the situation. The coronary-prone individual emits such behaviors as aggressiveness, competetiveness, and hyperactivity, because he perceives such situations as demanding that response, and he is unable to respond in the apparently more adaptive fashion that is characteristic of the non-coronary-prone individual. *Coping Processes* refer to biologic and psychologic responses to stress. At both the somatic and psychic level, these responses represent an attempt to restore the body to a state of homeostasis. Psychologically, these processes include unconscious defense mechanisms (e.g., denial, repression), conscious coping strategies (e.g., relaxation, physical exercise), various cognitive and perceptual styles (e.g., field dependence-independence, repression-sensitization) or even characteristic behavior patterns such as Type A. The *End Phase* of the process represents the eventual failure of psychophysiologic adaptation and is manifested by organ dysfunction or organic disease at the somatic level, and/or psychological maladjustment such as anxiety, depression, or psychoneurosis at the psychological level.

This model is consistent with the view that no single factor is solely responsible for the disease and recognizes that CHD represents a climax of physical and environmental forces. Some people may develop CHD primarily as a result of biologic conditions (i.e., genetics; enzymatic, metabolic or other biochemical disturbance; advancing age). However, for a majority of people, CHD is a result of the interaction of psychological, physiological, and biochemical processes.

Search for causative relationships is extremely difficult, since it is, from a practical standpoint, all but impossible to construct unequivocal causative relationships without experimental manipulation. The great number of positive findings in prospective and retrospective studies offer strong support for the possible role of personality in the development of CHD. However, these data remain indirect and do not offer conclusive evidence of the pathological mechanisms involved. One solution to the problem is that of preventative research. A number of programs have aimed at reducing biological risk factors such as lowering serum cholesterol levels, and reducing blood pressure. A logical extension of this approach is to conduct research aimed at modifying psychological and behavior patterns that apparently place individuals at higher risk for developing CHD. Should preventative research confirm that by intervening at the psycho-behavioral level, the incidence and prevalance of CHD is reduced, we can deduce that personality is related to CHD and then undertake more precise and intensive research to determine the underlying physiological mechanisms mediating the relationship between CHD and the psychological and behavioral variables.

It is only within the past decade that psychological factors have been considered important in the development of CHD. It would seem that a precise and objective evaluation of coronary-prone behavior patterns has methodological priority, since it is this variable that provides a basis for studying the underlying association of psychologic variables and CHD. It is also important to develop conceptual models for interpreting the effects of psychophysiological variables in the pathogenesis and expression of CHD.

References

Arlow, J. A. 1945. "Identification Mechanisms in Coronary Occlusion," *Psychosomatic Medicine*, 7:195–209.

Arlow, J. A. 1952. "Anxiety Patterns in Angina Pectoris," *Psychosomatic Medicine*, 14:461–67.

Blumenthal, J., R. Williams, Y. Kong, L. Thompson, C. D. Jenkins, and R. H. Rosenman. 1975. *Coronary Prone Behavior and Angiographically Documented Coronary Disease*. New Orleans: American Psychosomatic Society.

Bortner, R. W., R. H. Rosenman, and M. Friedman. 1970. "Familial Similarity in Pattern A Behavior," *Journal of Chronic Diseases*, 23:39–43.

Burnam, M. A., J. W. Pennebaker, and D. C. Glass. 1976. "Time Consciousness Achievement Striving and the Type A Coronary Prone Behavior Pattern," *Journal of Abnormal Psychology*, 84:76–79.

Caffrey, B. 1967. "Factors Involving Interpersonal and Psychological Characteristics: A Review of Empirical Findings," *Milbank Memorial Fund Quarterly*, 45:119–39.

Campbell, D. T. 1963. "Social Attitudes and Other Acquired Behavioral Dispositions." In S. Koch, ed., *Psychology: A Study of a Science*, vol. 6. New York: McGraw Hill.

Carver, C. S. and D. C. Glass. 1976. "The Coronary Prone Behavior Pattern and Interpersonal Aggression." In press.

Cleveland, J. E. and O. L. Johnson. 1962. "Personality Patterns in Young Males with Coronary Disease," *Psychosomatic Medicine*, 24:600–10.

Dunbar, R. 1943. *Psychosomatic Diagnosis*. New York: Paul B. Hoeber.

Epstein, F. H. 1965. "The Epidemiology of Coronary Heart Disease: A Review," *Journal of Chronic Diseases*, 18:735–74.

Friedman, M. 1969. *Pathogenesis of Coronary Artery Disease*. New York: McGraw-Hill.

Friedman, M. and R. H. Rosenman. 1959. "Association of Specific Overt Behavior Pattern with Blood and Cardiovascular Findings: Blood Cholesterol Levels, Blood Clotting Time, Incidence of Arcus Senilis and Clinical Coronary Artery Disease," *Journal of the American Medical Association*, 169:1286–96.

Friedman, M. and R. H. Rosenman. 1974. *Type A Behavior and Your Heart*. New York: Knopf.

Friedman, M., R. H. Rosenman, and S. O. Byers. 1964. "Serum Lipids and Conjunctional Circulation After Fat Ingestion in Men Exhibiting Type A Behavior Pattern," *Circulation*, 29:874–86.

Friedman, M., R. H. Rosenman, and V. Carroll. 1958. "Changes in the Serum Cholesterol and Blood Clotting Time in Men Subjected to Cyclic Variation of Occupational Stress," *Circulation*, 17:852–61.

Friedman, M., R. H. Rosenman, R. Straus, M. Wurm, and R. Kositchek. 1968. "The Relationship of Behavior Pattern A to the State of the Coronary Vasculature: A Study of 51 Autopsied Subjects," *American Journal of Medicine*, 44:525–37.

Friedman, M., S. St. George, S. O. Byers, and R. H. Rosenman. 1960. "Excretion of Catecholamines, 17-Ketosteroids, 17-Hydroxycorticoids and 5-Hydroxyindole in Men Exhibiting a Particular Behavior Pattern (A) Associated with High Incidence of Clinical Coronary Artery Disease," *Journal of Clinical Investigation*, 39:758–64.

Glass, D. C., M. L. Synder, and J. F. Hollis. 1974. "Time Urgency and the Type A Coronary Prone Behavior Pattern," *Journal of Applied Social Psychology*, 4:125–40.

Herndon, K. M., D. C. Glass, R. H. Rosenman, and R. W. Bortner. 1976. "Competetitive Drive, Pattern A and Coronary Heart Disease: A Further Analysis of Some Data from the Western Collaborative Group Study." In press.

Jenkins, C. D. 1971. "Psychologic and Social Precursors of Coronary Disease," *New England Journal of Medicine*, 284:244–55, 307–17.

Jenkins, C. D. 1976. "Recent Evidence Supporting Psychologic and Social Risk

Factors for Coronary Disease," *New England Journal of Medicine*, 294:987–94.

Jenkins, C. D., R. H. Rosenman, and M. Friedman. 1967. "Development of an Objective Psychological Test for the Determination of the Coronary Prone Behavior Pattern in Employed Men," *Journal of Chronic Diseases*, 20:371–79.

Jenkins, C. D., S. Zyzanski, S. Lefkowitz, M. Everist, and T. Ryan. 1974. *Psychological Correlates of Coronary Angiographic Findings*. Dallas: American Heart Association.

Jenkins, C. D., S. J. Zyzanski, and R. H. Rosenman. 1971. "Progress Toward Validation of a Computer Scored Test for the Type A Coronary Prone Behavior Pattern," *Psychosomatic Medicine*, 33:193–201.

Jenkins, C. D., S. J. Zyzanski, R. H. Rosenman, and G. L. Cleveland. 1971. "Association of Coronary Prone Behavior Scores with Recurrence of Coronary Heart Disease," *Journal of Chronic Diseases*, 24:601–11.

Kemple, C. 1945. "Rorschach Method and Psychosomatic Diagnosis: Personality Traits of Patients with Rheumatic Disease, Hypertensive Cardiovascular Disease, Coronary Occlusion and Fractures," *Psychosomatic Medicine*, 7:85–89.

Krantz, D. S., D. C. Glass, and M. L. Synder. 1974. "Helplessness, Stress Level and the Coronary Prone Behavior Pattern." *Journal of Experimental Social Psychology*, 10:284–300.

Mathews, K. A., and D. S. Krantz. 1976. "Resemblances of Twins and Their Parents in Pattern A Behavior," *Psychosomatic Medicine*, 38:140–44.

Meehl, P. E. 1954. *Clinical vs. Statistical Prediction*. Minneapolis, Minnesota: University of Minnesota Press.

Meehl, P. E. 1956. "Wanted—A Good Cookbook," *American Psychologist*, 11:263–72.

Menninger, K. A., and W. C. Menninger, 1936. "Psychoanalytic Observations in Cardiac Disorders," *American Heart Journal*, 11:10–21.

Osler, W. 1910. "The Humleian Lectures on Angina Pectoris," *Lancet*, 1:839.

Rosenman, R. H., and M. Friedman. 1959. "Association of a Specific Overt Behavior Pattern in Woman with Increased Blood Cholestrol and Clotting Time, Arcus Senilis and Incidence of Clinical Coronary Disease," *Circulation*, 20:759.

Rosenman, R. H., and M. Friedman. 1963. "Behavior Patterns, Blood Lipids and Coronary Heart Disease," *Journal of the American Medical Association*, 184:934–38.

Rosenman, R. H., M. Friedman, R. Straus, M. Wurm, C. D. Jenkins, H. Messinger, and R. Kositchek. 1966. "Western Collaborative Group Study: A Follow-up Experience of Two Years," *Journal of the American Medical Association*, 195:86–92.

Rosenman, R. H., M. Friedman, R. Straus, M. Wurm, R. Kositchek, W. Hahn, and N. Werthessen. 1964. "A Predictive Study of Coronary Heart Disease: The Western Collaborative Group Study," *Journal of the American Medical Association*, 189:103–10.

Rosenman, R. H., M. Friedman, R. Straus, C. D. Jenkins, S. Zyzanski, and M. Wurm. 1970. "Coronary Heart Disease in the Western Collaborative Group Study: A Follow-up Experience of 4½ Years," *Journal of Chronic Diseases*, 23:173–90.

Rosenman, R. H., C. D. Jenkins, R. Brand, M. Friedman, R. Straus, and M. Wurm. 1975. "Coronary Heart Disease in the Western Collaborative Group Study: Final Follow-up Experience of 8½ Years," *Journal of the American Medical Association*, 233:872–77.

Rosenman, R. H., R. H. Rahe, N. D. Borhani, and M. Feinleib. 1976. *Heritability of Personality and Behavior Pattern*. Rome: First International Congress on Twins. In press.

Zyzanski, S. J., and C. D. Jenkins. 1970. "Basic Dimensions Within the Coronary Prone Behavior Pattern," *Journal of Chronic Diseases*, 22:781–95.

✾11
Toward an Index of Emotional Drain: A Comparative Study of Coronary Patients and Controls

John G. Bruhn

THERE IS INCREASING evidence that mental and physical exhaustion may be closely associated with the occurrence of myocardial infarction (Jenkins, 1976). Wolfe and Theodore (1936) noted that psychological factors may cause an individual to undertake a greater physical burden than a strained cardiovascular system can handle; for example, an individual may work continuously or keep busy in order to reduce tensions created by problems he cannot handle. Weiss (1940) has said that a burden of repressed anxiety, resulting in prolonged muscle tension or other bodily changes, may place too heavy a strain on some organ or organs which in time develops a disorder that is diagnosed as functional. Some researchers have suggested that if the burden becomes too great, the individual may "give up" or lose his will to live, resulting in a heart attack or sudden death. (Wolf, 1967; Engel, 1968). Sociologic and psychologic data obtained from patients who later died from a recurrent myocardial infarction indicated that more of them had prolonged, unresolved emotional tension which resulted in physical and mental exhaustion or emotional drain than did their matched controls. (Bruhn et al., 1968).

In a study of 40,000 male students who were followed for 25

years after graduation from college, it was found that individuals who had died from coronary heart disease were more likely to have reported experiences of exhaustion in college and higher anxiety quotients in college as assessed by items such as nervousness, insomnia, palpitations, worries, self-consciousness and moodiness (Paffenbarger et al., 1966).

The phenomenon of emotional drain was tested among 330 multiphasic examinees who subsequently developed a first myocardial infarction. Items selected from a psychological questionnaire by outside experts were used to measure various "theories" of the causes of coronary heart disease, two of which were emotional drain and somatization. Items representing these two phenomena proved to be associated with subsequent myocardial infarction, but these relationships were no longer apparent when persons with coronary symptoms and diagnoses at the time of testing were removed from the study group (Friedman et al., 1974). The authors stated that even in prospective studies, symptoms of somatizing, emotional drain, sleep disturbances, and so forth may be manifestations of subclinical levels of cardiovascular disease and therefore may be prodromes rather than risk factors. The complexity of coronary heart disease makes discussions of which factors are prodromal and which are risk factors academic. The major objective is to identify individuals who have precursors or risk factors so that interventions may be suggested before a myocardial infarction occurs.

The purpose of the present paper is to present an index of emotional drain which can be used prospectively to identify individuals who are at high risk for a heart attack.

Methods

Twenty-six married men who had suffered a myocardial infarction were matched as closely as possible with 26 ostensibly healthy married men on age, education, occupation, height, and weight. The men were participants in a larger longitudinal study of factors thought to be causative of myocardial infarction. The men and their wives were separately interviewed in their homes by two female interviewers. The interviews were arranged at the couple's convenience and were identical for husbands and wives. The interviews lasted an average of two hours and consisted of many questions which permitted respondents to express their attitudes, feelings, and opinions. Each respondent was asked about his childhood, parents and siblings, educational experiences, attainments and aspirations, religious beliefs and attitudes, occupational history, finances, leisure activities, habits such as smoking, and life goals. The purpose of the interview was to construct brief biographies from which life-styles and life themes could be traced from childhood to the time of the interview.

The data were summarized in biographies by the interviewers, omitting the identification of the respondents as patients or controls. A medical student, who did not know the respondents, was asked to study the biographies of each marital pair and list factors that he thought were sources of conflict or emotional drain. Emotional drain was defined, for the student, as a conflict involving personal values which had been present since early life and created constant mental preparedness on the part of the respondent. The conflict was believed to be unalterable or unsolvable by the respondent, who experienced additional traumatic incidents which reinforced the original conflict. The respondent lacked meaningful or supportive relationships with others and saw his conflict as a personal burden—a draining experience.

Emotional Drain Items. The student listed 21 factors from his biographical reviews which he felt would distinguish patients from controls. The factors were felt to be indicative of value conflicts or to reflect unfavorably on a person's self-concept or self-esteem—for example, lack of education, lack of parental or marital support. Since it was not feasible to determine the relative importance of each of the items in the lives of the respondents, it was decided to give each item a weight of 1. The student scored each respondent, giving a point for each item present, and totaled the points. The possible scores ranged from 1 to 21. The higher the score, the greater the parameters of emotional drain.

Rater Agreement on Emotional Drain. In order to ascertain the degree of agreement in evaluating the presence of emotional drain, the same biographies were given to two raters, a cardiologist and an anthropologist, who were given the above definition of emotional drain and asked to rate its presence or absence in each respondent. Identification of the respondents as patients or controls was not provided to the raters. The raters were also asked to indicate each respondent's need for social and psychological support, whether or not support was given by the respondent's spouse and other sources outside of the family from which the respondent obtains support.

Social Characteristics of Respondents. The coronary patients were all Caucasian men whose mean age was 54.5 years, ranging from 36 to 76 years. The majority (62 percent) had lived at their present address for at least ten years and owned their own home (85 percent); hence they were quite stable geographically. The controls were all Caucasian men whose mean age was 53.0 years and age range was 31 to 72 years. The majority (65 percent) had lived at their present address for at least ten years and owned their own home (89 percent). The patients and controls were individually matched as closely as possible on education and occupation; there was an equal representation of both blue collar and white collar occupations among the two groups.

Results

Table 1 shows the distribution of total scores for the male patients and controls on the items relating to the Index of Emotional

Table 11.1 Distribution of Total Scores for Patients and Controls on Index of Emotional Drain

Total Score*	Patients (N = 26) Cum. %	Controls (N = 26) Cum. %
0	4	4
1	4.5	8
2	4.5	15
3	4.5	35
4	4.5	50
5	4.5	62
6	8	65
7	15	65.5
8	15.5	73
9	27	77
10	27.5	77.5
11	35	88
12	58	88.5
13	73	96
14	85	100
15	88	
16	88.5	
17	92	
18	100	

*Total possible score = 21.

Table 11.2 Distribution of Items on Index of Emotional Drain

Item	Patients (N = 26) (%)	Controls (N = 26) (%)	% Difference Patients minus Controls
Previous marriage	15	8	+7
Conflict with parents during childhood	81	31	+50
Education same or less than parents	27	7	+20
Education terminated or interrupted prematurely	73	48	+25
No well-defined educational goal	12	4	+8
Unable to achieve educational goal	81	46	+35
Education is same or less than wife	35	26	+9
Not a churchgoer	35	15	+20
Job superior to educational qualifications	15	22	−7
Job difficulties	77	46	+31
Frequent job changes	23	19	+4
Difficulties with employer	19	30	−11
Dependent role in marriage	46	15	+31
Admit to being tense	65	30	+35
Inability to communicate with others	54	33	+21
Moderate to heavy smoker	58	44	+14
Conforms to expectations of others	50	15	+35
Sensitive individual lacking in self-confidence	58	31	+27
Unable to achieve satisfactory marital relationship	19	11	+8
Introverted	50	8	+42
Evidence of emotional drain	92	31	+61

Drain. The table shows that more of the patients had higher scores than the controls; that is, the biographies of the patients contained more of the items felt to be indicative of long-term conflicts or were reflective of a negative self-concept or self-image. Table 2 lists the 21 items relating to the Index of Emotional Drain and the percentage differences between patients and controls on each of the items. It is noteworthy that the percentage of coronary patients exceeded the percentage of controls on all items except two. Fewer controls than coronary patients had difficulties with their employees and held jobs superior to their educational qualifications. The terms which were most common among the coronary patients—that is, on which there was a 30 percent or greater difference between coronary patients and controls—were: conflict with parents during childhood, inability to achieve educational goal, job difficulties, dependent role in marriage, admission of tension, conformity to other's expectations, introversion, and evidence of emotional drain. Collectively, these items would indicate long-term problems, many of which may have seemed unsolvable and thus overwhelming to the person who experienced a heart attack. It should be pointed out that most of the items comprising the Index of Emotional Drain are

not factors that would be altered by the experience of a heart attack. Hence, it would be difficult to argue that the coronary event
influenced the respondent's answers to the questions from which
the items were drawn.

Since emotional drain is a rather broad, complex phenomenon it is not likely that it can be fully measured. The 21 items
should be viewed as indicators of the presence or absence of emotional drain. It is advantageous, therefore, to assess the presence
or absence of emotional drain utilizing another method, that is,
the biographic review. Therefore, two additional reviewers independently read the biographies and rated the presence or absence of emotional drain in each of the respondents. Emotional
drain was judged to be present by both raters in 19, or 73 percent
of the coronary patients and in 10, or 38 percent, of the controls.
It is possible, therefore, to identify the phenomenon of emotional
drain from relatively brief biographies.

One biographical summary is presented here to illustrate the
absence of emotional drain and a second is presented to illustrate
its presence.

The A's have been married 16 years. He was 20 and she 18 when
they married. They have two living children, ages 12 and 10. Their
first child was killed in an automobile accident when she was 14
months old. They are buying a $13,500 house at present. Mr. A.
helps his mother occasionally, buys things for her and sometimes
gives her a little money. Both Mr. and Mrs. A work.

Mrs. A. was born and raised in a city. She remembers being
happy and contented as a child and that her parents had the "same
likes, morals, and standards." When Mrs. A. was 15, her mother died
of cancer and her father changed jobs so he could be with her and her
brother. My father was a wonderful person. He was both mother and
father to us. He was so good to us." Mrs. A's father worked for the
city water department as the driver of a "flusher," and died of a
stroke. Mrs. A's only brother is a problem. He drinks. He was married at 16, divorced, remarried, and divorced again. "It broke my
heart."

Mrs. A. completed high school and then quit because she
wanted to get married. She has been satisfied with her education but
"it would be nice to have more and it would offer better job opportunities." She also said that the main reason she is working is so her
two daughters can go to college.

Mr. A. was born and raised on a farm. He was one of seven
children, all still living and they "enjoyed life—had a good relationship with all of them." His father was boss, but he felt close to his

father because they worked together and were both interested in sports. He felt he was understood by his parents. "If they said no, we didn't argue. Dad was a man of few words." His father died of stomach cancer and his mother went to work. Mr. A. was critical of one brother. "He's divorced and not as dependable as the others. His word isn't always good."

At age 26, Mr. A. started courses in night school to complete a degree in engineering. He has 24 hours left and isn't planning on continuing, except that "the way this education is going, it seems almost like one degree is not enough." He hopes his daughters will also go to college "if they have the capabilities. That's one of the reasons we moved here, to be near the university."

Both the A's attend church more than once a week because they want to. "It's a pretty important factor to both of us."

Mrs. A. was a switchboard operator at the telephone company when she got out of high school. From there she went to a department store, first in the credit office, then as a keypunch operator. She quit work but returned at age 31 to a library, which she hated, and then as a keypunch operator. She likes keypunching, feels her job is important, challenging and a better job than most of her friends have. She earns $300 per month and expects to be promoted to supervisor.

Mr. A. did not want to be a farmer so he worked in the broomcorn fields, saved his money and came to the city job hunting. He got his present job by accident—an assistant engineer with the highway department lived next door and offered him a job. That was 18 years ago and now Mr. A. is an engineer in the highway department. He likes his job, can leave it at 5:00 P.M., thinks it's challenging and important, and a better one than he ever expected to have. He hopes to be promoted to a $8,550 per year job soon. He feels the job utilizes his potentials.

Both Mr. and Mrs. A. look after the money. They pool their salaries, she pays the bills and they share what's left.

Mr. and Mrs. A. state they have never really had financial problems. "There's always been enough to pay the bills."

Mr. A. said his wife is kind of nervous and can't sit still. "She gets angry quickly, gets over it right away. I may be angry for a week before anyone knows it." The A's appear very compatible. She had a hard time after her first baby was killed. A drunk ran into them, and she said it took at least six months to get over her grief. She was afraid to get in a car for awhile.

The family does things together, church activities, bowling, water skiing and football games. Sometimes they go camping and fishing. "We could spend our whole summer at the lake and never come in," he said. They both like television. If he had more leisure time he would watch more television and spend more time studying. She would sew more. Neither one belongs to any organizations except church. Mrs. A. smokes a package of cigarettes a day. He is a non-smoker. Both are nondrinkers.

If Mrs. A. could start over in life, she would "never start smoking. Other than that I wouldn't change anything." What she has always wanted was a happy marriage and she has one. Her only worry has been her brother's drinking. Mr. A. would "start after a college education sooner and with more determination." He wants to enjoy life and thinks he does. His greatest concern has always been "to be the type of person I think I should be."

Mr. A. received a score of zero on the Index of Emotional Drain. In addition, the two reviewers independently agreed that emotional drain was not evident in Mr. A's biographical summary.

The B's have been married 28 years. He was 29, she was 28 when they were married. They have one son, now in the military service and alienated from them. They have lived in their own home for the past ten years.

Mrs. B. was born in a small western town. Her family memories are all "happy." Once her mother was going to punish her with a little piece of kindling wood, but it broke and "we both ended up laughing." Mrs. B's father was killed in an accident when she was 19, crushed in a gate while driving a horse team. When her sister was 32, she and her whole family were drowned. She was disappointed in her brother because he "didn't accomplish much. He got married early and I was disappointed in him." Mrs. B has a bachelor's degree and had a chance to go on with a fellowship, but was $700 in debt and "in those days you paid off your debts." So she taught school instead.

Mr. B. was born on a ranch in the West. His mother and father fought a lot, "mentally and physically." When his sister was 20 months old, she was crossing the street toward her father's team. The team became frightened, bolted and ran over his sister. Mr. B's mother who was pregnant at the time, saw it all from the window. There was no doctor near the ranch, so they took the sister on a hand-car into the next town, but she died. His mother blamed her husband and never quite recovered from the tragedy. The parents separated several times and Mr. B's father once had his wife committed to a mental institution. He also claimed she tried to kill him. Finally they divorced. The mother remarried and divorced again. The father also married again.

When Mr. B. was a sophomore in college, his mother was found dead in bed in a hotel. There was a letter from him in her purse. Although the diagnosis was heart attack, Mr. B. wondered if it had not been partially starvation because she was so emaciated. She had no other relatives, so "we buried my mother."

Mr. B. was, therefore, reared mostly by his father and felt fairly close to him, more so than did his brother and sister. "Dad could depend on me. I tried to do things that were right." He said his father believed in physical punishment. "One winter I stayed home all winter except for school because I wouldn't apologize to a church group. Father was religious, he taught me that." In later years, Mr. B. grew to resent his father. "I don't think father paid much attention to us so long as we got our chores done. He didn't inspire me along lines I would have liked to have been inspired, what to accomplish in life and what is of value."

Mr. B. worked his way through college and completed a university premed course. He applied for medical school and was number 33. However, they only took 30 students and no vacancy occurred so he completed a year on his Master's degree. Mr. B. has felt bad about this ever since. "I think I'd have liked to be a doctor—doctors are financially independent and are admirable. It doesn't give you much satisfaction to not complete something." The B's son is a college graduate and has part of the work completed on a Master's degree. Mr. B. says his son is thinking about medical school. Mrs. B. is less optimistic. She doesn't want him to be just a "perennial student." "We both prefer to see him go on with his education, but we don't feel he's mature enough to be a doctor or dedicated." And, "when he reached the point of demanding money from us, we drew the line. Now we feel guilty because we won't help him."

Religion has been a problem among the B's. They are both Protestant, but of different denominations. "It's been a sore spot in our lives," Mr. B. said. "Our ideas are similar but my wife is a supersensitive person and can't forgive." He supports his church but goes to hers to "keep the peace," and claims they give more money to hers. She goes to church, she said, to get inspiration but doesn't believe she is very religious, although it is a "calming influence." Mr. B. said "if it hadn't been for our boy, my wife and I would have been divorced years ago. We think differently."

Mrs. B. taught school after leaving college. She has also been a bookkeeper, a general clerk, sold real estate, and has done personnel work. She quit personnel work because the management changed her job. She gave her qualifications to an employment agency but never heard from them. She did some substitute teaching but lately they "turn me down in place of a younger person."

Mr. B. is an air traffic controller. He has worked in his job for 23 years, the latter 10 years as an instructor. Mr. B. said he taught right after college, but "I didn't want to become attached to any girl. It would have meant not going to school. But I was getting older. I gave up and got married." He wanted a Civil Service job because it looked promising and more secure. Yet he was about to take another job when he was offered the Civil Service job. He still feels he'd rather have been teaching or in construction. "I had offers. I'm too easily satisfied. It's easy to become routine. I don't have too high aspirations." Mr. B. said, "the opportunities are there but not for me. I haven't made the most of them." He'd pay any replacement "much less" than he's earning.

The B's say they have not had financial problems. They both pay the bills. "We've always been frugal. He even moonlighted when we were first married. We never buy on time."

The interviewer's notes on the B's comments about their son are copious. In college, their son dated a girl of whom they disapproved. The B's sent their son to school in another state "to get her out of his system." However, the son came home to find that his parents had put his belongings in the attic. He started dating the same girl again, she became pregnant and they married. The new daughter-in-law never got along with the B's. The baby was born dead. A year later their son and daughter-in-law divorced. Mr. B. said that his son was ideal until he started going with the girl he married. A year after his son's divorce, Mr. B. had a heart attack at the age of 54. Besides the domestic trials of the previous two years, he was also having trouble at work. He thought he was being picked on unjustly and that his superiors were trying to block his promotion. He got the promotion, but he said the "damage had been done."

The B's don't do much together. They take a trip, often disagreeing about where to go. They visit infrequently because he said, "we don't have many friends." "We'd built our lives around our son and now we are alienated." Mrs. B. doesn't feel her husband is proud of her. He doesn't think she understands him either. Mrs. B. said twice she tried to take her own life and has thought about leaving him. What Mrs. B. wanted most out of life was for her family to be close. "I must try to be realistic. It is my greatest disappointment." Mr. B. said if he could do everything over he would like to find out "what I'm adapted for. I think I'd have gone into a mechanical line or medical school. I would marry a different person." What he wanted most out of life was happiness. When asked if he has achieved this he said, "No."

Mr. B. was given a score of 14 out of a possible score of 21 on the Index of Emotional Drain. The two reviewers both concurred that emotional drain was a characteristic of Mr. B's life. The reviewers comments were:

Reviewer 1: "lingering unhappiness and anxiety stemming from real insecurity during childhood; dissatisfaction with accomplishments; maladapted to type of work he's in; incompatible marriage partner; disappointment in son's lack of maturity and shotgun marriage."

Reviewer 2: "had horrible childhood and was not close to either parent. He was unable to obtain his educational goal of becoming a doctor. Had difficulty with his marriage and did not have a close relationship. He broke up his son's marriage and has not been close since. He is also very dissatisfied with his job. He wishes he had a multitude of other jobs."

The negative effects of emotional drain can be offset or minimized by social support. Social support can be obtained from a variety of sources, such as spouse, children, friends, relatives, job, religion, hobbies, social groups, or organizations. The biographies usually indicated the need for social support and the degree to which this need was met. The coronary patients commonly obtained their social support from their religion and job; there was usually little or no support from spouses, as is evident in the case of Mr. B. The controls usually secured support from a variety of sources, including their spouses and children. Hence, the assessment of emotional drain and the relative risk of a heart attack should be balanced by a consideration of the positive or supporting factors in an individual's life.

Discussion and Summary

Emotional drain is the result of a complex, long-term conflict of personal values; a conflict which the individual perceives as unresolvable. The accumulation of additional personal, familial, or work problems which extend or complicate already existing personal problems may leave the individual "drained" both physically and psychologically. This situation may be prodromal to a heart attack. Emotional drain can be assessed by using the 21-item Index or by review of a brief biography obtained through an interview. These two methods are best when utilized together to enhance the total predictive power of the assessment.

There is much criticism in the literature on coronary heart disease of findings reported from studies using retrospective methods. The methodology used in the present study, while retrospective, was based on biographical interviews with both husband and wife which elicited information prior to a coronary event. The data were obtained from husband and wife, enabling the dynamics of the marital situation to be assessed and information given by the marital partners to be compared. The biographical summary enabled independent reviewers to ascertain life-style and behavior patterns which were evident prior to a coronary event.

The Index of Emotional Drain and the biographic approach need to be applied prospectively by other researchers on a larger sample in order to determine its reliability and its usefulness as a predictive tool. Indeed, the techniques described here could be used to identify high risk individuals for a myocardial infarction who could be advised of the benefits of counseling, psychotherapy or value clarification.

References

Bruhn, J. G., K. E. McCrady, and A. du Plessis. 1968. "Evidence of Emotional Drain Preceding Death from Myocardial Infarction," *Psychiatric Digest,* 29:34–40.

Engel, G. L. 1968. "A Life Setting Conducive to Illness: The Giving Up–Given Up Complex," *Annals of Internal Medicine,* 69:293–300.

Friedman, G. D., H. K. Ury, A. L. Klatsky, and A. B. Siegelaub. 1974. "A Psychological Questionnaire Predictive of Myocardial Infarction: Results from the Kaiser-Permanente Epidemiologic Study of Myocardial Infarction," *Psychosomatic Medicine,* 36:327–43.

Jenkins, C. D. 1976. "Recent Evidence Supporting Psychologic and Social Risk Factors for Coronary Disease," *New England Journal of Medicine,* 294:987–94.

Paffenbarger, R. S., P. A. Wolf, J. Notkin, and M. C. Thorne. 1966. "Chronic Disease in Former College Students I. Early Precursors of Fatal Coronary Heart Disease," *Journal of Chronic Disease,* 83:314–28.

Weiss, E. 1940. "Cardiovascular Lesions of Probable Psychosomatic Origin in Arterial Hypertension," *Psychosomatic Medicine,* 11:249–264.

Wolf, S. 1967. "The End of the Rope: The Role of the Brain in Cardiac Death," *Canadian Medical Association Journal,* 97:1022–25.

Wolfe, M. D. and P. Theodore. 1936. "Emotions and Organic Heart Disease," *American Journal of Psychiatry,* 93:681–91.

Part III
Psychosocial Aspects of Cardiovascular Surgery

❦ 12
Interactions Among Patient, Family, Cardiovascular Surgeon, and Staff

Donal M. Billig

THE MYSTIQUE OF the heart, so woven into our language and culture, has made folk heroes of our cardiovascular surgeons and legends of their accomplishments. One has only to compare the media response to heart transplants as opposed to renal transplants to glimpse the emotional impact of cardiovascular surgery.

The fact that our surgical efforts are reconstructive, rather than ablative, combined with our great fortune to be treating diseases which admit of mechanical solutions with good overall results, has added to the mystique a sense of warranted optimism that pervades all of our attitudes toward the cardiovascular patient. The orientation is to life not death, to reconstruction rather than ablation. Bereavement and disability in this context have very different connotations than in the cancer patient.

Family guilt, fear of dying, fear of disability, the transference of godlike qualities to the surgeon, factors in the surgeon's attitudes toward his staff, affording familiarity with the hospital environment, and so forth, are parts of the family's and patient's adjustment to and preparation not only for surgery but also for potential or actual bereavement. These are common to all surgical situations, but must be considered in the light of the psychodynamic environment peculiar to the cardiovascular surgical patient.

I shall attempt to convey how one cardiovascular surgeon perceives these interactions. In highlighting some of the factors as I see them, it is my hope that the ideas presented may stimulate further research and investigation.

Dimensions of Life-Threat

The cardiovascular surgical patient, unlike most other surgical patients, is "life-threatened" in every instance. The dimensions of the threat vary.

There may be an immediate threat, as in the patient with a tender and expanding aneurysm of the abdominal aorta, implying impending or actual rupture.

There is the predictable 90 percent fatality rate within one year for untreated infants with severe congestive heart failure in the early weeks of life.

There is the less immediate threat for the patient with severe aortic stenosis, who has a median survival of four years but a constant possibility of sudden death.

There is the life threat two to three decades away as in the child with an ostium secundum atrial septal defect and a large intracardiac shunt.

The severity of the lesion, its natural history, the presence of associated abnormalities of pulmonary, cerebral-vascular, renal, coronary and other systems, all enter into the assessment of the severity of the life-threat.

The Surgical Solution

Surgical treatment itself imposes a potential life-threat. Mortality becomes related not only to the patient and his disease, but also to the judgment and skill of the surgeon and the entire staff.

In proposing a surgical solution to the patient and family, the surgeon potentially is disturbing a fine balance which may have been struck as an adjustment to the disease. The threat of death is, as a rule, vague and in the future. Impending surgery brings it into sharp focus, since surgical mortality is always a possibility that must be shared with patient and family. The surgeon is asking the patient and family to accept this reality of potential death in order to improve the quality and length of life, and assigns a definite time for its potential occurrence.

These various levels of life-threat are in most ways clear and definable. They are present to a greater or lesser degree in all cardiovascular surgical situations and are a measurable portion of the equation with which the surgeon has to deal. The surgeon initially sets up the dynamics of his relationship with patient and family with his assessment of these risks and time factors as the "known" in the equation. Two extreme examples will suffice.

In the patient with a tender and expanding aneurysm of the abdominal aorta, a catastrophic event, rupture, with rapid death, is certain to occur within minutes to days. All risks are acceptable for such a patient, who is often in excruciating pain. The result can be a not unexpected surgical mortality or a heroic salvage for a patient with no future unless surgically treated. These dynamics are simple to manage for patient, family, and staff.

In a child with a large shunt via an ostium secundum atrial septal defect, the life-threat is vague and a few decades away, as are the threats of morbidity from congestive heart failure and pulmonary arterial hypertension. But surgical mortality increases approximately 60 times once these occur, and if untreated, life may be shortened by more than 30 years. Optimal management is open heart surgery in childhood, at a time when the life-threat is a vague 25 to 30 years into the future. An entirely different dynamic dominates this situation, with parental guilt assuming a variable but important unknown in the equation. If they opt for no surgery, they must be left with the nagging guilt of not having done their best to ensure a healthy normal life for the child. If they opt for surgery, a perfect surgical result can shield them from guilt. Fortunately, the latter is almost always the outcome. The preoperative, operative, and early postoperative periods in these situations are always guilt-ridden moments for the parents, severely intensified by the infrequent complication or by the unusual surgical mortality. Only careful preoperative preparation of the parents, in order to bring them to a proper decision and allow them to understand the necessity for surgery so far removed from the life-threat, can soften these feelings. Most surgical patients lie between these extremes, and careful individual assessment of each situation combined with an attentiveness to emotional factors in each patient-family-disease complex is important in the preparation for surgery and potential bereavement.

It should be appreciated that the cardiovascular surgeon

deals largely with potential bereavement. In most instances, his patients survive, are improved, and have few serious complications. Those who die most often do so in the immediate perioperative period. This surgeon's actual involvement with dying patients and their families for long periods is unusual. In strong contrast is the cardiologist and primary-care physician who deal with many patients with inoperable or otherwise incurable cardiac defects over long periods. His main surgical involvement is in preparing the family for possible bereavement within the context of a more or less optimistic surgical outlook.

In my experience nothing of an ex post facto nature will substitute for an adequate preoperative understanding of the potential risks and complications of surgery and the potential risks and complications of nonsurgical treatment. In every instance, the surgeon is convinced that surgical therapy is the most effective means of ensuring rehabilitation, improvement, and increased longevity. His evaluation must be shared with patient and family. The manner in which one goes about this is extremely variable and depends upon the surgeon's assessment of how he may best handle a given situation.

Public Attitude Regarding Cardiovascular Surgery

A great many factors, some real, some imagined, some glorified in song and story by the media and media-conscious surgeons, combine to shape the public's attitude toward cardiovascular surgery. Of great importance is the inherited mystique which surrounds the heart in almost all cultures. To be sure we no longer eat the heart of our enemy to gain his courage. But we do use terms such as *good-hearted* for *kind, great-hearted* for *courageous, heartening* for *encouraging,* and many others. And while we no longer throw our victim down a pyramid after removing his beating heart, the removal of a "live" patient's heart and transplantation to another live patient in 1968 fired a medical shot heard round the world, while prior successful renal transplantation was from the outset a publicity "ho-hum," and subsequent liver and lung transplantation attempts have caused hardly a ripple.

The protagonists in the heart transplantation drama have written best sellers, been sued for millions, received unprecedented attention from the media, changed our definition of death in the courts, and utilized an experimental artificial heart in the race for another "first," resulting in loss of a professorship and a $4 million lawsuit. In fact, looking at the media coverage afforded many of us, one is reminded more of Valhalla and Siegfreid than of a hospital and a surgeon. Because of mystical emotional appeal, hearts and heart surgery simply sell more magazines, newspapers, and books than do other organs and their surgical treatment.

The technological explosion that followed after World War II saw the dream of miraculous surgical cures for heart disease become a reality. Valve prostheses, monitoring equipment, computerized intensive-care areas, coronary arteriography, hypothermic techniques for newborns, new methods for preserving homografts, and thousands of other advances now allow us to produce surgical results unprecedented for any other group of life-threatening diseases. This ever growing monument to surgical skill, motivation, and advancing technology has created a justified optimism in the mind of patients and families. The fact that almost all of our operative armamentarium consists of reconstructive rather than ablative surgery further enhances this feeling. These circumstances (as if we needed any encouragement) obligate us to a more aggressive surgical approach and justify it by even better surgical results in patients who are less far along in their disease.

These factors are largely responsible for the optimistic attitudes of surgeon, staff, and family. However, they make it even more important that the patient and family understand the possibility of death or complications resulting in disability, for they are an ever-present reality. Realistic appraisal of the risks is mandatory. In the final analysis, the patient and the family must make a decision based upon factual data received from the surgeon; surgeon, family, and patient must be prepared for bereavement within this context of optimism lest the emotional results be disastrous. Among the many pitfalls that the medicolegal problem has imposed upon us, an increased awareness of the necessity of informing our patients has come out of it: the right attitude for the wrong reasons.

The Patient, the Family, and the Surgeon

There are varying degrees of fear, guilt and hostility, mixed with gratitude and hope in all these relationships. The more threatening the problem, and the more complex the surgery, the more intense these feelings become. Each set of interactions is peculiar to each family environment, the seriousness of the life-threat, the manner in which the surgeon handles the situation, and often how well the medical physician has prepared the patient and family for the eventuality of surgery.

These interactions are usually deep-rooted in the makeup of the family interelationship, and the surgeon cannot possibly unravel this tangle nor can he alter its nature. Some surgeons seek to circumvent the problems entirely by fostering the illusion of infallibility. This may be of temporary solace. However, not only is it dishonest, it courts disaster in some instances, for a family ill-prepared for dire consequences and, on occasion, for the surgeon and his insurance company.

This "religious" solution has a very short useful span indeed. If the surgical outcome is excellent, it was hardly necessary. If the result is poor, the bubble is broken, along with the myth of infallibility. "If he couldn't pull him through, who could?" is not always the postscript. Immeasurable guilt, hostility, and self-recrimination are liable to occur, beyond salvage, in a surgeon who has relinquished his credibility. The price is far too high.

More suitable solutions which permit a confident but realistic optimism are available. They allow the patient and the family to adjust to the threat of surgery and to possible or actual bereavement, and permit the surgeon to help the family in an hour of need. They can be summed up in a series of position statements.

"This operation has been done many times by myself and other surgeons throughout the world with reproducibly good results. It is neither new nor unique. The techniques are fairly standardized. There are complications which may occur. They are infrequent. Most patients survive the surgery and are improved by it. Almost no complications result from poor technique, since the operation has been done so often that we have come to learn the pitfalls and to avoid them. Most deaths are due to what severity of disease and what other organ involvement the patient has."

For most operations, these conditions are true. Where the risks are greater, the risk of nonsurgical treatment is always greater still. "There is little choice but to operate at this time. Eighty percent of infants with this disease will die by six months of age, 90 percent by their first birthday. We can save more than half of them with surgery. I know this is a large risk, but it is far less than the risk of treatment without surgery."

What parent would not opt for surgery when faced with this honest appraisal, and what surgeon would be so heartless and mindless of the potential grief just a few hours away as not to add, "You must not hope for too much. But this is the only, reasonable course, and we are often successful."

Many patients and families will equate surgical treatment with "cure," and nonsurgical treatment with "hopelessness." This is in strong contrast to other areas of medicine where patients are usually relieved to find that the problem is so mild that surgery will not be required, and more like the attitude of cancer patients who recognize that no surgery means incurable disease.

Since both circumstances exist in cardiovascular disease, it is extremely important, in a nonoperative situation, to take great care in explaining to a patient why one has opted for nonsurgical treatment. Great relief naturally occurs when a patient can be told that his disease can be controlled without surgery, and that surgery is not necessary and may or may not be necessary in the future. In the patient whose disease is so far along that surgical treatment is far too risky with little chance of improvement, one must often be more circuitous. It is important to leave certain things unsaid in the first go-round and to provide an emotional escape route. Those who wish more concrete information will ask for it. Those who do not will ask few additional questions. Little will be gained from pursuing the matter to a crushing conclusion in such patients.

In general, honesty tempered by sensitivity and judgment will bring most relationships into as favorable a frame as may be with the least risk of inflicting emotional harm on all participants. The surgeon must be as thoughtful of these psychodynamic interactions as he is in planning his operative approach.

The Surgeon and His Staff

The "team" approach has been greatly stressed in cardiovascular surgery. Actually, it extends to almost all major surgical situations, but because of the great number of personnel and the sophisticated equipment necessary in cardiovascular surgery, the team concept is extremely important.

The surgeon spends less than 5 percent of the day with any individual patient except for the day of surgery. During more than 95 percent of the day, the patient is in the hands of resident staff and nurses.

The surgeon must foster an attitude of respect for the other health-care professionals on his staff, and they and the patient and family must be aware of this attitude. Not only does this ensure that they will take pride in their performance, be more diligent, and care more about the patients in their care, but it is extremely comforting to family and patient to sense this confidence. The family and patient need to feel that everything that is necessary is being done, that the staff is working with skill and care under the direction of the surgeon. This becomes more and more important as the postoperative situation becomes more and more complicated. In case of death, the feeling that the total care was as thoughtful and effective as it possibly could have been will do much to alleviate the family's guilt and sorrow.

Familiarity with the Hospital Environment and the Staff

No fear is so great as our fear of the unknown. An explanation by the surgeon of the events on the day of surgery, including rough time estimate, is important.

Of equal or greater importance is a preoperative intensive-care-unit (ICU) orientation for family and patient. An explanation of waiting room protocol, monitoring, chest tubes, respirators, and so on, prepares them for the day of surgery and, if properly handled, creates confidence by the sheer weight of instrumentation. The sight of many patients recovering from surgery and doing well is more than comforting. The purpose of this activity is to familiarize and prepare the family for the initial shocking visit after surgery, with tubes and lines attached to their loved one, lights flashing, respirator sighing, and so forth.

Whether this actually aids them in bereavement is hard to say, but, in my opinion, anything which reduces fears and engenders confidence in the staff is of extreme importance.

Pediatric Problems

Parental guilt is a real factor in most pediatric cardiac surgical patients. Its most frequent cause is guilt because of imagined responsibility for the defect. Guilt is always enhanced by the child's death and softened by an excellent surgical outcome. Explanations that the disease is not hereditary, and therefore has little to do with the parent, are of little avail in my experience; unless parents broach the subject, I tend to stay away from it.

Guilt over deciding to have the child undergo surgery is more amenable to help by the surgeon. A proper perspective on the necessity for surgery is mandatory, as discussed above. The only sure relief is a good outcome.

Children themselves understand little of risks or chronic disability. Their fear is of the unknown, of death, and of separation from the mother.

The preoperative visit to the intensive care unit is very important for parents and child. We have developed a coloring book for the child which explains the unit, operating room, and hospital course. Today's children are extremely visual rather than verbal, and this has made for better understanding. Not surprisingly, a more composed child makes for a more composed and better prepared parent.

Family-participation units, where mother sleeps in, are excellent facilities. My initial reaction to this was skeptical, feeling that separation was inevitable on the day of surgery and for one to several days thereafter of ICU care, and that it was best to prepare the child for this. Years of observation have taught me that this is wrong. Two days of separation will not cure the years of protection and dependence that most mothers lavish on the child with heart disease. If the mother requires the few days (that in her mind may be the last) with her child, it is far more unsettling and creates far more hostility and guilt to separate them.

Children with birth defects such as Downs' syndrome are a very special case. Overwhelming parental guilt and the protective behavior pattern it inspires are a recurring theme. Bereavement is always associated with a sense of relief, immediately turned into even more overwhelming guilt. Many surgeons decline to operate upon such patients, feeling that far too much medical manpower and national and state resources are already being spent upon them. This is a political decision, and in my opinion not within the province of the surgeon. My experience with them is that both they and especially their parents need all the emotional support we can give them. To reject them for care is to force an already tortured parent to face society's rejection, and is an inhuman and uncivilized attitude. Here, as perhaps nowhere else in surgery, is the surgeon forced to the realization that he is truly "operating upon an entire family."

Conclusion

The subject admits of no conclusions and no simple solutions. Although I have attempted to stress a few of the psychosocial features which enter into the dynamics of these relationships, the coverage is admittedly far from complete.

At present the surgeon can draw only upon his own experience and sensitivity to help him through some of these serious situations. An in-depth multidisciplinary analysis may well reveal new directions and guidelines for dealing with these sensitive situations.

❋ 13

Psychosocial Implications of Surgery for the Life-Threatened

Frank Glenn

IT IS NOT unusual for a surgeon to expose at operation a lesion grossly suggestive of a terminal condition. Its seriousness is often confirmed by the pathologist who examines a microscopic slide he has immediately prepared. Perhaps 75 percent of these patients are operated upon on an elective basis and less than 25 percent are emergencies.

There are a multiplicity of factors that may arise when an individual is demonstrated to have a condition that under ordinary circumstances is considered to be terminal. Sudden revelations of an irreversible situation often precipitate panic and depressing hopelessness that inhibits efforts and innovations to lessen the impact for all involved. Potential disability and curtailment of life become evident.

Pre-operative examinations and evaluations may have clearly indicated the findings. The doctors involved may have been fearful of the suggested diagnosis. The possible findings are often discussed with the patient and his or her family. All, including the surgeon, naturally await the actual demonstration of the pathological changes, both gross and microscopic, before discussing the potential course. All are hopeful that the operation will reveal "something not too bad" and that the surgeon can remove it or pave the way for x-ray or chemotherapy. It is with this background that the surgeon is regarded as the one who may discover "good news or bad."

In the period that is required for the operation and the preliminary pathological examination, facts become available that are the basis for realization on the part of all involved—patient, family, and attending physicians and surgeons. The interpretations of findings by these individuals are variable. They may be over-pessimistic, overoptimistic and, in other instances, as actual and accurate as they can be. In any event, the latter is to be hoped for and actually sought by the doctors. If they can keep close to this objective, the future of the problems that the disease imposes will be more readily dealt with. These are illustrated by an actual case history and discussed in their broad aspect.

Case History

Eric Scott, a middle vice-president of a bank, was 42 years old when he sustained a massive coronary thrombosis. His wife was 38, they had three children in high school. The family was a close one with many common objectives pursued with enthusiasm. Life up until this point had been a series of successes for all. Scott had been in remarkably good health throughout his life. His hospitalization was a shock to all, including him. The internists and the cardiologist told him that he had had a "massive thrombosis involving the left heart" and that it would be necessary for him to be immobilized for some time. He probably would not return to work for several weeks. His business associates were most solicitous and generous. They assured him that he could return to work at any time that he was up to it and that it would not impair his chances for becoming first vice-president, the next step in the hierarchy. His hospital course was quite satisfactory, and he was discharged home earlier than had been anticipated. His spirits were good. The family were greatly relieved and then two weeks later (after having followed instructions most carefully at home) he developed a new trend of symptoms that led to a diagnosis of possible ventricular aneurysm. In spite of rather rigid conservative measures they increased. He was readmitted to the hospital and, following further evaluation, a decision to excise the aneurysm and close the defect in the heart wall was decided upon by the surgeon, cardiologist, and internist. A frank and somewhat detailed description of the problem was presented to the patient. Many questions were answered directly and then the major one, "What is the prognosis for the future?" The surgeon said he hoped that it was good but that at that time he was unable to say more than that. The findings at operation would add additional information. The family internist, the cardiologist, and the surgeon were in agreement. On the day before the operation Mrs. Scott and the children talked about the operation with their father. He was optimistic but serious as he talked with them, leaving them with the impression he was apprehensive.

At operation, the ventricular aneurysm was readily resected but unfortunately there was evidence of marked coronary sclerosis. Nevertheless, the operation was well tolerated and the immediate postoperative course satisfactory. The patient and his family were greatly relieved that he had done so well and within a few days were slightly euphoric—as was the patient. About 10 days after operation, however, the cardiologist and the surgeon discussed the operative findings with the patient, and although they were as optimistic as they could be, the conclusion was evident to the patient and to his wife that his life expectancy was reduced and that the future course was unpredictable.

In the quiet hours of the night the patient thought a great deal about the probability of his death and what it would mean to his family. The dreams of his earlier life and what he had hoped now seemed unlikely. On his return home following the operation when the children were at school, he repeatedly reviewed his thinking with his wife. With a minimum of tears they mutually and enthusiastically agreed to make the best of it. The doctors had said that they could not predict the future and probably, they hoped, his would be an exception and that he would have a satisfactory recovery. His progress was slow and within a period of two to three weeks it was evident that his cardiac reserve was minimal. He spent most of his time in bed. It was during this period that he turned first to his surgeon, telling him that he was making no progress and felt that he was merely holding on. With this change, when would he die? Would he have pain, as he had had at the time of the primary coronary attack? The surgeon could answer some but not all of his questions but he could listen, and he did listen. He was also quizzed by Mrs. Scott seeking respite and reassurance. The children, all in high school, having been asked repeatedly every day about the progress of their father who was well known in the community, became increasingly apprehensive. All were fearful about what would occur next. Apprehension was gradually followed by depression. The internist, who was the family doctor, made frequent visits answering and reanswering increasing numbers of questions. The cardiologist, who adhered rather closely to the facts as he knew them, assumed an attitude of guarding against any deception. This probably influenced Mr. and Mrs. Scott to think and discuss with each other what they could do to make things as easy as possible for all concerned when he died. The close relationship between husband and wife caused both of them great pain. They discussed whether or not she should ever marry again. The financial aspect, discussed with the company, and the insurance seemed reasonably secure so far as the education of the children was concerned. What she should do was of great concern to him.

Amidst all this, the previously unconsidered way of thought developed, namely, what was the source of life, how rapidly had his 40-odd years passed, the many happy experiences of accomplishments and then to look into the future and see the termination of it all? If there was a beginning and an end of all previous events, so he looked at death as the beginning of something he knew not what. Nor could he visualize the end of it. His question to the internist and, indeed, the cardiologist and the surgeon, who were quite attentive, was in essence: How long is death? Is there another world after death?

Although members of the local church, their association with the clergy had been limited to the events of baptisms, weddings, and funerals of their family and friends. Now he sought counsel of the pastor. During their discussions the pastor was reassuring, but afterward Mr. Scott was left feeling that there was a lack of tangible evidence that there was anything but oblivion in his future. After a period of some six weeks at home and with increasing limitation of activity, various circulatory deficiencies developed and required additional medication, and with this additional medication, there were periods of confusion, almost always followed by apprehension when they cleared. The increased visits of the doctor, increased medication, assistance by visiting nurses, emphasized the unsatisfactory course of the patient.

It was most apparent to him and almost equally so to Mrs. Scott and the children. The doctors and the pastor basically portrayed the concept as there was a beginning of life so there was an end, and that he had been fortunate to have had so much satisfaction in his life. He gradually but finally accepted this philosophy and, disappointing as it was to him and in spite of his physical disability, he radiated an attitude of cheerfulness and extended as much comfort as he could to the family.

Mrs. Scott, on the other hand, became more and more depressed and because of the vigor of many of their friends, both younger and older, she felt that life had dealt quite harshly with them. Many discussions they had tended to convince her further that she would prefer to die herself rather than embark upon a period of the unknown which she must experience after his death. The counselors kept her from indulging in details as much as possible, as Mr. Scott's condition worsened. Medication to correct it tended to obscure his awareness and diminish the concern and apprehension that he had had. His expressed attitude was one of hope that he could remain alive as long as possible and that now he had no fear of death and that he might welcome it to avoid the penalties of his disabilities. He gradually deteriorated further and died, some eight months following the resection of his ventricular aneurysm, the cause of death being gradual myocardial failure.

Activities associated with the funeral, solicitations of friends, and the quietness that followed and the realization of both Mrs. Scott and the children of their immediate situation resulted in their seeking help and counsel. This was indeed a painful experience for Mrs. Scott. She was advised to marry as soon as possible, to seek a position, or to become interested in some kind of business venture. Her B.A. provided no preparation for entrance into a self-supporting position. The eldest boy, a senior in high school, obtained a scholarship for the first year of college. With enthusiasm he embarked upon it. The two younger children found the household difficult to become accustomed to in the absence of their father. They talked too with their friends, neighbors, teachers with a very limited understanding which was eventually best neutralized by their mother.

. . . .

The future of the members of this family is unknown and unpredictable at the particular phase of the illness that has been described. The doctors in this instance followed what many of us consider to be the ideal procedure. They provided the best possible medical care. There was no deception, there was frank discussion, understandable to all involved. Some might think that its harshness was too great and that there should have been longer delay in establishing the probable course following the operation which demonstrated the impairment of the coronary circulation. Workings of the human mind concerning one's origin and destination are brought quickly into focus under these circumstances. The active life of the individual remains the center of hope to the patient and all intimately related to him. His ability to cope with the approaching events and their implications to his family require counsel that is factual but with some practical solution that is feasible. Just as important in the counseling is the careful listening to the patient and to the family, because such discussions do a great deal to clarify the situation insofar as what may be considered inevitable is concerned. The counselors must bear in mind always that they do not know the future and that certain events are highly probable but not always inevitable. Slender though this hope may be, it should not be destroyed. Not only should the counselors, the doctors, the clergy be willing to listen, they should also provide the opportunity to those involved to discuss it fairly frequently. This is particularly of therapeutic value in the terminal phases, not so much to the patient as to the family. Reflection on the part of those who counsel patients as to what they would do under the same circumstances and what they would want done for them would be of material help though no two situations are alike.

Patients with conditions that appear to require emergency surgery have additional problems that vary according to circumstances. Generally speaking, these occur most frequently among the elderly. In this group, the risk with or without operation is greater than in the younger and more robust. The apprehension of potential death is extenuated by the patient's realization that many of his peers have died over the previous 10 years or so. The comparison of the patient's symptoms to those of his or her acquaintances is often the basis for hesitancy in accepting recommended therapy. Many but not all of the patients are willing to discuss this frankly. Actually, many relish an opportunity to substantiate or negate the conclusions that they have reached in their own mind. These include the possibility of death with the desire to know more about what is involved. They are concerned about the matter of pain and whether or not it can be controlled. Operations are always associated with risk and patients understand this. They are best reassured by explaining that with facilities, personnel, and care in the hospital these can be minimized. It is often effectual to emphasize that the risk of doing nothing may be greater than the risk involved in the therapeutic procedure. The uncertainty of prediction requires explanation in terms that the patient can understand. Dependent upon the patient's experience with his acquaintances and observations in hospitals, death has often been related to surgery. Perhaps the most common statement to be made after such a discussion is inaugurated by the question: What will dying be like? They seek the doctor's opinion for specific details that center around pain, disability, and eventually the matter of what occurs after death. The more thoughtful and informed the patient, the more numerous may be the questions concerning the matter of life after death. Many have religious convictions that are accepted and satisfy them. But perhaps a greater number are concerned about such questions as to whether or not cremation of a body destroys the likelihood of its being reassembled in the next world.

It is not suggested that the professional answer these questions. They are included to emphasize their wide existence in the minds of the elderly patients who present themselves for medical care. The patients want to be listened to.

Those who reach the age of 65 are subject to a wide range of disorders, many of which are best treated by surgery. A few decades ago, there was a tendency to withhold indicated surgery because of the anticipated risks that accompanied this form of therapy. However, medical knowledge in general has increased, as have ways and means to meet the problems that are peculiar to the aged. These have evolved from research laboratories and the careful recording of experiences with patients, as well as the dedicated and unrelenting efforts of the medical profession, together with the nurses and paramedical groups. The most important advancements in the recent half century have been related to anesthesia, water and electrolyte balance, methods of measuring impaired function to determine the capacity of an individual to withstand a surgical procedure, and within the past decade, the replacement of organs that are beyond repair by transplantation or mechanical devices.

The aged, like the very young, have a rather slim margin of physiological functional reserve, even in a good state of health, and when they are ill from any disease process, it is further narrowed. An awareness of this on the part of the medical profession has been of fundamental importance in first estimating the reserve and then selecting the surgical procedure that meets the immediate critical situation, in order that life may be prolonged, leaving definitive correction to be carried out on an elective basis. The increase in hospital beds, wide distribution of hospital facilities in communities, and the presence of well-prepared physicians who have had the benefit of postgraduate training, have had a profound influence upon the care that the aged are now receiving. An appreciation of this on the part of the public at large, and those over 65 in particular, is reflected in their attitude toward hospitals. For example, many of those now over 65 recall that in their youth, hospitals were institutions where people went to die. At present, hospitals are looked upon more often as a place of refuge. All types of illness are so well cared for that only a small percentage of patients fail to return to the community.

The disease entities in the elderly requiring surgery are even more varied than those in the younger age groups. Examples of such disease entities include: changes in the vascular system associated with the aging process (such as obliterative vascular disease and cardiac insufficiency); carcinoma of practically every structure; impaired function of specific organs (the lungs, pancreas, or kidneys). In the process of evaluating these patients and seeking to help them, procedures have been evolved that are

very valuable but that always impose a burden upon the individual. These include visualization of the vascular system by x-ray,
pulmonary function studies, direct tissue biopsy, and metabolic
evaluations of critical processes in the digestive and excretory
mechanisms of the body. Thus, not only are the number and extent of surgical procedures for the elderly increasing, but also the
methods of evaluating these individuals in preparation for these
procedures. Together this constitutes an increase in the daily
work of the general hospitals throughout the country, which are,
almost without exception, participating in the care of the elderly
group.

The magnitude of the problem relative to the care of those 65
and older becomes more distinct when it is approached in proper
perspective. On the one hand, those 65 and older make up approximately 10 percent of the population; on the other hand,
requirements of the elderly for medical care—and for surgery in
particular—require almost 50 percent of the facilities of hospitals.
According to data from the Metropolitan Life Insurance Company
and the Associated Hospital Service of New York, an individual
who is 65 years of age or older is much more likely to be admitted
to the hospital than a person who is under 65 years of age. The
duration of their stay, because of the complexity of the problems
associated with their care, is twice as long as for those in the
younger and more robust period of life.

The surgical principles to be applied to the aged individual,
while not unlike those applied to all other age groups, have many
associated ramifications that require recognition and consideration
and meticulous management. While these may primarily involve
disease and the aging process of the physical being, which are
often readily defined, thought and action are also required to recognize the factors of the environment from which the patient
comes, and the circumstances to which he will be exposed when
the required surgical services of a general hospital have been sat-
isfactorily fulfilled. It is the recognition of these on the part of the
patient that frequently detracts from the benefits that surgical
therapy may have provided. The will to live, the desire to plan for
the future, the participation and enjoyment of events in ordinary
life on the part of the aged tend to be drastically reduced in comparison to those of younger individuals.

There linger still among older laypersons—and even among
older medical professionals—definite inhibitions about embarking
upon surgery in the elderly. These are based largely on past expe-

rience from a lay point of view. This over-65 age group recalls that hospitalization for surgery was associated with complications and death. The hospitals of that era too often unwittingly became institutions of terminal care.

On the other hand, individuals—even those now 65 years and older—who know about hospitals through personal experience or experience of members of their families, now usually exhibit a different attitude and regard the hospital as the proper place to take care of major illness, whether medical or surgical. In addition, the increased availability of hospitals has had a definite effect upon the thinking of the lay population, so that this is also bringing about change. Thus, it is well to bear in mind the attitude of many of the elderly and the background that has given rise to it.

The attitude of the medical profession has been changing concomitantly, and perhaps more rapidly—particularly among the segments directly associated with hospital practice. They have had an opportunity to see what can be accomplished when steps are taken to reduce the risk of any surgical procedure. Unfortunately, there still remains a small proportion of the profession who, because of limited experience with hospitals, are prone to consider that it is perhaps better to let an elderly patient die of complications at home than to send him to a hospital where—despite a relatively short life expectancy—he will be subjected to prolonged examination and perhaps an operation. This too has been influenced by past experience. Surgeons in large hospitals, in particular, would do well to understand sympathetically the position of the general practitioner who carries the elderly along during the period that they are having symptoms from a condition that might be corrected by elective surgery, and who sends the patient to the hospital only when an emergency arises.

Insofar as the patient's attitude is concerned, the activities of the individual greatly influence his reaction when confronted with illness that carries an indication for surgical procedures. If the elderly individual is engaged in some activity that holds his interest, or if he is participating in other problems so that he is well occupied, he generally accepts surgery without hesitation. This is a manifestation of the current desire of the elderly to be active and to continue to live as long as they can, in contrast to the past, when they were restricted from ordinary activity either by illness or by so-called retirement.

Pertinent to this also is the appreciation on the part of the patient that many of his peers have died. This often influences him to consider that "his time is approaching" and that interference with the process by surgical measures, which he holds to be rather heroic, is not for him. Elderly patients are usually much more interested in continuing their activities than they are merely in prolonging their lifespans. Death in the minds of many patients is an event in the vague future. They would rather not consider it and seek to avoid thinking about it. It is rare for a patient to decide to have an operation because he believes he can live an additional specific length of time.

References

Altemeier, W. A. and R. P. Hummel. 1965. "Antibiotic Agents in Colon Surgery," *Surgical Clinics of North America*, 45:1087.

Associated Hospital Service of New York (Blue Cross). Personal Communication.

Bahnson, H. T. 1976. "Thoracic Aneurysms." In D. C. Sabiston, Jr. and F. C. Spencer, eds., *Gibbon's Surgery of the Chest*, Philadelphia: W. B. Saunders.

Cowdry, E. V. 1971. "The Physician and the Patient." In E. V. Cowdry and F. U. Steinberg, eds., *The Care of the Geriatric Patient*. St. Louis: C. V. Mosby.

DeBakey, M. E., E. S. Crawford, D. A. Cooley, G. C. Morris, H. E. Garrett, and W. S. Fields. 1965. "Cerebral Insufficiency: One to 11-year Results Following Arterial Reconstructive Operation," *Annals of Surgery*, 161:921.

Glenn, F., S. W. Moore, and J. Beal, eds. 1960. *Surgery in the Aged*. New York: McGraw-Hill.

Glenn, F. and A. J. Okinaka. 1964. "Surgical Problems and Pulmonary Function in the Geriatric Patient, including Observations on a Man Purported To Be 167 Years Old," *American Geriatric Society*, 12:632.

Kirsh, M. M., D. M. Behrendt, M. B. Orringer, O. Gago, L. A. Gray, Jr., L. J. Mills, J. F. Walter, and H. Sloan. 1976. "The Treatment of Acute Traumatic Rupture of the Aorta: A 10-year Experience," *Annals of Surgery*, 184:308.

Powers, J. H., ed. 1968. *Surgery of the Aged and Debilitated Patient*. Philadelphia: W. B. Saunders.

Randall, H. I. 1968. "The Treatment of Cancer in Older Patients." In J. H. Powers, ed., *Surgery of the Aged and Debilitated Patient*. Philadelphia: W. B. Saunders.

Stone, H. H., C. A. Hooper, L. D. Kolb, C. E. Geheber, and E. J. Dawkins. 1976. "Antibiotic Prophylaxis in Gastric, Biliary and Colonic Surgery," *Annals of Surgery*, 184:443.

𝔄🌿14
Heart Disease, Heart Surgery, and Death

Richard S. Blacher

MOST THANATOLOGICAL RESEARCH has focused on "chronic illness" and we associate the concept of dying with the slowly deteriorating patient. Yet in patients with heart disease, "acute dying" is often the central issue.

From the dawn of history, the heart, with its dramatic all-or-nothing quality, has been considered the central organ of the body, the seat of emotions, feeling, and even intelligence, and the end of life has been measured by cessation of its beat. Despite the recent medical use of a flat electroencephalogram (EEG) as an indication of death, most laypersons feel that death occurs when the heart stops. Cardiac resuscitation is still reported in the press as a patient dying and then being brought back to life, and this reflects the general view of our culture, illogical as the idea may be. The close connection between death and the heart touches all aspects of our work with patients with heart disease. Nowhere is this more evident than in cardiac surgery.

Most patients facing *general* surgery and anesthesia struggle with their fears of dying. Being anesthetized itself is experienced as a major threat. The passive surrender to a fellow being, who will then have total charge of your body and indeed your life, is an act of great trust. In the face of a life-endangering illness, where the threat of death is already present, the extinction of consciousness reminds us of the "putting to sleep" of a pet. The operation itself is experienced as an invasion of the body with the possibility of mutilation and discovery of malignant processes.

For the cardiac-surgery patient, these anxieties are compounded by anticipation of the handling and incision of the heart. In addition, reality and fantasy merge concerning the time during an open-heart procedure when the heart is indeed stopped. Patients talk of the "moment of truth" when the doctors await the resumption of the heartbeat. The commonly held belief that the stopping of the heart means death lends itself to the feeling that the procedure is in essence a dying, followed by a rebirth. Thus, for the general-surgery patient, the fear is that the heart will stop; for the cardiac patient, the worry is that the already-stopped heart will not resume beating. The latter's concern is that although he has already accepted the preliminary state of absence of heartbeat, he won't be revived.

This concern over death and rebirth in heart surgery has broad theoretical and practical consequences. It helps explain some observations concerning the patients' view of various procedures. For example, many patients consider that their chance for survival is 50-50, despite a thorough explanation by the surgeon of the actual statistical risks (Blacher, 1972). Clearly the patients' odds represent the idea that one either lives or dies, that is, that the heart will beat or not beat.

Large numbers of patients conceptualize their valves as outside the heart despite the surgeon's careful description of the procedure. The physician may use a model and drawings, yet the patient distorts the matter when he tries to discuss the anatomy (Blacher, 1975). This transmural migration of the valves to the outside of the heart and into the blood vessels is directly linked with an attempt to deny the incision of the heart. The need that the organ remain intact becomes almost desperate. Several patients, in describing the procedure of valve replacement, have suggested that the heart and lungs are removed intact and placed on a pump. Despite this seemingly extreme picture, the same patients blanch with anxiety when it is suggested that the heart might be incised in order to replace the valve.

Concerns with death, in my view, have much to do with postcardiotomy psychosis. The background and etiology of this condition have been widely discussed in recent years from the viewpoint of both organic and psychological factors, and the threat of death has not been ignored (Blacher, 1972; Abram,

1965). There has been relatively little emphasis on this, however, as a factor. This is not surprising precisely *because of* the danger of death that overhangs the heart-surgery situation—both for patient and staff.

Given this unspoken but omnipresent presence of the threat of death, it is not surprising that psychosis erupts at a time when the patient's sensorium is clearing—about the third postoperative day. The reaction seems to be one that only a few patients can articulate: "I began to realize what they'd done to me—opening my heart and all, and wow! I became unbelievably frightened," commented one man. One might translate this as meaning, "When I realized I had died and come back to life, it was an overwhelming thought." When the defense of denial breaks down and the patient is confronted by his *own* view of reality, that reality becomes intolerable and psychosis becomes, in a sense, a refuge. The organic substrate resulting from time on the cardiac-bypass pump, and the metabolic disruption in surgery create a background situation for the patient's drifting off into the psychosis. While organic elements have been emphasized—especially pump time (Tufo et al., 1970), it is clear that coronary bypass patients who spend much more time on the pump than valve—so-called open-heart patients—suffer a much lower rate of psychosis (Rabiner et al., 1975). Thus, postcardiotomy psychosis can be considered a psychosomatic entity, with organic elements interdigitating with the psychic dealing with death and invasion of the heart. A striking support for this idea is the observation, in several intensive care units, that the patient with an apparent organic delirium does not attempt to pull out tubes the way his counterpart after abdominal surgery might.

Coronary Patients

Clearly, issues of death and denial of death pertain to the reactions of patients and staff in a coronary unit and to post-cardiac-arrests as well. Coronary patients have been described from the viewpoint of denial by Hackett, Cassem, and Wishnie (1968). Such a situation is evident to any observer on a coronary unit who can note that most patients, after the immediate time of hospitalization, appear to be casually resting at a spa, rather than being closely observed because of the imminent danger of death. We have observed remarkable manifestations of denial in such patients (Blacher and Joseph, 1972). One man stared constantly at the oscillograph of his monitor and explained that he had "always wanted to see what a normal EKG looked like." Yet, clearly death is a constant threat and this is illustrated by a number of patients who would awake in the middle of the night, see the flashing monitor, and reason that since the monitor light still blinked, they must still be alive.

It seems reasonable to assume that the denial seen in the coronary patient may have profound protective advantages. Anxiety in coronary patients may cause increased catecholamine production, arrhythmias, and death (Klein et al., 1968). Without denial such patients would have to face the grave threat of their illness while forced to lie in bed immobilized and unable to discharge some of the anxiety via activity.

Cardiac Arrest

Cardiac arrest evokes the same responses as does open-heart surgery but with the added stress of its occurring in a less controlled situation. Little has been written about its sequelae but it clearly is not taken lightly.

In a study of ten such patients, Druss and Kornfeld (1967) found major changes in their subjects, all of whom had major difficulties in adjustment. Many were anxious and irritable. Insomnia was the most common persisting symptom. This is suggestive of a continuous process of self-monitoring, with the patient fearing to sleep lest he die. Their tranquil appearance was belied by frequent frightening and violent dreams.

An extraordinary case in my own experience involved an educated and proper matron who heard the cardiac-arrest announcement made on the hospital loudspeaker while she was passing out (her nurse had called someone on the phone). "My God, that's me!" was her last conscious thought. Upon recovery she amazed her family and her sedate, suburban community by speeding around town in a new motorcycle, her hair streaming behind. Her husband insisted upon a consultation, during which she was able to describe her dealing with her fear of death by confronting it. It was as if she were saying counterphobically, "I won't be a passive victim; I'll go out and *seek* death." After this clarification, she gave up the motorcycle with evident relief.

If one follows cases of cardiac arrest, one is struck by the total amnesia for the surrounding time period, when the patient is questioned shortly after the event. If one sees a patient for several weeks and establishes a relationship, memories start emerging and many details, often horrifying, are filled in by the victim.

Staff Reactions

It is clear that physicians, nurses, and other medical attendants are never fully comfortable with dying patients, yet they must deal with the danger involved in heart disease. While cardiac surgeons may insist, at times a bit too insistently, that the heart is nothing but a large muscular pump, there is reason to believe that they too are touched by their cultural heritage and may feel a sense of awe in the touching, manipulating, and incising of this special organ. One eminent surgeon has told me that when he begins to operate, he must divorce himself from the realization that he knows the patient as a person and deal only with a heart-lung preparation. Another surgeon tries to avoid any intimate contact with the patient before the operation.

The nurses in the Surgical Intensive Care Unit may choose this work because of a fear of death. This is not so much a counterphobic attitude as one of intolerance for the passivity and helplessness of waiting for a chronically ill patient to deteriorate. Rather, they actively fight off the enemy in an often successful battle in the ICU. Different groups in different ICUs may use their own successful methods for warding off anxiety—methods, incidentally, that ultimately help the patient, since an anxious nurse would add an intolerable burden to an endangered patient. Quite often the approach can be summarized by one head nurse's comment, "We treat the enormity of the patients' situation with irreverence."

The staff of coronary and cardiac-surgery ICUs are called upon to invest heavily in patients who may well die—indeed, the devotion may spell the difference between life and death. Unlike the attendants of patients who are slowly dying, the staff in the ICU cannot withdraw interest in order to soften the possible loss of the patient. Rather, everyone takes an emotional risk in hopes that the patient will survive. Not surprisingly, death, if it comes, can stir up stormy reactions. Nurses may cry in an ICU much more frequently than do nurses in other parts of the hospital when patients die.

The staff in a coronary unit has a different task from that of the cardiac surgery group. The latter can occupy itself in constant ministrations to the patient, his equipment, and surgical situation. The postcoronary state requires the nursing staff to spend a great deal of time in hyperalert waiting and watching, taking life-saving action when the monitor signals danger. This may be a more difficult task for action-oriented colleagues than constant "doing." The means of dealing with the tension, I am sure, varies from unit to unit. I have seen nurses in such a unit deal with death by denial, whispering in the presence of the deceased, so as not to awaken him. This illustrates how seemingly inappropriate behavior may be called into play in an attempt to master the enormous emotional pressures of the ICU.

The staff faces the greatest anxiety in dealing with cardiac arrests, as witness the high level of tension of resuscitation attempts and the dealing with such anxiety by means of jokes. Several eminent cardiologists describe how patients undergoing arrest found it to be a pleasant experience (Burch et al., 1968), according to the description given by their patients. Clearly, Druss and Kornfeld's extensive interviews on follow-up revealed a very different picture, with much anxiety beneath the surface. Actually, we have a model for subjective responses to cardiac standstill in the Stokes-Adams attack. Here the patient experiences nothing. "I was walking along the street. The next thing I knew I was opening my eyes and lying on the ground." What one does see are patients slowly losing consciousness and floating gradually off into an hypoxic state. In such transitional states of consciousness, a pleasant mild euphoria may be present. While the cardiologists were merely describing the data they had obtained, their conclusion is one which all of us would wish to entertain, namely, that dying is a pleasant experience. They state that death is "only a deep eternal sleep."

Conclusion

Clearly the danger of death is present as a backdrop in every case of heart disease. The unique role the heart plays in our psychic life and the realistic dangers involved with heart disease and surgery combine to create an emotional hazard for the patient with which his medical attendants must be concerned. In certain surgical procedures, the fantasy of dying and coming back to life provides an understanding of a number of patient-reactions, and indeed provides a thanatological model. Despite the patients' understandable reluctance to discuss the fantasy, future research may well be able to utilize this situation in studying reactions to death and dying. Previous studies have focused on what one might call "chronic dying." The adaptations to "acute dying" are no less important.

References

Abram, H. S. 1965. "Adaptation to Open-Heart Surgery," *American Journal of Psychiatry* (December), 122:6.

Blacher, R. S. 1972. "The Hidden Psychosis of Open-Heart Surgery: With a Note on the Sense of Awe," *Journal of the American Medical Association* (October 16), 222:3.

Blacher, R. S. 1975. "The Meaning of Heart-Valve Surgery to the Patient," *International Journal of Psychiatry of Medicine*, 6:4.

Blacher, R. S. and E. D. Joseph. 1972. "Psychological Reaction to A Cardiac Monitor," *Mt. Sinai Journal of Medicine*, (July-August), 39:4.

Burch, G. E., N. P. Depasquale, and J. H. Phillips. 1968. "What Death Is Like," *American Heart Journal* (September), 76:3.

Druss, R. G. and D. S. Kornfeld. 1967. "The Survivors of Cardiac Arrest," *Journal of the American Medical Association* (July 31), 201:5.

Hackett, T. P., N. H. Cassem, and H. A. Wishnie. 1968. "The Coronary Care Unit," *New England Journal of Medicine*, 279:1365–70.

Klein, R. F., V. A. Klinger, D. P. Zipes, W. G. Troyer, Jr., and A. G. Wallace. 1968. "Transfer from a Coronary Care Unit," *Archives of Internal Medicine* (August), 122:104–8.

Rabiner, C. J., A. E. Willnes, and J. Fishman. 1975. "Psychiatric Complications Following Coronary Bypass Surgery," *Journal of Nervous and Mental Disease*, 106:5.

Tufo, H. M., A. M. Ostfeld, and R. Shekelle. 1970. "Central Nervous System Dysfunction Following Open-Heart Surgery," *Journal of the American Medical Association* (May 25), 212:8.

ℵ15
Psychological Preparation
of the Cardiac Surgery Patient
W. J. Keon and R. K. Coombs

THERE IS AN increasing awareness among professionals of the need for a greater understanding of the emotional stress of a patient facing cardiac surgery. This is not a surprising development since there is "highly creditable evidence, from several sources, that leaves little doubt that the frequency of symptomatic psychoses [in open-heart surgery] is far higher than is the case with other types of surgery" (Freyhan et al., 1971).

A number of factors contributing to these postoperative psychoses have been studied. Age appears to be a positive factor (Nahum, 1965; Kornfeld et al., 1965). In virtually no cases did children under 14 to 16 years of age experience signs of delirium. This has been attributed to this younger age group's lower anxiety level and better quality of sleep, their anxiety stemming from a fear of unrelieved pain rather than from fear of death. It has also been found that there is a direct correlation between severity of the heart condition (as measured by the American Heart Association's Functional Classification) and the incidence of psychiatric symptoms postoperatively (Blachly and Starr, 1964).

Another factor which is directly related to the postoperative psychological status is the presence of a psychological problem preoperatively. One study has demonstrated that 54 percent of those patients having preoperative psychological problems displayed postoperative organic delirium, as compared to 17 percent of those patients with no preoperative psychological problems (Rubenstein and Thomas, 1970; Kennedy, 1966). Continuous activity in the postoperative environment also has been found to play a role in the increased incidence of postcardiotomy delirium (Hay and Oken, 1972). When considering recovery, Heller and co-workers (1970) found a decrease in psychoses was related directly to the day of discharge from the ICU. Other factors found to contribute to an increased incidence of delirium are sleep deprivation (Dim et al., 1971), duration of cardio-pulmonary bypass (David et al., 1969), and decreased cardiac output (Blachly and Koster, 1966).

Some of these factors are medically based and are not within the scope of this paper. What we will deal with, however, is how these patients can be psychologically prepared preoperatively and supported postoperatively in an attempt to reduce postoperative psychoses. A grave illness, necessitating cardiac surgery, makes the patient very dependent on the cardiac team. This state of dependency sets the stage for the development of uncertainty, suspicions, and anxiety. The level of anxiety is a major consideration in the psychological preparation for surgery. Therefore, we are challenged to come to know each patient within a limited time, and to the extent it is possible, to perceive his needs and act to meet them in an attempt to alleviate or prevent this distress.

To meet this challenge the staff of the University of Ottawa Cardiac Unit have developed a flexible patient-care plan providing continuity of care. The cardiac team is composed of many different personnel who come into direct contact with the patient: surgeons, cardiologists, anesthetists, nurses, aides, orderlies, technicians, physiotherapists, dieticians, and social workers. One person must be available to assure continuity of care and promote communication between patient, staff, family, and clergy. This is the function of the clinical nurse specialist and the nurse clinicians. A nurse clinician is a registered nurse with demonstrated expertise in the technical and professional practice of a clinical nursing specialty. The clinical nurse specialist trains the nurse clinician in the patient-teaching program. Preoperative nursing histories are taken by one of these nurses and added to the medical histories to gather base-line data preoperatively. This is communicated to those persons caring for the patient throughout his or her hospitalization. This gathering of base-line information can serve several purposes (Lasater and Gusanti, 1975):

1. To help establish a rapport and lend support to the patient. By setting up a reliable, trustworthy personal relationship and preoperative rapport, the likelihood of developing psychological symptoms postoperatively is reduced (Lazarus and Hagens, 1968).
2. To provide a guideline for careful postoperative observations.
3. To plan nursing-care activities outlining present problems.
4. To identify possible postoperative problems and enabling the nurse to take appropriate measures to alleviate or avoid the anticipated problems.

The nurse then coordinates the services of the paramedical staff. A schedule of visits by the paramedical staff to the patient is arranged preoperatively including the following:

Day of Admission	1500–1700	Social Worker
The following day which is the day of surgery	0730–0800	Nurse Technician—fasting, blood work and coagulogram
	0800–0830	E.C.G.
	0830–0900	Physiotherapist
	0900–0930	Breakfast
	0930–1015	Preoperative teaching by Nurse Clinician or Clinical Nurse Specialist
	1015–1045	IPPB teaching
	1100	Nurse Technician–p.c. blood work
	1045–1130	Shave prep
	1300–1400	Lunch and rest
	1400–1430	Chest X-ray
	1430–1500	Nurse Clinician or Clinical Nurse Specialist
	1500–1515	Physiotherapist
	1515–1700	Social Worker
	1900	IPPB teaching

The nurse also acts as a liaison with the patient's family, meeting with them prior to surgery to talk with them and to answer their questions and supporting the doctor's explanation about the medical-care plan. Arrangements are made to accompany the family on their first few visits postoperatively and a half hour every morning is set aside when she is always available to receive telephone calls from the family members of inpatients, as well as those who have been discharged.

On the day of surgery, the nurse accompanies the patient to the operating room and then receives him in the recovery room where she assists in the nursing care. She follows his progress throughout his stay in the Intensive Care Unit and the convalescent surgical ward. When the patient is ready for discharge, the patient, spouse (or close relative), and nurse meet to review the discharge plans for activity, diet, and drugs. (See Appendix 1). This program reduces the stress that a patient encounters by promoting continuity of care and maintaining a trustworthy patient-nurse relationship. The results of this approach are best summarized in the words of one patient:

> From the test necessary prior to surgery to the preoperative instruction class through surgery, intensive care, postoperative and recuperation periods, everything possible is done to make sure that the patient and, equally important, the family feel that the whole team— surgeons, doctors, nurses and technicians—has a personal involvement and concern.
> During surgery the members of the family are taken in hand by an efficient and understanding group who relieve their anxieties and minister to their needs. Open lines of communication are maintained between the family and the unit all through the period of hospitalization.
> Even home aftercare is arranged for through the district health and welfare nurse.

It is obvious, of course, that the nurse clinician is an added dimension to the overall care of the patient. This dimension is not meant to remove the need for careful coordination of patient care between medical specialists and nursing and paramedical personnel. Medicine and society, in general, have become so complex that frequently patients find themselves requiring the services of some 15 or 16 distinct medical and paramedical specialists in the management of their problem. To many patients, this can represent a taxing and frustrating situation, and they are frequently unsure as to who is responsible for a specific phase of their care. The nurse clinician is capable of rendering invaluable service to these patients by discussing their problems with them, alleviating their anxieties, and helping to make appropriate arrangements with the various key personnel involved in their treatment.

Another proven way of reducing stress is by education. Meyers' study (1974) demonstrates that less anxiety is created when the patient is given specific information so that he can prepare himself for the impending stress. An effective way to start teaching is to ask the patient to explain what he already knows, if anything, about the surgery. The staff can then fill in the gaps and correct misconceptions. It is important also, at the beginning, to ask the patient what questions he has. Otherwise the patient with a "burning" question may not hear the instructions because he is looking for the answer to his question.

In this way, a teaching program is developed tailored to each patient's need, his desire to have knowledge, and his anxiety level. It includes information: concerning his specific heart problem and the proposed surgery; explanations of procedures and equipment used; explanations of what he will see, hear, and do in all phases of his recovery from preoperation to discharge. A description of information covered in a cardiac-surgery teaching plan is found in Appendix 2.

A number of teaching aids are employed in patient education—for example, scale models of the heart, information booklets, and a preoperative class for in-city patients awaiting their surgery date, where a videotape of a typical cardiac patient's hospital experience is presented. It has been observed by the staff that those patients attending the classes displayed less anxiety before surgery than those patients who did not attend. Information is given in small amounts to avoid overwhelming the patient and to enable the staff to get feedback about earlier teaching. All staff are involved in this teaching program, whether formally or informally, although it is coordinated by the Clinical Nurse Specialist. Family members are included in patient teaching to help allay their anxiety and to enable them to play a supportive role in the patient's recovery.

The staff also has the opportunity of reducing postoperative psychological distress. Improving the postoperative environment by decreasing unnecessary stimuli, discontinuing special equipment and tubes as soon as medically possible, carefully planning care to allow maximum time for rest, and maintaining semblance of a day and night pattern (Walker, 1972) can contribute to a reduction of postoperative psychological symptoms.

The nurses, in their preoperative discussions, warn the patient that he may experience "strange dreams" and that these will pass. If psychotic symptoms do occur, their lasting influence may be relieved by sharing them with some other individual (Burgess et al., 1967). If a relationship is established preoperatively, the nurse, utilizing verbal and nonverbal cues, can help the patient deal with this experience.

All the measures taken are to assist in providing an atmosphere of security established by professional competence, warm understanding, and genuine concern to help reduce the patient's fear and anxiety. This can improve the psychological preparation of the individual and reduce postoperative complications.

Appendix 1: Information Included in the University of Ottawa Cardiac Unit Patient's Discharge Manual

1. Risk factors in heart surgery
2. Instructions on postoperative treatments; pain; "strange" dreams
3. Physical activity
4. Diet
5. Medications
6. Wound care
7. Visits to doctors
8. Convalescence
9. Smoking
10. General information for patients taking anticoagulants
11. Special instructions for children undergoing heart surgery
12. Remedial exercise program
13. Phone numbers of all relevant people associated with the follow-up care and an EMERGENCY number where someone can be contacted at all times.

Copies of the Patient Discharge Manual can be obtained from:
University of Ottawa Cardiac Unit
Ottawa Civic Hospital
1053 Carling Avenue,
Ottawa, Ontario
Canada, K1Y 4E9

Appendix 2: Cardiac Surgery Teaching Plan

A. The Heart Problem

1. Find out what patient knows.
2. Review anatomy and physiology.
3. Diagram of type of surgery.

B. Preparation for Surgery

Tell patient he will:
1. Have blood tests, chest x-ray, electrocardiogram.
2. Have a skin preparation (phisohex baths and shave).

3. Pack his belongings and send them home or to Admitting (false teeth and glasses kept on ward).
4. Meet chest physiotherapist and learn coughing and limb exercises.
5. Meet inhalation therapist and learn use of respirator.
6. Meet cardiac anesthetist and be told he will order sleeping pill and a needle before surgery.
7. Meet the clergyman—at patient's request.
8. Not smoke at least 24 hours pre-op.
9. Talk with another patient who has had cardiac surgery (at patient's request).
10. (If a child) be brought with his parents to see recovery area.

Talk to patient's family to:
1. Decide where to be contacted postsurgery.
2. Answer questions re: surgery.
3. Give instruction sheet for visits to Recovery Room and ICU.
4. Arrange for phone calls to family.

C. The Operation

Tell patient:
1. Where incisions will be (chest, radial, femoral).
2. He leaves ward for O.R. at 7:30 A.M. or a half hour before surgery.

If patient asks, tell:
3. What he will see in Operating Room.
4. What is done before he is anesthetized.
5. Other details (e.g., how pump works, number of staff).

D. Recovery Room

Tell patient he will feel:
1. Tube in his throat and be unable to talk. Tube out morning after surgery. Teach 5 hand signals.
2. Respirator to help inflate lungs.
3. Dry tongue and mouth (may have ice chips).
4. Pain in incision or backache (drug for pain will be given into I.V. tubing—no needle prick; given as necessary, not every four hours).
5. Foley catheter (may cause feeling of pressure and urgency).
6. Flat chest x-ray; lie on hard x-ray plate for 1 to 2 minutes; repeated at least three times in first 24 hours.
7. Frequent taking of blood pressure.
8. Frequent use of stethoscope on chest.
9. Feeling pulses in arms and legs.
10. May feel chest tubes (only mention if patient asks).
11. Levine tube to stomach and no food or drink until bowel sounds.

12. Sheepskin under back.
13. E.C.G. leads and monitor.

Tell patient he will see:
1. Intravenous equipment: blood, clear solutions, plastic tubing.
2. White corrugated tubing from respirator.
3. Clock up on wall.
4. Nurse and doctors (his own nurse for first 24 hours—never left alone).

Tell patient what he will hear:
1. Bubbling sound of chest drainage equipment.
2. Puff-puff of respirator.
3. Telephone.
4. Noises of children and other patients in Recovery Room.

Tell patient what he will do:
1. Use signals.
2. Deep breathe and cough.
3. Move and exercise limbs as nurse suggests.
4. Pay no attention unless staff talk directly to him.

E. The Intensive Care Unit

Tell the patient:
1. Move to ICU—in same bed, along same floor—done morning after the operation.
2. Share room with other patients.
3. Progressive ambulation: sit up in bed–side of bed–stand by bed–sit in chair–walk.
4. I.P.P.B. used q1-2-3h as necessary.

F. The Surgical Ward

Tell the patient:
1. Return to same ward (level 3) usually two to three days after surgery.
2. Activity is gradually increased under nurse's supervision; walking in room–later in hall up same number of stairs as at home or one flight.
3. Take part in daily hygiene.
4. Hospital stay is, *on the average,* 14 days from day of surgery.

G. Discharge Teaching

Full discussion of posthospital way of life is not done until patient is three or four days from discharge. If the patient *asks* any of the following points, brief answers are given in the preoperative period. Points to teach include:
1. Receive a manual with discharge instructions.
2. No smoking (mandatory after coronary artery surgery).

3. No heavy lifting (bags of groceries, babies, laundry).
4. Length of convalescence (two months to three months) depending on type of surgery.
5. Not to be left along at home for first two weeks.
6. See surgeon and cardiologist on appointments arranged by their secretaries.
7. Diet is usually a standard full diet unless otherwise ordered.
8. Drugs are ordered the day before discharge. Patient gets prescription filled at own pharmacy or if clinic patient at O.C.H. pharmacy. Drug teaching is done by pharmacist and patient is familiar with names and actions of drugs.
9. Anticoagulants: taught the dangers, whom to report to regarding bleeding and where to go for weekly blood tests. Arrange with cardiologist.
10. Ambulation: advised he may walk outside depending on weather and may gradually increase within limits of fatigue, chest pains, and shortness of breath. Plan with patient.
11. Return to work on surgeon's and cardiologist's advice.
12. Drive car on surgeon's and cardiologist's advice (after one month).
13. Resume sexual activity two weeks after discharge.

H. Problems After Discharge

1. Understands social worker is available.
2. Referred to Public Health Nurse (no charge).
3. Nurse available every morning, 8:30 A.M. to 9:00 A.M., Mon. to Fri.
4. May call surgeon.

I. Instructions Included in Discharge Manual

1. Rheumatic heart disease
2. General information for patients taking anticoagulants.
3. Medicines.
4. Instructions after heart surgery—adults
5. Instructions after heart surgery—children
6. Instructions after coronary-artery surgery
7. Medi-alert-bracelet application
8. General instructions re diet, activity, drugs, and sex.

References

Blachly, P. H. and A. Starr. 1964. "FE, Post Cardiotomy Delirium," *American Journal of Psychiatry*, 121:371.
Blachly, P. H. and F. E. Koster. 1966. "Relation of Cardiac Output to Post-cardiotomy Delirium," *Journal of Thoracic and Cardiovascular Surgery*, 52:422.

Burgess, G. N., J. W. Kirklen, and R. M. Steinhelber. 1967. "Some Psychiatric Aspects of Intra-Cardiac Surgery," *Mayo Clinic Proceedings*, 42:10.

David, H., H. M. Tufo, H. Najafi, et al. 1969. "Neurological Abnormalities Following Open-Heart Surgery," *Journal of Thoracic and Cardiovascular Surgery*, 58:502.

Dim, B. W., H. Rosen, K. Dickstein, et al. 1971. "The Problems of Sleep and Rest in the Intensive Care Unit," *Psychosomatic Medicine*, 12:155.

Freyhan, F. A., S. Giannelli, R. A. O'Connell, et al. 1971. "Psychiatric Complications Following Open-Heart Surgery," *Comparative Psychiatry*, 12:181.

Hay, D. and D. Oken. 1972. "The Psychological Stresses of the Intensive Care Unit," *Psychosomatic Medicine*, 34:109.

Heller, S. S., K. A. Frank, J. R. Malm, et al. 1970. "Psychiatric Complications of Open-Heart Surgery: A Re-Examination," *New England Journal of Medicine*, 283:1017.

Kennedy, J. A. 1966. "Importance of Emotions on the Outcome of Cardiac Surgery," *Bulletin of the New York Academy of Medicine*, 42:811–49.

Kornfeld, D. S., S. Zimber, and J. R. Malm, 1965. "Psychiatric Complications of Open-Heart Surgery," *New England Journal of Medicine*, 273:287–292.

Lasater, K. L. and D. J. Gusanti. "Post-Cardiotomy Psychosis: Indications and Interventions," *Psychological Aspects of Critical Care* (September–October 1975), 5(4):724.

Lazarus, H. R. and J. H. Hagens. 1968. "Prevention of Psychosis Following Open Heart Surgery," *American Journal of Psychiatry*, 124:1190.

Meyers, M. M. 1974. "Effects of Types of Communication on Patients' Reactions to Stress," *Nursing Research* (Spring), 13:126.

Nahum, L. H. 1965. "Madness in the Recovery Room from Open-Heart Surgery, or 'They Kept Waking Me Up,'" *Connecticut Medicine*, 29:771.

Rubenstein, D. and S. K. Thomas. 1970. "Psychiatric Findings in Cardiotomy Patients," *AORN Journal*, 11:77.

Walker, B. B. 1972. "The Post-Surgery Heart Patient: Amount of Uninterrupted Time for Sleep and Rest the First, Second, and Third Post-Operative Days in a Teaching Hospital," *Nursing Research*, 21:164.

16

Surgery and the Congenital Cardiac Patient

George H. Humphreys II

BABIES ARE NOT afraid of dying, and small children have no concept of death relating to themselves. But there is an elemental emotional tie between parents and child that is deeply disturbed when the child's life is threatened. If the threat is sudden and unanticipated—an accident or acute-crisis illness—the child reacts by a physiologic struggle for survival in which fear of death plays little or no part. However anxious or fearful the parents may be, their normal response is to comfort and support the child in his struggle. This strong emotional support is as important to the child's recovery as is much of the physical care and medical therapy given. As the child improves and parental anxieties abate, the child gains confidence in those caring for him, and the stage is set for reinforcement of trust in his family and in the professional people who have helped them.

When, on the other hand, the threat is a continuous or episodic one, parental fear and anxiety may be unconsciously transmitted to the child. Without knowing why, he senses an unknown and therefore deeply disturbing threat. His fear is not of death, but of the unknown reason for his parents' attitude toward him, and this constant fear of an unknown threat has a far more powerful effect on his emotional stability than any immediately perceived danger.

The latter condition is too often the case when a congenital cardiac anomaly is present. A newborn baby may hover on the brink of death for days or weeks, then gradually improve. But the parents find it difficult to forget their initial shock and anxiety, and cannot forget that their child is not normal. In other cases, sudden alarming episodes may recur unpredictably, in which the baby may die, or may appear to have died, only to recover until the next episode. No parent can escape anxiety under these circumstances. The more frequent the attacks, and the longer the period during which they have been occurring, the deeper the fear and anxiety become imprinted in the parents and the more emotionally disturbed the child becomes in response.

Even if the threat of immediate death is not so obvious, it is hard for parents to treat the child normally. Many children with congenital heart defects do not have alarming episodes, are not cyanotic, and have a normal interest in activies. Yet if, as is often the case, there is a considerable overload on the heart, they may grow and develop slowly, become easily tired and querulous, and eat poorly. The puny child is a constant reminder to his parents that he is not normal. Even when this is not the case, parents, aware of the murmur and its evidence of "heart disease," often are afraid to permit normal activity and suffer from a deep underlying anxiety that there is an eventual threat to life or longevity with which they do not know how to deal.

Parents, of course, vary in their emotional stability. A naturally anxious parent is likely to overreact, especially if the anomaly is one causing variable cyanosis. A child may appear nearly normal when quiet and happy, but cyanosis deepens with exertion or distress, and when he cries hard, his arterial blood becomes so lacking in oxygen that he becomes very dark and loses consciousness from cerebral anoxia. These alarming episodes are called "blackouts." Parents do everything in their power to forestall them. On the one hand, they pamper the child so he won't cry; on the other they deny him even such activity as he may be able to sustain, thus making him unhappy and inviting another crisis. It takes an unusually stable person to maintain normal discipline, and these children learn early to exploit their parents' anxiety.

The same problem is present, varying with the physiologic burden of the anomaly and emotional response of the parents, with less obviously serious conditions. Understanding parents who truly love their child may be able to create a relatively normal pattern of life around his handicap, in spite of the burden and underlying anxiety. Too often, however, parents are overprotective, either through genuine concern about unknown and imaginary threats, or as overcompensation to deny a guilty hate for the child and the burden he imposes. There is also guilt in having brought the child into the world in the first place. Notions of hereditary fault from one side or the other strain relations between parents, or incidents during pregnancy may be held responsible. The child is a stigma as well as a burden. In unsophisticated societies he may actually be hidden and his existence denied. Even in ours, a guilty wish to be rid of the problem, by the child's death if need be, is a barely suppressed thought that underlies much overprotection. For certainly, whatever the cause, it is not the child's fault.

Operations to correct some cardiovascular anomalies have been possible for nearly 40 years. The earliest, which seemed miraculous when first introduced, are now considered almost routine. These procedures do not involve opening the heart, or temporarily stopping its beat, and now carry a relatively low risk of death or complication. During the past quarter century operations for more and more complex intracardiac anomalies have been devised. They have been made possible by increasingly sophisticated technical developments to support the circulation with heart-lung machines, or to prevent anoxic damage during cardiac arrest by lowering body temperature. In these procedures, the heart is opened, its interior is manipulated, and then it is closed. The risk of death, either at operation or later, is far greater than with the simpler procedures, and many more complications may occur. These may result in brain damage, paralysis, or loss of a limb, even when the heart anomaly is corrected. And total correction does not always prove possible.

When, then, the possibility arises that a cardiac anomaly may be corrected surgically, a surge of reinforced parental emotion is inevitable. Suddenly the predicament of the parents becomes a dilemma. They must decide whether to consent to a procedure which may kill their child or to deny him a possible cure. Because of its inherent drama, heart surgery has been unduly exploited in the lay press and television. As a result, hopes are often raised beyond reason. Expectation of cure obscures the real risk of death, especially if the lesion itself seems life-threatening. Yet, even then, guilt is present if there is an alternate possibility that, without surgery, the child might improve. If death occurs, this guilt is reinforced. Was it, perhaps subconsciously what the parents wanted?

If there is not an immediate threat, decision is often extremely difficult for parents. They may not comprehend the seriousness of the risk. In their minds, it may seem greater than it is, or they may block out the possibility of death in the expectation of cure. It is even harder to accept a risk of death in the hope of a longer and healthier life for their child, when he has no obvious handicap. Yet some anomalies progress, and symptoms even improve, while the risk of operation becomes greater, ultimately to a point at which correction can no longer be done. Young adults who find themselves in this situation can hardly be blamed for resenting their parents' previous timidity.

It is the obligation of all of the professional staff who care for these children to support all reasonable hope while making clear the risks and the reasons for taking them. The surgeon, especially, must never forget or minimize the risk, even of the simpler procedures. Often he must take time, even several years if the lesion is not progressive, to get to know parents and child and to gain their complete confidence. During this period he, or the pediatric cardiologist, can do much to offset parental anxieties and to bring parents and child to the stress of the operation as emotionally prepared as possible.

The doctor should explain to parents that the term "congenital heart disease" is unfortunate and improperly alarming. For these hearts are not "diseased," like hearts injured by rheumatic fever or coronary disease. They are often hypertrophied, which can be interpreted as "stronger than normal." Their anomaly makes them work harder and less efficiently than normal. Hence, there is a definite handicap—a limit to what the heart can be expected to do. But it does the heart no harm to go to that limit— and the limit is best determined by what the child can do without difficulty. Arbitrary limitations do no good and are psychologically damaging, both to parents who try to enforce them against their child's will and to the child, who becomes resentful, defiant, or acquiescent in a conviction of a greater handicap than is actually present.

"When he rests, his heart works as though he is walking; when he walks it is as though he is running; when he runs on the level it is as though he runs uphill; and he cannot run uphill" is one way to explain a handicap. By themselves, children with cardiac anomalies will not do more than they should; only if shamed, exhorted, or challenged by competition will they be pushed beyond their capacity. So competitive sports are best avoided. With such explanations from the doctor giving greater under- standing of the nature of their child's problem and limitations, both parents and child will lose much of the emotional strain be- tween them. They will also gain the confidence in their medical advisers that, when otherwise frightening diagnostic procedures like cardiac catheterization are suggested, minimizes the anxiety of consent.

When the time then comes to decide on surgical correction, both parents and child are prepared. Actual signed consent must be, by law, "informed." Theoretically, every possible complica- tion, from death in the operating room to survival with irrevers- ible organ damage or simply without effective correction of the lesion, should be explained to and understood by the family. But this is not practicable. In the first place, every complication will not occur in any one case. In the second, the family cannot com- prehend statistical chances and, however well prepared, are sel- dom in a frame of mind to get from such a discussion more than a frightening concept of a confusion of horrible possibilities. It is no service to the family, the patient, or the professional staff to in- crease the natural fears of parents or to undermine their con- fidence in the people who are caring for their child.

A secure relationship between parent, child, cardiologist, and surgeon is enhanced by the familiarity with the ancillary team associated with heart operations. Social workers, nurses, tech- nicians, house staff, and students may already be known to the family from outpatient contacts or previous diagnostic admissions. If not, care should be taken, during the preoperative period, that they are. Previously unknown people, such as anesthesiologists, operating room nurses, orderlies, technicians, and recovery room personnel should not be strangers. It may even be expedient, if the child is very apprehensive but old enough to understand, to take him to the anesthesia area and the operating and recovery rooms, so that these areas will not be strange to him in his period of greatest stress.

For the child wants and expects to be made well. He will approach the operation eagerly if his parents can transmit the calm confidence they should feel. While fully aware of the dangers, their confidence is reinforced by the competence and composure of the team. They are hypersensitive, however, to hurried, flustered, or thoughtlessly callous behavior even of minor members, and any evidence of professional disagreement in management is most disturbing. The patient reflects his parents' behavior. His fears are related mainly to separation from them, and are dispelled by familiarity with the hospital setting and confidence in the people taking care of him.

During and in the early hours and days after operation, especially if the procedure is a long and complex one, parents must be kept constantly aware of their child's condition. When his condition is critical, provision must be made for them to remain close and even visit him for brief periods, if possible, so that he will not feel abandoned or unduly isolated. If he dies or suffers a serious life-threatening or permanently incapacitating complication, the parents need special attention and support from the surgeon and senior team members. No matter how well balanced and well prepared, they cannot then escape not only grief but a lingering guilt, and almost remorse, for having consented. The surgeon must relieve them of this to the best of his ability by emphasizing the reasons for accepting the risk and taking full responsibility not only for the technical aspects of the tragic outcome, but also for his decisions and advice. He will rarely be blamed by truly understanding parents.

A final service to the parents should never be omitted or treated lightly. When a child dies, even more than when he is about to undergo a dangerous operation, parents may seem to listen to and understand what the doctor says, but deep emotional turmoil interferes. They may think they hear what they want him to say, rather than really listen to what he is saying; they may misunderstand him completely, or they may simply listen without hearing. Autopsy may be wanted, permission may be given reluctantly or it may be refused, but every effort should be made to obtain it. Not only will autopsy often be informative to the doctors (a fact intelligent parents will understand), but also it will permit the doctor to write a letter of condolence and explanation that will go far to assuage the parents' grief. Even in the absence of autopsy findings, such a letter is imperative, and often a postmortem visit may be useful to settle the afterthought questions that are sure to plague them.

Ideally, surgical correction of a cardiac anomaly converts a sick or handicapped child into one who will live a long and normal life. This happy outcome, fortunately, is the most frequent. When the result is death, the tragedy can be dealt with by the family and ultimately accepted without prolonged regret if professional attention has been what it should be. But when, after accepting grave risks and the expense, pain, and anxiety of an operation, the result is not successful, though not fatal, it may be harder to bear than death. This is true especially if a complication results in permanent injury that leaves the patient worse off than before. Under these circumstances even the greatest preoperative preparation and confidence may not suffice and long-term, understanding follow-up is essential. Whatever the outcome, there is no substitute for a strong bond of empathy between doctor and family.

❧17
Assessing and Expanding the Coping Abilities of the Child Hospitalized for Cardiac Surgery

Adrienne Baranowitz and Joan Chan

HOSPITALIZATION FOR CARDIAC surgery may provide the child with one of the most valuable learning experiences of his life. Experiencing a peak period of disequilibrium, the child can benefit by utilizing and expanding his coping abilities during this period of crisis. A crisis is a situation causing a change in feelings so that elements surface that were not previously understood, presenting an opportunity for the positive building of strength (Hardgrove and Dawson, 1972). Immediately then, these newly acquired or enlarged adaptational techniques can enable the child to improve his psychosocial situation, while providing a concrete basis of action for other adaptations in the future.

It is our responsibility as Child Life Health Professionals to channel the child's crisis energy into positive activities for learning and growth. In order to do so, we must have a flexible yet accurate method of assessing what the crisis is and how this particular child is experiencing it. An accurate assessment, however, must necessarily involve a knowledgeable survey of what is causing the child's anxiety. The support we provide depends on the child's age, intelligence, emotional maturity, and any special vulnerabilities.

The child's primary vulnerability lies in his special cardiac condition, for it exacerbates all of life's crises and tribulations. If he faces a crisis about his hospitalization, he does so in addition to facing his normal developmental crises. Erikson (1970) said "Life is a sequence of not only developmental but of accidental crises. It is hardest when both types of crises coincide."

In children with cardiac problems, there is an exaggeration of their need for coping mechanisms which allows us to recognize and delineate these mechanisms. Thus, we can recognize the subtle crisis stages that all children may undergo when facing and experiencing hospitalization. Therefore, we hope this study can be extrapolated to the crises confronting all hospitalized children, so that caregivers may recognize and help assuage the severity of hospitalization and surgery when it arises.

Background

Today, the child born with a cardiac impairment has a much better chance of surviving with this disability than he would have had in any other period in history. The child who has undergone cardiac surgery often shows expanded physical as well as social and intellectual capabilities. Yet despite these gains, the child's emotional growth is often hindered by the views of the very society which has sought to nurture and protect him.

Attitudes change slowly. Attitudes toward patients with cardiac impairments have not kept pace with medical fact; for indeed, any impairment of the heart is often regarded as life-threatening. As youthful mortality becomes less frequent, the aura of mystery and anxiety surrounding a pediatric death intensifies. Often, hospital staff unknowingly attempt to mask their own insecurity with mortality by perpetuating a cryptic, uncomfortable aura surrounding death and fear of death for the patient. Under the stress of impending surgery, the child's tenuous situation is often worsened by this evasive action.

This crisis is spawned or fed by the perception of cardiac surgery as a life-threatening situation in which the body is invaded by strange and painful stimuli. While some children may be able to express their fear, others may be able to react only with anger or withdrawal. With some children, denial may become so great, that verbalization of any feelings may become impossible. In order to express his fears, the child needs realistic support from those around him.

Children who are aware of the condition of "their most vital organ" will often experience a culmination of fears and family pressures during their hospital stay. Children from whom the reality of the situation has been hidden will experience a shock-born crisis when their presence in the hospital can be reconciled in no other way. All children, then, will experience some type of crisis in which they feel their very vitality threatened.

Parents, charged with the care of a child perceived to have a tenuous hold on life, often undergo a change of life-expectations for their child. They become so concerned with the possibility that their child will have a diminished life span that they tend to neglect the quality of the child's life.

Parents not only fear their child's attitudes about surgery, but also feel indecisive about it themselves. Their fears are corroborated by the child's poor eating and sleeping habits and his difficulties in breathing and performing physical tasks. Often they blame themselves for the child's failure to thrive. This causes an inconsistency of expectation and discipline in regard to the child.

Parental overprotection is often a fact which determines the child's coping level. Overprotected children usually enter a given situation with a lower level of coping ability than would be predicted for their developmental stage. They can remain at this low level for a long period of time, and, indeed, some may never move out of it. This demonstrates how previous coping abilities may determine future ones. The child who has never had an opportunity to demonstrate and experiment with his own potential is often unable to utilize it when it is most important that he do so.

The child does not function in a vacuum, and the sum of this pressure must at some point bear upon him. He may feel he is ill because he has misbehaved, or when he does not feel ill, he feels victimized by those who treat him. If his handicap is visible, he may feel socially and intellectually inferior. He may feel deserted in this time of need, for he is unable to express his fears of death. He feels constrained to bear his burden stoically, maturely, and optimistically, feeling that an admission of fear would disappoint parental expectations.

It is this expression of inner turmoil anxiety that we will be able to treat by activating the child's adaptive coping abilities. The anxiety consists of both interpersonal and perceptual components. The child is undergoing longer periods of separation from his parents and other trusted figures while being forced to interact with unfamiliar staff and patients, to leave a familiar environment for an untried or untrusted one. His perception of the hospital environment is influenced by his past experiences with medical staff, situations, and illness. While his fears are aroused, he has less opportunity to release his anxiety in the confines of the hospital. Here the normal channels of play which dispel anxious energy are not available. The Child Life Worker, through the medium of therapeutic play, may help discharge this energy, and in doing so may alter this experience into a positive, growth promoting one that aids the child in acquiring situational mastery.

Coping Assessment

We have found our assessment of the child's coping abilities to fall into four major categories. These categories correspond to the nature of the child's awareness of his own concerns about his hospitalization and cardiac surgery. They are:

Stage 1: *Nonparticipation.* Here the child must be encouraged to participate in the surrounding environment as a way of reawakening his dormant coping mechanisms.

Stage 2: *Tentative Emergence.* Here the child is beginning to elucidate feelings to which previously he may not have had access.

Stage 3: *Emerging Awareness.* Here the child is encouraged to explore activity as a way of exposing his active coping mechanisms.

Stage 4: *Awareness and Participation.* Here the child has obtained a realistic awareness of his crisis and is learning to participate actively in releasing the tensions he feels about it.

While the child at the Awareness and Participation level is approaching mastery of his situation, the child at the Nonparticipation base-line level is showing poor coping abilities. These areas are not exclusive, however, for a child may or may not exhibit all the stages, and he may not progress through them in an orderly sequence. We have found each stage to be characterized by the predominant use of certain coping mechanisms, yet the same mechanisms to different extents may be exhibited in other stages. It is the degree and the subtle shadings within the stages that determine where the exhibition of the individual's capabilities lie. We have found these levels useful, however, for they provide the accuracy yet flexibility required for a composite of the child's situational level.

Stage I: Nonparticipation

The child at the level of Nonparticipation is frozen in his situational responses. This stage is usually exhibited by severely maladjusted children with other problems prior to hospitalization. This child can barely adapt to external stimulation, for his interests are totally self-contained. Burdened by weak ego development, he is not coping. This may impair his intellectual and social function. He can be described as withdrawn, immobile, anorexic or listless. These children are poor-risk patients.

Paul would not interact with staff or children when he entered the playroom. His development was delayed and his motor skills uncoordinated. When unobtrusively observed, he exhibited ritualistic and hoarding behaviors. Eventually we got Paul to play with balls, by first playing for Paul when he was not playing for himself. When Paul's mother entered the playroom, however, Paul resumed his maladaptive isolation. It took many more weeks of work to get Paul to resume his previous play.

Paul was utilizing isolation, regression, and denial. By isolating himself from his new situation he denied his new environment. By regressing, he obtained more parental attention, so it became unnecessary for him to adapt. Paul's coping abilities were so limited that in critical situations, such as his ride down to the operating room on the day of his open-heart surgery, he was unable to cooperate.

We encouraged Paul to expand his interests to the outer world by directing his attention to the play around him and by playing for him. We interested the nonparticipant in the world around him by providing materials he could touch, hold, and manipulate. Water play, in particular, is valuable with this child because it presents so little resistance to his uncertain approaches to play.

We reached Paul through the use of a transitory object, a ball. By rolling a ball to Paul and having him roll the ball back, we established contact with him. Through play then, the child can move from passivity to activity.

Thus, we must first demonstrate this activity by playing for the child who cannot play for himself, for "play" can only occur when the child can impose on reality his own conceptions and complaints (Ellis, 1973). As the child becomes the controlling agent, he can begin to take further initiative. This minimizes the use of maladaptive mechanisms of withdrawal and immobility, so that the child can later be encouraged to use other, more adaptive methods.

Stage II: Tentative Emergence

The child who has reached the level of Tentative Emergence has begun to explore his own actions, yet is only beginning to utilize his adaptive coping abilities. Most children enter the playroom at this stage, as shy and quiet, yet cooperative and tentative. Children here often fear abandonment yet are unable to verbalize their fears.

To express his anger, a child has to feel accepted in his relationship with the therapist. The shy, quiet, cooperative child exhibits a limited ability to recognize and, thereby, express anger. This child tends to be forgotten because he is not disruptive, but actually he needs great attention in order to activate his adaptive coping methods. It is our responsibility as Child Life Health Professionals to recognize the needs of the tentatively emerging child.

> Susan was a shy, quiet, cooperative girl. When her parents were in the playroom she exhibited fearful, passive dependence on them. She was extremely shy with unfamiliar children and adults and exhibited lack of confidence in her dealings with them. Her manner of play was restrained, and she never gave vent to feelings of either anger or joy. She spent most of her time arranging small blocks in a meticulous sequence or mimicking telephoning games she had seen other children perform.

Susan was repressing fear and anger while denying the seething anger within her by her scrupulous, meticulous overtidiness. By copying other's activities, that is by participating in imitative or contagion play, Susan used others as models to express her feelings and learn new modes of behavior.

Here we helped Susan gain confidence in herself and her therapist. We engaged in this acceptable behavior with her until she felt free to express her feelings. We helped Susan to express and expand through the use of nonthreatening tactile explorations such as play-dough, paints, clay, and sand play. This helped her to further gain confidence in herself through initiating activity.

Stage III: Emerging Awareness

The child who has reached the level of Emerging Awareness has entered the exploratory stage of interpersonal relationships and has begun to express his emerging confidence in his therapist while relaying his disturbances. Anger is a common emotion at this level.

> Robert was a very angry little boy. Told he would remain in the hospital for a day, he felt deceived when he had to remain there for a week. Often Robert showed aggression toward his peers. When Robert was given a drum he pounded on it long and hard, and eventually was able to verbalize his frustration. Slowly, he began to interact with his peers, and indulged in their fantasy games.

Projection, fantasy formation, and misinterpretation of surrounding events are common mechanisms at this level. Projecting his anger onto the drum allowed him to release it. Anger was a cathartic for Robert, which released him to further communicate. In this way he was able to indulge in fantasy play that dulled the pain of his reality without obscuring it. As Robert gained a more rational hold on his reality, he became better able to cope with it.

Here we help the child by providing unhurried explanations of all unfamiliar and painful procedures. At this stage, the child will often misconstrue such events as an external threat to his vitality, for he is displacing his internal fears of death. We alter this misconception by emphasizing that we do not wish to hurt him.

Children often participate in parallel play at this level. They will play alongside each other while participating in either different or similar activities. Fighting may erupt, and the therapist may be of aid by channeling the child's aggression into appropriate play channels. Hammering drums, pounding clay, and punching bags are a good way for the child to work out anger. By learning to come to terms with himself and the world around him, the child is then ready to move onto more adaptive coping patterns. With the attainment of this, he can become more congenial in his interpersonal relationships.

Stage IV: Awareness and Participation

A child coping at Awareness and Participation has embarked on the route to attainment of situational mastery. While puppet therapy imparts information, the child–therapist relationship blossoms as it assists the child in expressing realistic responses to impending surgery. The play gains validity because of adult participation, yet the child is learning to communicate as an intact individual, without withdrawal, denial, or fear. For the child at this level we provide a miniature mock-up cardiac operating room, complete with dolls on which to demonstrate. When the child handles unknown instrumentation through the puppets, he can verbalize anxiety while being supported by an understanding adult. He is helped to gain mastery over his new surroundings and at the same time is prepared for forthcoming events.

> Carolyn was a child who had utilized adaptational mechanisms in working through her impending surgery. She often used needle play in the context of the hospital setup. She used the doctor doll to request clarification of what her own doctor had said. She interacted well with her doctor and with her peers.

The mechanisms of sublimation and identification are common. Carolyn transformed her feelings about needles and treatment into a play that allowed her to request information about past or potential procedures. This assuaged her anxiety, and so she was able to interact with her peers. She identified also with her aggressor, the doctor, in the guise of the doctor doll, and this allowed her to accept his explanations while interacting with him.

For the child at this level, the ability to request an explanation or reassurance is an important achievement. Thus, even at the most threatening times, the morning and night before surgery, the child can communicate needs for clarification of what is happening and obtain accurate and reassuring feedback from staff and therapists. The child, by learning to cope with and interact within his threatening situation, has strengthened his coping abilities for future situations as well as gaining mastery over his present one.

We can help the child by providing materials for healthy exploration of his new surroundings. This gives the child feelings of power or mastery and allows him to investigate this environment at his own pace. He can also participate with others in a cooperative play around a common theme such as the hospital. This helps to control the previous regression experiences he has begun to master. He can learn and expand by role-playing within a comfortable, noncompetitive group. The child gains control and discipline by waiting his turn, yet he can work out some of his qualms about hospitalization by being the doctor, giving shots, being the nurse or the patient. This, in conjunction with imaginative activities, can provide a meaningful learning experience for him.

Fluctuational Response

Children fluctuate in their coping abilities. Therefore, regression of coping abilities is often exhibited with the addition of an unexpected stress. Robertson's theory of response to separation is an illustration of this (1958). The child makes an initial angry protest at his parent's departure. This verbal communication of anger denotes the Emerging Awareness level of coping. Next, the child undergoes a regression to despair, exhibited by increasing disinterest in the outside world. This regression is completed with denial, for by denying the problem, the child is denying his external situation, and is thereby not coping with it.

A Word About Puppet Therapy*

We have found puppet therapy, the therapeutic vehicle most often utilized with children hospitalized for cardiac surgery, to be a viable alternative mainly for those children whose coping abilities have reached the level of Participation and Awareness. Puppet therapy implies the need for both child–therapist interaction and an intellectual awareness of an ability to deal with the crisis.

Since it is our contention that play must be initiated at the child's coping level, we believe that not all children will benefit from puppet therapy, since they may not have reached the coping level at which they will be able to utilize its cathetic value.

Instead, by utilizing the assessed coping level, we can utilize the delineated therapies which better suit the stage. By playing out the child's cathexis in this particular stage, we can expand coping abilities while playing out anxieties. Eventually then, these children will be able to benefit from puppet therapy, by therapeutically growing into the stage where they will be able to utilize it and expand through it.

*We are here utilizing puppet therapy designed to play out feelings. Puppet therapy utilized to explain procedures has some value for all therapeutic levels, but retains optimum value only at the stage of Participation and Awareness.

Summation

Children enter the playroom at different levels of coping ability, which have been determined by the totality of their previous experience. We have been successful in helping children cope with their hospitalization for cardiac surgery through the use of therapeutic play materials. We do this through assessment, planning, and intervention. First we assess the child's coping levels through his interpersonal interactions and his use of play materials. Then we plan how we can best help the child expand and utilize his coping abilities. Finally, by intervening in a positive way at this time of his development, we as health professionals can help the child overcome regression and function as a healthy individual.

References

Erikson, E. 1970. In F. G. Blake, "Open Heart Surgery in Children," p. 76. *Public Health Service Public*, no. 2075.

Ellis, M. J. 1973. *Why People Play*. Englewood Cliffs, New Jersey: Prentice-Hall.

Hardgrove, C. and R. Dawson. 1972. *Parents and Children in the Hospital*. Boston: Little, Brown.

Robertson, J. 1958. *Young Children in the Hospital*. London: Tavistock Publications.

❧18
Nursing Care of the Cardiosurgical Patient

Rita K. Chow

OVER THE PAST two decades, we have witnessed the birth of significant open-heart surgery and its dramatic growth to astonishing maturity. Understandably, cardiac patients who are admitted to the hospital for surgery to abolish severe anginal pain or to overcome disability, such as two-pillow orthopnea and dyspnea on exertion, are apprehensive and anxious about the possible outcome. After surgery, patients, especially those who have undergone cardiopulmonary bypass during the intracardiac procedure, require monitored care in the Surgical Intensive-Care Unit (SICU). From the viewpoint of the cardiopulmonary nurse, the work is demanding. It requires vigilance to detect such emergent complications as postoperative hemorrhage, water or electrolyte disequilibrium, pulmonary edema, renal or cerebral dysfunction, and the like. Yet, in spite of the demands on their energies, many SICU nurses apparently experience great satisfaction from giving intensive care to patients, even in the stressful milieu. The purpose of this paper is to describe the milieu of the SICU; to give some examples of reactions of patients to the SICU; and to suggest some ways nurses can continue to humanize their care.

SICU Environment

Intensive care units have advantages for administering safe, efficient care, which must be given by nurses who have had special preparation for handling complex equipment and coping with vital problems. For example, nurses measure arterial and central venous pressures. They detect an arrhythmia such as premature ventricular contractions (PVCs) on the oscilloscope and document the tracing on electrocardiogram (ECG) rhythm strips. Upon distinguishing various ECG patterns, nurses anticipate the therapy that may be required. Moreover, they prepare equipment to administer synchronized precordial shock to terminate atrial flutter or fibrillation. They also prepare the patient and equipment for transvenous cardiac pacing. Also, through serial arterial blood gas studies, the physician–nurse team can evaluate the extent of a patient's condition of metabolic acidosis.

On the other hand, there has been much expressed concern about the antitherapeutic atmosphere of the SICU. Although intensive care units without partitions enable patients to be under constant surveillance by experts, these units may be the setting for psychological trauma. Busy units with a large number of critically ill patients can be noisy and disturbing. At times, odors, such as from patients suffering from physiological dysfunction, may be disagreeable. In addition, a patient may develop the complications of disturbance of acid-base balance and cardiac arrhythmias. A case in point is Mr. W., who developed cardiac arrest about three hours postoperatively. As a part of the cardiopulmonary resuscitation effort, the patient-care team of physicians and nurses administered external cardiac massage, electroshock, and intracardiac epinephrine. Nevertheless, the patient expired. The situation in which death may be imminent may temporarily disturb the psychic equilibrium of unit personnel and sentient patients in adjacent beds. A helpful interaction concept is the "awareness context," as developed by Glaser and Strauss (1965). Undoubtedly, there is a profound impact of each type of awareness context upon the interplay of patients and personnel.

SICU Sound Levels

It has been found that the human ear can detect sound-pressure variations down to 0.0002 of a microbar, which is even less noisy than a quiet whisper (Goldsmith and Jonsson, 1973). Therefore, it may be worthwhile to study the nature and measure the "loudness" of sounds in intensive care units in microbars (one-millionth of 14.7 pounds per square inch). The study should systematically examine the psychological and physiological effects on SICU patients of the noise level of frequently used equipment (for example, bedpan flushers, patient-identification-plate stamping machine, mechanical respirators, pulsating "beeps" from the cardiac monitoring system); and methods of communication (for example, frequent professional specialty-team bedside conferences, use of telephones in the unit, paging systems). It would be important to discover from the patient's viewpoint how he perceives not only the interprofessional discussions that he may overhear, but also the voices from anxious postoperative patients who, for example, call out for succor, "Mother, help me." During an interview, some patients have told me, "I can't stand it; get me out of here."

Types of Families

The differences in families and the individual needs of patients require special consideration by patient-care personnel. Much depends on the complex interplay of forces affecting the patient admitted to the hospital for cardiac surgery. For discussion purposes, we shall describe three types of families: the deceptive, the overprotective, and the religion-oriented.

The Deceptive Family. It does not make true statements to a child about his hospitalization. Instead of explaining to a child with an atrial septal defect, for example, that he has "a hole in the heart," and that the doctors are going to "open the heart and sew up the hole," a parent may tell four-year-old Bobby that he is going to the hospital "to get some pills." The deceptive actions of parents can affect a child severely. To illustrate, when I first met Bobby in his preoperative hospital room during mealtime, he was all alone and appeared uneasy and confused. His dishes were completely empty, but he had just finished pelting tiny missiles of his entire meal all around the room. After conferring with the nursing staff, I phoned his grandmother to discuss my concern about Bobby's immediate need for security and better knowledge of his physical condition. The very next day the parents came to visit Bobby. They seemed to appreciate the staff's viewpoint that the child needed a sense of trust and to know the truth that he was going to surgery. They changed their stance and discussed with the child what to expect in the hospital.

The Overprotective Family. It overindulges the young preoperative cardiac patient. Petrillo and Sanger (1973) have observed that tense, anxious, achievement-oriented parents may have a latent hostility toward a child for interfering with what they wish for him. To alleviate the family's anxiety, it may be best to emphasize the competence and willing spirit of the postoperative staff. Postoperatively, the young patient seems demanding and aggressive. For instance, to prevent postoperative atelectasis, a SICU nurse urged a young man to "cough and take some deep breaths." His challenging response was, "You can't make me."

The Religion-Oriented Family. It of course has beliefs and values which must be respected. The devout, gentle, and industrious Amish, for example, are one of the many religious groups among the Pennsylvania Dutch. Since the Amish have a high regard for the customs and beliefs of their forefathers, the hospital personnel, in turn, should be cognizant and considerate of the Amish way of life. As an example, from the time a man is baptized or married, a beard is usually required of all men of the church. Therefore, when Mr. W. was admitted to the hospital for open-heart surgery, he had a beard. When I observed him again in the intensive-care unit, he had none. While Mr. W. was dying, an unsettling question came to my mind as to whether it was absolutely necessary that Mr. W. should have been required to shave off his beard.

Humanizing Health Care

The nurse's extremely human role in the midst of the tense, sometimes distressful environment of the SICU is rather an uneasy one. Yet, in spite of the trying circumstances, well-prepared nurses who have the requisite skills and knowledge and who engender reciprocal respect and positive concern for others form the stable foundation of the intensive-care unit. Such nurses do everything they know and can to identify the special needs of individuals; to detect and treat physiological imbalances; and to communicate a humanistic caring attitude.

Special Needs

The key to the quality of "humanness" is the ability to personalize cardiosurgical nursing care even though the patient is usually attached to a chest drainage system, urinary drainage and measurement system, a source of oxygen, a strain gauge to measure pressures, and an instrumentation system for continuous monitoring of ECG and heart rate. One of the first postoperative efforts is to call the patient by his own name to help him regain a feeling of personal, distinctive identity. The patient will also need reassurance and an explanation of what the machines do for him. Even with the monitoring sensors attached, a child will plead for love and security by crying out to the nurse, "Pick me up . . . lift me up."

Specific needs of adult patients can be identified during a SICU nurse's preoperative patient interview. In such an interview, the nurse ascertains the patient's attitude toward his impending surgery and his self-awareness of his cardiac condition. After sessions of sympathetic listening, she may discover that the patient is inclined to deny reality, that is, to avoid a painful perception; have acceptance; or be in depression, and so forth. The nurse extends psychological support to her patient to help him face the future days with reason, courage, and hope.

The nurse, to sum up, has a continuous, unending task. It demands gathering accurate information and making astute observations that will serve as a basis for sagacious decisions to attain hoped-for goals. Administering empathic, knowledgeable patient-centered care is our professional commitment and a great and privileged service to humankind.

References

Glaser, B. G. and L. Strauss. 1965. *Awareness of Dying*. Chicago: Aldine Publishing Company.

Goldsmith, J. R. and E. Jonsson. 1973. "Health Effects of Community Noise," *American Journal of Public Health* (September), 63(9):782–793.

Petrillo, M. and S. Sanger. 1973. "Eight Types of Families . . . And How They Affect Your Job," *Nursing '73* (May), 3(5):43–47.

Additional Bibliography

Kubler-Ross, E. 1970. "Five Stages A Dying Patient Goes Through," *Medical Economics* (September), pp. 272–91.

170   Rita K. Chow

Kubler-Ross, E. 1969. *On Death and Dying*. New York: Macmillan.
Mitchell, M. 1973. "Heed The Silent Cry," *Supervisor Nurse* (March), 4(3):62–64.
Robinson, L. 1972. *Psychological Aspects of the Care of Hospitalized Patients*. Philadelphia: F. A. Davis.
Shusterman, L. R. 1973. "Death and Dying," *Nursing Outlook* (July), 21(7):465–471.
Vaillot, Sister M. C. 1970. "Living and Dying," *American Journal of Nursing* (February), 70(2):268–73.
Veatch, R. M., W. Gaylin, and C. Morgan, eds. 1973. *The Teaching of Medical Ethics*. New York: Hastings Center.
Vernick, Joel J. *Selected Bibliography on Death and Dying*. Washington, D.C.: U.S. Government Printing Office.
Weisman, A. D. 1972. *On Dying and Denying: A Psychiatric Study of Terminality*. New York: Behavioral Publications.
White, L. P., ed. 1969. "Care of Patients with Fatal Illness." *Annals of the New York Academy of Sciences* (December), 164(3):635–896.

❧ 19
The Rapid Rise of Heart Clubs

Raphael L. Wittstein

LAYMEN-RUN, HOSPITAL-BASED heart clubs started with a handful of founding heart veterans in 1973 when the "Nassau Task Force for the Psycho-Social Rehabilitation of Persons Suffering from Cardio-Vascular Disease" was established in New York State's Nassau County, on Long Island. The title is long but every word is a working and meaningful word. A few laymen heart veterans who had regained their health and were grateful for their good fortune, including the writer, were aware of what their less fortunate brothers, sisters, and families were going through. From our own experiences, we knew of the traumatic physical and emotional shock to the individual, and the lonely problems that the patients and their families tried to solve in finding their way back to stability, resuming a place in the mainstream of life, and meeting successfully its trials and obligations. The original Task Force membership included, besides laymen, a scattering of psychologists, nurses, physicians, and a social worker. Help came from the Nassau County, New York Heart Association.

The first heart club was opened at South Nassau Communities Hospital in Rockville Centre, New York, in January 1974. Three more clubs were opened in rapid succession with memberships of 100 to 200 heart veterans and their spouses. Accordingly, we set up the Nassau Heart Clubs Coordinating Council,

made up of the chairman of each club or his or her representative, to act as a clearing house for exchange of materials, club
publications, reemployment references, job training, and rehabilitation programs.

By 1976, 18 such clubs, meeting in hospitals, had been
opened in the Greater Metropolitan New York area. Five more
were in the discussion stage—three in the Metropolitan area and
one each in Connecticut, and in Syracuse, New York, with more
planned for two other New York State counties, Suffolk and Rock-
land. Membership totalled over 3,000.

Clubs meet (usually monthly at 8:00 P.M.) in local hospitals.
Guest speakers are usually drawn from the hospital staff or from
adjacent areas, including New York City. The speakers may be
cardiologists, psychiatrists, nutritionists, pharmacists, coronary
and nurse educators, work physiologists, representatives from Social Security, Blue Cross, and weight-reduction programs. The
program subjects run the gamut of the interests and educational
needs of the membership, aimed at increasing their knowledge
about themselves, and, through group and self-help, boosting
their morale and making them better able to cope with and master the problems of recovery.

Speakers are asked to talk for about 15 minutes, since educational discussion, replete with questions and answers, is the main
purpose of the group's being brought together. Every effort is
made to keep the average size of meetings small—to afford
members the time to respond in a question-and-answer-period.
We aim to bring together those with heart problems and their
families with other heart veterans, so that they can receive information, ask questions, and express themselves freely, exchanging
problems and experiences, both giving and taking from each
other and professionals. They give support to each other in recovering both physically and mentally (where does one end and
the other begin?) from the shocking, life-upsetting experience of
heart attack. Many find assurance, comfort, wisdom, renewed
strength, and courage in developing a more reasonable, more
workable, more enjoyable, and more healthy outlook and way of
life.

The writer has worked with laymen with a history of heart
trouble and a variety of hospital, medical, and health professionals, by getting clubs started, talking to staffs, getting hospital
approvals, supplying formats, literature, and public relations materials to open clubs; by aiding in soliciting laymen leadership,

evaluating and training of same, giving personal support in forming steering committees, and at following meetings at fledging
clubs until they developed their own adequate club steering committee and leadership. Tremendous gratitude is due the coronary
nurses for their deep, humane understanding and the unselfish
dedication of their own time and wisdom to help start and develop these clubs.

After the first few clubs were established, requests for aid in
forming new clubs began to come to us from other hospitals with
increasing frequency. The club development and support work is
time-consuming and, up until now, conducted by less than a
handful of lay volunteers. If we were to reach out to new hospitals
on our own, we know from experience that clubs would be
opened rapidly right across the country. The need is that great.

Another purpose of the clubs is to develop an awareness
among hospitals and the medical profession of the psychosocial
causes and reactions of the heart patients before, during, and
after their hospitalization. A paramount purpose of the heart clubs
is not only to educate their own members, but also to work with
physicians and hospital personnel for the improvement of the
treatment of the heart patient as a *whole person*. By aiding the
patient to learn to help himself, we hope to reduce the sad statistics of repetitive heart attacks and high mortality rates.

The clubs are looked upon as a form of communicative channel between patients and physicians. The lay chair and cochair
serve as dedicated volunteer liaisons bringing both groups
together and representing the lay point of view, problems, and
wishes.

Meeting formats are varied. Not only have we had guest
speakers with question and answer programs, but we have, from
time to time, separated those attending into workshops lasting approximately an hour, with four, five, or six participants in each
group. We then participate in a simple, direct discussion and
exchange, after which all groups come together in a one-hour
forum discussion. We have also had meetings with cardiac pulmonary resuscitation demonstrations, hypertension and diabetes
blood testing, aided at times by nurses, physicians, and Heart Association personnel.

The heart clubs are primarily for those in need of moral support from their peers. We look upon the clubs as "open end
clubs," for ex- and present cardiac patients who come occasionally
or regularly. We do not try for numbers or for bigger and bigger

meetings. Rather, we work on saving and rehabilitating *individuals*. We work to rebuild confidence and courage in their future and faith in themselves, so that armed with new valuable knowledge and the support of their peers, they can face their futures and take their place once again in the mainstream of life.

On the request of physicians, nurses, or families, some of us with extended experience visit needful or troubled patients at home or in the hospital. By the very presence and appearance of recovered heart veterans, by aiding and responding to *our* incapacitated brothers' problems, drawing upon the memory of our own, we are able to give humane, concerned, judicious help. Our phones are open at all times to our peers and their families. In addition, some clubs, every two weeks, run small "person-to-person" discussion groups for those members and/or their wives, who wish to discuss intimately their private problems, thoughts, fears, and are in need of counsel, encouragement, or just the sounding board of other fellow heart veterans.

Those in the physical trades, and often on a lower educational level, who have been hit by a heart attack are particularly in need of morale building, rehabilitation, and reemployment. Too many of them, as they recover, are advised by their cardiologists that they "will do okay" but that they cannot go back to the strenuous physical work they have done all of their lives. Helping them is a most difficult challenge. Help them we must, and help them we do, with much more to be done.

There are many more problems and needs, which, within the limits of time and our personal resources, we endeavor to meet and help with. We turn no one away. There are millions of Americans with a variety of heart problems, whether medical, surgical, or psychological. We are grateful that millions have been able to recover physically and emotionally to become once more useful, confident members of society. The heart clubs are there to aid all of our brothers who need help, regardless of the length or the nature of their illness, whether it be physical or emotional.

❧ 20
Changes in Family Interrelationships Following Cardiac Surgery

Maurice H. Greenhill and
Robert W. M. Frater

IN 1974, 96,000 cardiac surgical procedures were performed in the United States. Of these, 16,000 were for emplacement of pacemakers, 23,000 for replacement of valves and 57,000 were coronary bypass operations. In 1976, it was expected that 100,000 bypass procedures would be done. A number of reports exist on psychological predictors for outcome and psychological behavior of patients during the immediate postoperative period (Burgess et al., 1967; Egerton and Kay, 1964; Elsberry, 1972; Frank et al., 1972a, 1972b; Freyhan et al., 1971; Kornfeld et al., 1965; Rabiner et al., 1975). Very few exist on the medical status and psychological accommodation of patients in the months and years following surgery (Blachly and Blachly, 1968; Frank et al., 1972; Lucia and McGuire, 1970; Willner et al., 1976). Articles on aftercare planning and follow-up treatment are scarce. In our experience, we could find no reports of family interrelationships following cardiac surgery.

This paper represents an exploratory study on the outcome of cardiac surgery up to four years after operation, with emphasis upon the psychosocial parameters, particularly those related to family interrelationships. It was made possible as a result of a working association between the authors (a psychiatrist and a cardiac surgeon) and Mended Hearts, Inc., a national organization of individuals who have had cardiac surgery, and their spouses. It became evident through numerous formal and informal contacts that behind a cheerful, optimistic demeanor, most "open heart" patients and their spouses were experiencing adaptational difficulties of a characteristic type not encountered before, which should be taken into consideration in their comprehensive health care. Altered marital and child-parent relationships were striking.

Method

Mended Hearts, Inc. is an organization which has 8,000 members in the United States and consists of 75 chapters connected with specific medical centers. Members and their spouses are recruited following cardiac surgery. The work of the chapter is meaningful to its members through group association in workshops on cardiac disease and surgery, through social events, and in particular, through the procedure of visiting cardiac surgical patients preoperatively. Specific members, if they so elect, are trained to be such "visitors" to help preoperative patients accept and accommodate themselves to impending surgery. The visiting program has been eminently successful.

This study was done with the help of Chapter 85 of Mended Hearts, Inc. connected with the Hospital of the Albert Einstein College of Medicine in Bronx, New York. Chapter 85 consists of 120 members. It became apparent to one of us, while conducting workshops on the psychological aspect of cardiac surgery for visitor training established by the Division of Thoracic Surgery, that medical aftercare was not emphasized. Although improved, patients continued to have cardiac symptoms, and emotional difficulties were being experienced by both patients and spouses. As a result, the chapter encouraged more workshops with the psychiatrist-leader and 10 percent of the chapter spontaneously requested and received individual counseling. These illustrations, combined with many informal contacts with Mended Hearts visitors on the surgical floors and in the Intensive-Care Unit, led the authors to the conclusion that the area of extended aftercare for cardiac surgery was largely neglected, was highly important as an aspect of treatment from the individual and family aspects, and was an epidemiological phenomenon in view of the large population undergoing cardiac surgery. It furthermore suggested to Chapter 85 of Mended Hearts that it potentially had as large a role in aftercare as it did on preoperative visiting.

As a result of this, the collaboration of the two investigators and subjects from Mended Hearts was easily arranged. Fifteen operated patients and their spouses volunteered to meet in group sessions at regular intervals so that material could be obtained for study. The patients had been operated on in seven New York City hospitals by eight cardiac surgeons. All sessions were tape recorded, typed, and analyzed for clusters of data related to medical symptoms, psychological defenses, levels of anxiety, emotional characteristics of patients and spouses, and reported and demonstrated interactions between patient and spouse. Material was obtained in this way from three large group sessions in workshops held before the decision to make this study (N = 40–60) and eight sessions of the volunteer group. Each session was 90 minutes long. Five sessions were held with patients alone, two with spouses alone, and a final meeting occurred with both patients and spouses present.

It is recognized that the number of subjects is small and the sampling is limited, so that an attempt at statistical analysis cannot be made. However, the volume of data appeared to be large enough to categorize some findings as part of an exploratory investigation.

Medical Findings

There was general agreement among the subjects that anginal pain and/or dyspnea had been reduced by surgery. Twelve had had bypass surgery alone, two valvular surgery alone, and one both bypass and valvular surgery. Anginal pain was still experienced by all 13 bypass patients but only occasionally and in a mild form. However, because of anginal pain, four patients had to undergo cardiac catheterization again, five had to be hospitalized briefly for observation, and one experienced occlusion of a small coronary vessel. The anginal pain was usually associated with physical or emotional stress. Two patients complained of residual symptoms of hepatitis and one patient underwent bypass surgery for occlusion of iliac vessels.

Although all patients agreed that their cardiac status was

decidedly better than before surgery, no patient in this series was free of cardiac complaints. It may be said of this group that all bypass patients experienced some degree of coronary insufficiency.

Fatiguability was a complaint made by nine of the eleven bypass patients. It was a troublesome symptom and may be an aspect of the coronary insufficiency. They claimed they tired easily and could not do as much as before surgery without tiring. The obvious fatigue of these patients was a source of concern to the spouses. The two valve patients did not complain of fatigue, but both had changed occupations to more sedentary jobs.

All bypass patients complained of periodic generalized pruritus (itching). This is a symptom which, as far as we know, has not previously been reported. We do not know its cause.

The complaint heard most often by far, was memory defect for recent memory. Both patients and spouses complained of this problem in 12 of the 15 subjects. It was an annoying symptom which did not interfere vocationally but troubled the patients and their families. This seemed to be particularly true with the bypass patients. It did not seem to be correlated with age. Typical examples included forgetting why one had walked into another room to obtain an object, not recalling why one had called a coworker into one's office, and losing thoughts in the middle of them. Attention has been called to memory defects particularly after valvular surgery by Freyhan (1971), Kimball (1969), Quinlan (1974), and Willner (1976), who refer to random cases in connection with the relationship of preoperative cerebral disturbance, postcardiotomy delirium, and operative outcome. No one before this has uncovered the high incidence of memory defects in patients who have undergone bypass surgery. When we add together our volunteer subjects with those who attended Mended Hearts chapter workshops, it is possible that 80 percent of patients who have undergone cardiac surgery have mild residual memory problems. Whether or not we can refer to this state as brain damage we cannot say, but we are currently investigating physiological changes while patients are on the heart-lung pump and preoperative and postoperative intellectual functioning.

Psychological Findings

In a medical center in which Mended Hearts has a chapter, only about 15 percent of operated patients join the organization. The reasons for this are not clear, except that some individuals want to avoid further contact with cardiac considerations. The most common characteristic of those who did join, as we have seen it in meetings and group sessions, is a buoyant, cheerful optimism. The general tone of gatherings is that of euphoria. This is mixed with an intense adherence to the subject of visiting preoperative patients. There is little question but that the overriding attitude is one of denial. The note that is sounded is, "We are lucky to be here, all of us, patients and spouses, and we are going to live happily ever after." It is our experience that it takes two or three group sessions to dispel this and to find what is really underneath.

Within the patients, as reported by them and their spouses, is considerable impatience and irritability, far beyond what they had prior to surgery. It seems to be linked—at least partially—with the experience of fatigability. Tolerance and endurance are not the same and sudden impulsive outbursts are not uncommon. This obviously places strain on marital relationships, although spouses tend to engender it with solicitous overconcern.

Work records make a reasonable index of degree of accommodation to disability. One-third of our patients were not working and one-fifth had taken less demanding jobs. All were attempting limitations on hours worked. Blachly and Blachly (1968) have reported that 41 percent of their postoperative patients felt unable to work, and Lucia and McGuire's findings (1970) in a group of similar patients showed that 30 percent had different jobs and 53 percent had lower incomes after surgery. It seems apparent that although cardiac surgery affords relief of some cardiac symptoms, work accommodation can be a serious matter which should be taken into consideration.

One final psychological factor which seems to play an important role in psychosocial adjustment is the hyperactivity of cardiac patients who have undergone corrective surgery. About one-half of our small group of patients became overactive to a degree greater than demonstrated before surgery. As far as we could tell they appeared to be Type A individuals who "took off the wraps" after having bypasses. This became an important feature of family disruption, as will be discussed presently.

Family Interrelationships

Patients and spouses meeting separately in groups gave both the opportunity to ventilate freely. Meeting together the interplay between patients and spouses brought out hitherto unexpressed emotions about the cardiac condition and doubts of survival. The considerable body of material in this aspect of the study will be divided into the following sections: attitudes of spouses, attitudes of patients, interactions between husbands and wives, and attitudes of patients and spouses toward their children. Within the volunteer group, all patients were over 50 years of age and thirteen of the fifteen patients were men.

Attitudes of Spouses

The spouse group, seen alone, consisted entirely of wives. Of the two women patients, one was a widow, while the husband of the other attended only the mixed group.

The predominant feelings expressed by all wives was concern, fear, and anger. The anger extended from outright statements of hostility and ridicule toward the husbands to veiled criticism or sarcasm. Solicitude was so great as to be resented by the husbands. There was an overriding vigilance kept by the wives. They watched the color of the skin, the rate of movement, the expressions of the face for discomfort, and the breathing. A frequent activity discussed by the wives in the group was the habit of watching the husbands as they slept to see if they were still breathing. Within the group process, expressions of fear emerged, centered around *sudden death*. Such statements were voiced as, "He could get an occlusion or another coronary." "The bypass vein might break loose." "Something might happen to the mechanics of the operation."

The spouses were very aware of the common factor of fatigue experienced by the patients. Because of this and their general concern, they attempted to hold the patients back in their activities. With the obvious Type A individuals (the female patient with the living husband was one of these) this became an almost impossible task, which produced marked tension within the marriage. Almost all of the wives questioned the good judgment of the husbands concerning health since the operation.

The dominance idea among the wives was noteworthy. All but one considered that she was the dominant member, the leader, of the dyad, who always ended up guiding major decisions. They considered their judgment was better and they were more intelligent. They admitted that the current obstinacy of the husbands tended to change this balance. The relationships since surgery exposed marked degrees of dependency on the part of the wives, which had been covered over and denied in previous years. Troublesome ambivalence became an obvious theme. Anger over cardiac illness and concern for life kept coming through. Loss of dominance was a factor.

Attitudes of Patients

Patients were softer in their attitudes toward spouses. In the early sessions, guilt was expressed over what suffering mates had experienced at the time of operation. There was universal praise of the behavior of spouses during that critical time. They tended to want to make up to the spouses for that difficult period.

They seemed annoyed rather than hostile over the solicitude of the spouses. This they complained about frequently. "We don't want to be babied" was often stated. The only criticisms of wives' current behavior was in this area. Taking an insistent and dominant stand with mates on this issue appeared to be more than satisfying to them.

Patients insisted on their rights in judging the degree of activity of which they were capable. Most used good judgment; two did not. Degrees of activity seemed to be a necessity for "testing out" their integration, safety, and masculinity. There was strong denial of anxiety over cardiac danger, although with any sign of trouble, patients reentered the hospital with alacrity. Fear of dying was denied. An interesting feature expressed by several was that death was nothing to fear since they had been through it on the heart-lung machine during surgery.

Real hostility was never expressed toward wives, but there were instances of displacement toward wives of preoperative patients being visited.

Interactions Between Husbands and Wives

The ambivalences, concerns, and attempts at dominance were consistent aspects of the interactions when patients and spouses were together. The marked open criticism of spouses toward patients, witnessed at times in the large workshops, was greatly diminished by the time of the final meeting of the mixed volun-

teer group. But concern and hostility were there on the part of
spouses, and insistence on control on the part of patients.

In discussion concerning marital interaction prior to cardiac
disease in bypass patients, the impression came through that
dominance, control, and pressure on the part of spouses had been
a problem, either because of intrapsychic problems on the part of
the spouse or in reaction to dealing with Type A behavior in the
patient-to-be. It appears that this struggle is still extant after
surgery, with the patient having gained the ascendancy.

Attitudes of Patients and Spouses toward Their Children

It was noticeable that, in all sessions held, neither patient nor
spouse ever brought up the subject of their children. The overriding concern was for themselves. After this omission was pointed
out, the reaction was that since, in all instances but one, the
children were grown, they were out of it. One patient stated,
"We haven't got our children at home anymore; we concentrate
on each other." Most couples spoke and acted as if they were
childless. All said that, of course, the children were concerned at
the time of surgery, but unless the grown children lived at home,
they were somewhat detached regarding the illness of the parent.
It seemed as if the parents had been successful in projecting their
own denial on to the children.

This set of circumstances seemed to underscore the strong
ambivalent alliance between patient and spouse which tended to
exclude others. In the one instance where a patient had young
children at home, the attitudes seemed appropriate—both patient
and spouse were concerned mainly that the patient survive until
the children were on their own.

Case Examples

A closer look at four situations might add to the characteristics of
family interrelationships after cardiac surgery.

Case 1 The patient and spouse are in their early fifties. He is a Type
A businessman, who suffered a myocardial infarction upon returning
from a strenuous vacation. This led to a double coronary bypass, and
in the recovery stage he came down with hepatitis. He is now three
years postoperative, and is as active as ever, playing paddle tennis,

skiing, and swimming. This is of constant concern to his wife and they have frequent arguments over it. She is more verbal and intellectual, but she can no longer influence him as she once did. He is more headstrong and irritable. She watches his color and breathing. Once she awakened him in the middle of the night because she thought he had stopped breathing. He, of course, was startled and exclaimed, "What do you want to do, make love?" His activity is so great that he tends to clear the dinner table before his wife has finished her meal. If he is physically uncomfortable playing singles in paddle tennis, he shifts to playing doubles, rather than stopping. Nothing was ever mentioned about a problem son who was about to get married.

Case 2 Six months after a triple bypass operation this 50-year-old man did not think he could work on his job again, but went to work on his house. It was his idea to make all necessary repairs and improvements before he died from heart disease, although his prognosis was good. He paneled several rooms, jacked up one side of the house to correct a fault in the foundation, remade several floors, put siding on the house—all by himself. The wife was frantic, attempting to slow him down. She enlisted the aid of six daughters and together they compelled him to see a psychiatrist, who put him on tranquilizers. He finished what he wanted to do, and then got depressed.

Case 3 The wife has been a dominant, controlling professional woman who "wore the pants" until after the patient had a double bypass operation. He can now become irritable and pugnacious and can succeed in holding her down. In the group sessions, she made hostile derogatory statements about him but these softened after a time. She watches him constantly and analyzes much of what he does. Their children were not discussed in the group sessions, but it is known that the wife attempts to dominate them as well.

Case 4 The patient had a single bypass operation and has adjusted well since. He sensibly moved into a more sedentary occupation. He is a man of good judgment and leadership. He has had to be rehospitalized on one occasion for catheterization after coronary insufficiency. His wife is severely concerned about him and watches him breathe. She has begun to have occasional anxiety attacks under the strain. He is concerned for her, but will not let himself be invalided.

Conclusions

It is obvious that the care of the patient does not end with cardiac surgery. There is some evidence to show that in one chapter of

Mended Hearts, Inc., in which patients have been involved with several surgeons and hospitals, aftercare is spotty. Very few operated patients see cardiologists or cardiac surgeons on a planned basis, but only on need. In the meantime, the patients are continuing with a clinical condition which is troubling to them and to their families. This assumes epidemiological proportions inasmuch as there are in the neighborhood of 100,000 patients in this category each year.

Although mortality for cardiac surgery is low, survivors experience the following symptoms: occasional angina, fatigability, irritability, generalized pruritus, and mild memory defects. These they tend to struggle with alone. Memory defects tend to trouble almost 80 percent and are noticed by both patient and spouse. Occupational modifications have been noted in all patients, ranging from decrease in working capacity to change in occupation, to no work at all.

Family relationships were changed by the catastrophic experience of this critical surgical procedure. Patients and spouses were drawn together into troublesome ambivalent alliances. Both expected that the results of surgery were tenuous and that sudden death could take place. A type of euphoric denial is pathognomonic for the whole group, covering enormous anxiety regarding death. The patients deny concern for death, claiming they have experienced it on the heart-lung machine. Their denial extends itself into spurts of startling hyperactivity going beyond Type A expectations.

The spouses are oversolicitous to a point of being a burden to the patients. There is a deeply built-in hostility on the part of wives of patients, who almost universally considered themselves to be dominant over their husbands. Such patients have in almost every instance taken the leadership away from their wives by their high activity, irritability, and aura of possible death. A strange corollary to this death-threat symbiosis is the virtual elimination of children from emotional involvement in the problem. The exceptions are children living at home, who are enlisted by spouses to aid in control and vigilance. Children living elsewhere express only superficial concern as part of family denial.

Sex after surgery was freely discussed, but after the first six months, does not appear to enter into the death concerns as it had previously.

The aftercare indications seem distinct. The euphoric denial need not be disturbed where it is helpful, but periodic follow-up visits to a cardiologist would allay concern that diffuses through family relationships. Certainly it seems self-evident that patients and spouses could be told by surgeons what they might expect in aftercare symptoms. Our patients and their spouses seemed to have gained some relief from tension in their ambivalent alliance by their experience in the group sessions. A small number of such sessions would seem indicated as part of aftercare in cardiac surgery.

It is recognized that in this study we have been dealing with a small sample—thirty subjects in the group-process sessions, and 120 subjects in the workshop meetings. The question arises as to the validity of the sample. Is it a group of subjects truly representative of cardiac surgery patients generally or is it a select sample? The opinion of Cardiac Surgery at the Hospital of the Albert Einstein College of Medicine, where this study was done, has been that 75 percent of patients are alive and symptom-free one to seven years postoperatively. The results of study with the Mended Hearts portion of that operated group does not bear this out. On the other hand, this particular Mended Hearts sample comes from seven medical centers and may be more generally representative than the Einstein group. However, in view of the strong factor of denial found in our series, a reevaluation of the Einstein cases reported by Cardiac Surgery would be indicated.

References

Blachly, P. H. 1967. "Open Heart Surgery: Physiological Variables of Mental Functioning." In H. S. Abram, ed., *International Psychiatry Clinics*, vol. 4, no. 2.

Blachly, P. H. and B. J. Blachly. 1968. "Vocational and Emotional Status of 263 Patients After Heart Surgery," *Circulation*, 38:524–32.

Burgess, G. N., J. W. Kuklin, and R. M. Steinhelber. 1967. "Some Psychiatric Aspects of Intracardiac Surgery," *Mayo Clinic Proceedings*, 42:1–12.

Egerton, N. and J. H. Kay. 1964. "Psychological Disturbances Associated with Open Heart Surgery," *British Journal of Psychiatry*, 110:433–39.

Elsberry, N. L. 1972. "Psychological Responses to Open Heart Surgery," *Nursing Research*, 21:220–27.

Frank, K. A., S. S. Heller, and D. S. Kornfeld. 1972a. "A Survey of Adjustment to Cardiac Surgery," *Archives of Internal Medicine*, 130:735–38.

Frank, K. A. et al. 1972b. "Long Term Effects of Open Heart Surgery on Intellectual Functioning," *Journal of Thoracic Cardiovascular Surgery*, 64:811–15.

Freyhan, F. A. et al. 1971. "Psychiatric Complications Following Open Heart Surgery, *Comprehensive Psychiatry*, 12:181–95.

Heller, S. S. et al. 1970. "Psychiatric Complications of Open Heart Surgery," *New England Journal of Medicine*, 283:1015–20.

Heller, S. S. et al. 1974. "Psychological Outcome Following Open Heart Surgery," *Archives of Internal Medicine*, 134:908–14.

Henricks, T. F., J. W. Machinzie, and C. H. Almond. 1969. "Psychological Adjustment and Acute Response to Open Heart Surgery," *Journal of Nervous and Mental Disease*, 148:158–64.

Henricks, T. F., J. W. Machinzie, and C. H. Almond. 1971. "Psychological Adjustment and Psychiatric Complications Following Open Heart Surgery," *Journal of Nervous and Mental Disease*, 152:332–45.

Kilpatric, D. G. et al. 1975. "The Use of Psychological Test Data to Predict Open Heart Surgery Outcome: A Prospective Study," *Psychosomatic Medicine*, 37:62–73.

Kimball, C. P. 1969. "A Predictive Study of Adjustment to Cardiac Surgery," *Journal of Thoracic Surgery*, 58:891–96.

Kornfeld, D. S. et al. 1965. "Psychiatric Complications of Open Heart Surgery," *New England Journal of Medicine*, 273:287–92.

Lucia, W. and L. B. McGuire. 1970. "Rehabilitation and Functional Status After Surgery for Valvular Heart Disease," *Archives of Internal Medicine*, 126:995–99.

Quinlan, D. M., C. P. Kimball, and F. Osborne. 1974. "The Assessment of Open Heart Surgery IV. Assessment of Disorientation and Dysphoria Following Cardiac Surgery," *Archives of General Psychiatry*, 31:241–44.

Rabiner, C. J., A. E. Willner, and J. Fishman. 1975. "Psychiatric Complications Following Coronary By-pass Surgery," *Journal of Nervous and Mental Disease*, 160:342–84.

Tufo, H. M., and A. M. Ostfeld. 1968. "A Prospective Study of Open Heart Surgery Abstracted," *Psychosomatic Medicine*, 30:552–53.

Vasquez, E. and R. W. Chitwood, Jr. 1975. "Postcardiotomy Delirium: An Overview," *International Journal of Psychiatric Medicine*, 6:373–83.

Willner, A. E. et al. 1976. "Analogical Reasoning and Postoperative Outcome: Predictions for Patients Scheduled for Open Heart Surgery," *Archives of General Psychiatry*, 33:255–59.

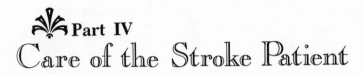

Part IV

Care of the Stroke Patient

⚜21
The Stroke Patient

John C. M. Brust

A PATIENT WITH a stroke is not always "terminal." Defining stroke as a sudden focal neurological deficit caused by pathology in blood vessels allows for wide variability in etiology, degree of deficit, and course. Strokes can be divided into ischemia/infarct and hemorrhage. They can also be classified according to their underlying cause, including such diverse diseases as atherosclerosis, hypertension, sickle-cell anemia, berry aneurysm, subacute bacterial endocarditis, migraine, recent myocardial infarction, systemic lupus erythematosis, atrial myxoma, and so forth. Strokes can be described further by their location; lesions in the distribution of particular vessels often produce rather stereotyped symptoms and signs, and very small lesions in critical regions sometimes cause more severe or longer lasting deficits than larger lesions in other areas.

The difficulty in predicting prognosis in a patient with a recent stroke is well-known. Certainly a patient comatose when first seen is more likely to do badly than one alert, and the longer a limb remains flaccid and paralyzed, the less likely it is to recover strength. Surprising improvements have occurred weeks or months after a stroke, but a patient seemingly doing well may suddenly worsen. Moreover, a patient functionally incapacitated may remain medically stable for months or years. In addition, several studies have reported that the most common ultimate cause of death in stroke survivors is not recurrent stroke but heart disease (Matsumoto et al., 1973). Thus, a stroke patient is seldom labeled definitely "terminal" in the way a patient with, for example, metastatic disease might be. After a variable period of time, one can approach a patient with a stroke in terms of his ability to function—for example, is he unable to work; or does he require institutional care; or has he because of aphasia or dementia lost the ability to communicate with others; or is his deficit so devastating that the physician recognizes that the most vigorous measures being taken to prolong life are likely to fail or even questions whether persistence in such measures is ethically justified? While many milder strokes alter life-style severely and can cause depression over loss of function or fear of recurrent episodes, it is the group of stroke victims with already catastrophic deficits who will be considered here as being life-threatened.

Case Report

A 77-year-old left-handed woman was admitted to the hospital because of sudden left-sided weakness and difficulty in speaking. She had been known to be hypertensive for at least 30 years, but treatment had always been sporadic. At age 55, she had a stroke which left her with a moderate right hemiparesis and slurred, but otherwise normal, speech. A major motor seizure at age 75 was associated with elevation of blood pressure to 260/160, and was treated with antihypertensives and anticonvulsants. At that time, she was inattentive and had poor recent memory, but the only other neurological abnormalities were her moderate right hemiparesis and slurred speech. She was then stable until her abrupt left hemiplegia on the day of admission.

Examination showed a supine blood pressure of 210/120; her pulse was 84 and regular, respirations were 15 and regular, and temperature was 99°F (37.2°C). She was lethargic, mildly inattentive, and showed impairment in recent memory. Speech was not only slurred but hesitant and nonfluent; naming, speech comprehension, and reading were intact; writing was impossible because of bilateral limb weakness. There was a left homonymous hemianopia, left facial weakness, left flaccid hemiplegia with a left Babinski sign, and left hemisensory loss, plus the old moderately severe right spastic hemiparesis. Cerebrospinal fluid was clear and colorless with normal pressure, no cells, and a protein of 57 mgm/100 ml.

Over the next week, she worsened, especially in language function: speech became more nonfluent, at times nearly mute, and she lost the ability to name, comprehend, or read. A number of medical problems arose: renal insufficiency with serum creatinines 4–7 mgm/100 ml; congestive heart failure requiring digitalis (which in turn led to first-degree heart block); urinary tract infection; electrolyte disturbances with hyponatremia and hyperkalemia; pneumonia and/or atelectasis; anemia with hematocrit 25 (considered "anemia of chronic disease"); and blood pressures fluctuating from 220/130 to 100/70. Difficulty swallowing required continuous intravenous feeding, and fluid balance became variable as there seemed to be a narrow zone between dehydration with increasing azotemia and overhydration with congestive heart failure.

Neurologically, she became stable but severely impaired. Six weeks after admission (and at the time of this writing) she is alert and moves her eyes toward whoever is speaking to her. Speech consists of nonconsonant grunting sounds, and she shows little language comprehension. The other neurological signs present on admission are still there: her left arm and leg remain flaccid and paralyzed, and her right limbs are weak and spastic.

One cannot be certain this woman will not regain some motor or intellectual function, but it seems unlikely that much significant recovery will occur. On the other hand, if she continues to receive adequate nursing care, she may live for months or even years. How can a physician make such a dreadful situation more tolerable to the patient or the family?

It is crucial for the doctor to try to understand the nature of any mental deficit present. This woman has aphasia (Geschwind, 1971), which can be defined as a disorder of language caused by cerebral disease and not explained by impaired primary sensory receptors or by decreased muscle power or coordination or by dementia. That is not to say that she does not have some loss of intellectual ability in addition to her language deficit, but aphasia can exist with apparently intact mentation as tested outside the sphere of language. This is especially likely with Broca's aphasia, in which there is nonfluent, labored, seemingly dysarthric speech but intact speech comprehension on the patient's part, and with anomic aphasia, in which there is difficulty naming and often paraphasic substitutions but, again, preservation of the ability to understand the speech of others. When aphasia involves loss of speech comprehension, especially when so severely that a patient's own speech feedback is lost and he speaks incomprehensible "jargon" (so-called Wernicke's aphasia), it is likely that higher intellectual function in addition to language has also been impaired. Such a patient often performs badly on nonlanguage testing and may also show total lack of awareness that he is unable to understand others or that they are unable to understand him.

Writing is usually impaired in any aphasia, and reading is often abnormal. There may also be apraxia or, especially in non-dominant hemisphere lesions (not causing aphasia), bizarre agnosias, for example inattention to space, including the patient's own body, on the contralateral side.

These aphasias, apraxias, and agnosias may look like psychoses; a patient may be considered insane by his family, or he himself may feel he is losing his mind. Aphasic patients have been mistakenly admitted to mental hospitals. A physician can perform a major service by trying to penetrate a patient's language disorder (however difficult this may be, as for example with Wernicke's aphasia) in order to show that he understands the nature of the problem. The situation can be explained to relatives and friends, who may be able to increase their communication with the patient once they have an idea of his limitations. Of course, communication may still be impossible, or nonlanguage dementia may be the real barrier following a stroke, but such a conclusion can be reached only after a patient has been carefully tested and the true nature and extent of aphasia and/or dementia determined.

A stroke can inflict a myriad of other neurological deficits: hemiplegia, quadriplegia, limb or gait ataxia, chorea, hemiballism, "thalamic pain," vertigo, sensory loss, dysphagia, blindness, seizures, coma and so on. Although seizures can be controlled, and neurosurgery has been performed to relieve hemiballism or thalamic pain, and contractures can be prevented in a paralyzed limb by physiotherapy, therapy to restore specific neurological loss is seldom available. Again, the doctor can help by explaining the nature of the deficit and the realistic hope for its long-term improvement.

Stroke therapy is multifaceted. Acutely, one might consider anticoagulation (often used for transient ischemic attacks, strokes-in-evolution, and some embolic strokes, with the intention of preventing further deficit rather than relieving that already present) (Millikan, 1971), corticosteroids or other antiedema agents (the efficacy of which remains unproven in stroke) (Bauer, 1973), vasoconstrictors or vasodilators (similarly controversial and of uncertain value) (Browne and Paskanzer, 1964), or emergency surgery (for example, evacuation of a cerebellar hemorrhage) (Fisher et al., 1965). There is also preventive therapy, including treatment of hypertension, hyperlipidemia, arrhythmia, or other underlying diseases; or discontinuation of, for example, birth-control pills (*New England Journal of Medicine*, 1973); or, in selected patients, surgery on neck vessel atherosclerotic plaques (Bauer et al., 1969).

Then there is the often long and difficult time of rehabili-tation, embracing physiotherapy, occupational or speech therapy, social service, and sometimes psychiatry, all geared toward pro-ducing maximal independence of function despite persisting neurological deficit. (The struggles and terrors of this period have been wittily and movingly described by Eric Hodgins [1963] in *Episode*, an account of his own cerebrovascular accident.)

When, however, a patient is as disabled and failing to im-prove as the woman described above, in whom acute therapy has failed to prevent the patient from becoming "terminal," and in whom, consequently, measures designed to prevent further strokes become practically an academic exercise, one is relying largely on palliation and supportive therapy, the purpose of which is not simply to prolong life but to provide maximal comfort to a dying patient (New York Academy of Medicine, 1973). Preventing or treating medical complications—for example infection, conges-tive heart failure, pulmonary emboli, or anemia—may serve this end, not only by decreasing symptoms caused directly by such complications, but also by possibly lessening neurological deficit: it is well-known that focal neurological signs may worsen with a superimposed metabolic insult. Physiotherapy continues to be important. One may no longer realistically be expecting return of function, but prevention of contractures or a frozen shoulder means increased comfort for the patient, even if bedridden. Vig-orous nursing care is similarly necessary to ensure adequate ali-mentation, bowel and bladder evacuation, and prevention of bed-sores, and to allow the patient that maximal degree of activity from which he appears to benefit—for example, sitting in a chair, watching television, and so forth.

These principles are really the same applied to terminal ill-nesses of diverse cause. So are the questions of whether life-supporting measures such as a respirator or a cardiac pacemaker are indicated, of whether heroic therapy such as cardiac resuscita-tion is justified, and of whether medically supportive measures should be discontinued, either because they are ineffective or be-cause the patient meets the criteria for cerebral death (Beecher, 1968). Where a stroke perhaps differs from many other life-threatening illnesses is, first, in the length of time a patient can

194   John C. M. Brust

sometimes remain medically stable after a sudden devastation, and, second, in the difficulty an observer may have in gauging the degree of viable mind behind the barrier of aphasia or dementia. Understanding the special unpredictability of the course of illness and the nature. of the neurological deficit can make it easier for the patient, the doctor, and the family to cope with this particular disease.

References

Bauer, R. 1973. Open discussion: *Clinical Management of Cerebral Ischemia, in Cerebral Vascular Diseases.* Eighth Conference. F. H. McDowell and R. W. Brennan, eds. New York and London: Grune and Stratton.

Bauer, R. B., J. S. Meyer, W. S. Fields et al. 1969. "Joint Study of Extracranial Arterial Occlusion. III. Progress Report of Controlled Study of Long-Term Survival in Patients With and Without Operation," *Journal of the American Medical Association,* 208:509–18.

Beecher, H. K. 1968. "A Definition of Irreversible Coma: Report of the Ad Hoc Committee of the Harvard Medical School to Examine the Definition of Brain Death," *Journal of the American Medical Association,* 205:85–88.

Browne, T. R. and D. C. Poskanzer. 1969. "Treatment of Strokes," *New England Journal of Medicine,* 281:594–602, 650–57.

Geschwind, N. 1971. "Aphasia," *New England Journal of Medicine,* 284:654–56.

Fisher, C. M., E. H. Picard, A. Polak, P. Dalal, and R. G. Ojemann. 1965. "Acute Hypertensive Cerebellar Hemorrhage: Diagnosis and Surgical Treatment," *Journal of Nervous and Mental Disease,* 140:38–57.

Hodgins, E. 1963. *Episode: Report on the Accident Inside My Skull.* New York: Atheneum.

Matsumoto, N., J. P. Whisnant, L. T. Kurland, and H. Okazaki. 1973. "Natural History of Stroke in Rochester, Minnesota, 1955 through 1969," *Stroke,* 4:20–29.

Millikan, C. H. 1971. "Reassessment of Anticoagulant Therapy in Various Types of Occlusive Cerebrovascular Disease," *Stroke,* 2:201–8.

New York Academy of Medicine. 1973. "Statement on Measures Employed to Prolong Life in Terminal Illness," *Bulletin of the New York Academy of Medicine,* 49:349–51.

New England Journal of Medicine. 1973. "Collaborative Group for the Study of Stroke in Young Women, Oral Contraception and Increased Risk of Cerebral Ischemia or Thrombosis," *New England Journal of Medicine,* 288:871–78.

❀22
Stroke Symptoms and Their Implications

Morris E. Eson and Boris J. Paul

THE UNDERLYING ASSUMPTION of the literature in Thanatology is that the individual, such as the terminal cancer patient, facing a clear indication of the end of life, can be helped to deal with this overwhelming awareness. When, however, thanatological concepts are transposed from the realm of the terminal cancer patient to that of the cardiovascular patient, the goals of care, instead of adaptation to dying, become adaptation to living. It is not altogether clear that the goal of care in the stroke patient is adaptation to living, in the usual sense of the word. The goal may well be conceived as adaptation to a transitional state between full living and death. Even though such a starting point may appear pessimistic, it will serve to enlighten us in providing a clearer perspective on the life-death polarity.

Because of our experience in Rehabilitation Medicine, we have chosen to define the Life-pole of the Life-Death polarity in a less sharply distinct way than is usually the case in thanatological discussion. Those patients whom we see are generally not those who die shortly after the cerebrovascular episode but those whose lives are seriously changed and perhaps diminished as a result of it. The particular psychosocial consequences to the patient, to the family, to the staff, and to the community will depend on a host of factors—for example, the patient's premorbid status, economic factors, the severity of the symptoms, the resources available to the family and the community. We have chosen here, for the purposes of analysis, to focus on three common residual symptoms resulting from stroke. Our selection of these three sequelae is based upon the following considerations: they are pervasive, and they have significant impact upon the patient and those who become involved with his care. Most important from the standpoint of our discussion here, however, is that these sequelae impinge upon fundamental characteristics of behavior that most clearly define human life. These fundamental functions that, in a limited sense, define human life are: The delicate functional asymmetry around which our perceptual-motor interaction with the world proceeds; the initiation of activity, both mental and psychological, that enables us to be spontaneously productive; and the quality of speech which has been taken as the distinctive mark of human life. If any of these basic features of life is seriously disrupted, or, as is often the case, all of them are involved, then the state of existence has become so radically altered as to require what may be a more difficult adaptation than adapting to death itself. It may be an adaptation to a transitional state between life and death. We shall take up each of these sequelae briefly and consider the psychosocial aspects of each in turn.

Disturbance of the Delicate Functional Asymmetry

In the ontogenesis of behavior, the development of lateral dominance plays a significant role. Locomotion, skillful tool use, visual pursuit, and perceptual scanning are all dependent on an integration of the dominant side with the support of the nondominant side. Once this dominance is established in the latter part of the first half-decade we witness an onrush of motor skill development; bicycle riding, writing, managing a musical instrument, refined hand-eye coordination, athletics, and generally refined kinesthetic adjustment. We underestimate the extent of organization that underlies all of these until we observe the disruption of this balanced functional asymmetry. The person who has sustained a cerebrovascular accident will have this delicate balance distorted. We can imagine what it might be like to live the life of a blind person; with greater difficulty we can put ourselves in the place of a deaf person; but it is well nigh impossible to transpose oneself into the distorted dynamic world of the stroke patient.

Little wonder, then, that we observe denial of the impaired side in some hemiplegic patients. It is almost as if the patient is hoping to establish a new equilibrium without the encumbrance of the side that used to support his fluent movements and is now failing him. It is not only that the patient is clumsy, as all of us are on occasion, but every movement has lost its tacit and implicit control and must be guided deliberately. The patterned activities that we as human beings acquire are designed for the normal range of functional asymmetries and for the coordination of the two sides of a bilateral structure. Many of them are beyond the capacity of the distorted asymmetry resulting from stroke.

We have seen instances of stroke in which the motor impairment of one side appears relatively minor, or where considerable recovery of motor function has occurred on the affected side, only to observe continued denial of the weak or clumsy limbs or mounting frustration on the part of the patient when he becomes aware that he is no longer whole. We have been struck by the marked difference in adaptation to the loss of the use of an arm between the patient who has suffered an amputation of an upper extremity and the patient who loses function after a stroke. Both patients can be observed to mourn their losses but the amputee will adapt—with or without a prosthesis—much more quickly and completely than the stroke patient. A more profound and subtle loss has occurred with the disruption of this equilibrium.

The Initiation of Activity

The general passivity and lack of initiative frequently observed in the stroke patient has generally been interpreted as a reactive depression due to the patient's recognition of his loss. This is no doubt a reasonable interpretation when one considers the impact of the loss of an accustomed role and the frustration resulting from psychomotor disturbance that we have just described. We also observe more extreme forms of motivational inertia and personality change which have been attributed to lesions in the corticobulbar systems bilaterally (Ferraro, 1959). Essentially such lesions appear to interfere with voluntary control. At a more theoretical level, we can ask what is involved in voluntary control. Voluntary control is manifest not only in the ability to inhibit undesirable activity; it is also a manifestation of volition, will, and purposive behavior—all of which are essential in the initiation of action. When viewed in this way the diminution of voluntary control appears to mean diminution of will and purpose.

Schopenhauer said that we can do what we will but we cannot will what we will. One view of the stroke patient might be that not only does he have diminished capacity to do what he wills but that he may also have diminished capacity to will. We have observed a number of stroke patients (particularly males engaged in the professions) who have retained the abilities to read, play cards, and use a typewriter, but who seem to have lost the capacity to initiate or sustain such activities or to engage in them with any enthusiasm or pleasure. Patients who manifest this disturbance of initiative make us aware of how important is this subtle feature of our human existence. At the same time they arouse in the health-care provider, in the family, and in the extended family a sense of anxiety, frustration—almost agitation—related to the inability to arouse this manifestation of living. We recall the case of a 72-year-old physician who suffered a mild stroke with right hemiparesis and dysphasia. After three or four weeks the symptoms had apparently resolved completely. He had essentially complete motor control of all extremities with only a minimal impairment of very fine coordinated movement of the right hand. His speech was clear and appropriate. His remote memory was excellent. He was able to use his right hand to write legibly, although his handwriting was less attractive than prior to the stroke. He had been a scholarly person who, in addition to functioning very well as a family physician for about 40 years, was an ardent scholar of literature and the humanities. However, following his stroke he lost all interest in reading, writing, and teaching and withdrew almost completely from human interaction except for the minimum required to live at home. We do not know how to deal with this phenomenon of slow dying in contrast to our trained response in the emergency of resuscitating a patient with cardiac or pulmonary arrest or even with the cancer patient who has arrived at a terminal state. Somehow, to us, the stroke patient is capable of indefinitely long life, even in his incapacitated state.

A diminished capacity to will is indeed a diminished capacity to live. We are not making judgments here about what it is that different individuals may will to do—even the will to do what, by our particular estimate, is the doing of evil is a manifestation of life. What we are emphasizing is that a person whose will is diminished is partially dead and to face up to this reality is a gigantic challenge, particularly for those like caretakers whose will and initiative have to be coordinated with the hardly existent will and initiative of the patient.

The Quality of Speech

The power of words is inestimable. The philosopher Cassirer takes the symbolic form to be the core of the genuinely human aspects of life. He writes:

> In the human world we find a new characteristic which appears to be the distinctive mark of human life. The functional circle of man is not only quantitatively enlarged; it has also undergone a qualitative change. Man has, as it were, discovered a new method of adapting himself to his environment. Between the receptor system and the effector system which are to be found in all animal species, we find in man a third link which we may describe as the *symbolic system*. This new acquisition transforms the whole of human life. As compared with other animals man lives not only in a broader reality, he lives, so to speak, in a new *dimension* of reality. (Cassirer, 1944, p. 24)

The literature on aphasia is extensive. The particular manifestations of the disorder have been described so that the diagnosis can be made with specificity. However, the diminution of this uniquely human dimension of reality, which occurs in relationship to the impairment of language function associated with stroke, has received less attention. The innumerable subtle variations of impairment in the use of language symbols are frequently underestimated or inadequately appreciated.

Here again we note that the loss of language in any significant sense results in a state of being that is altered so as to threaten life, not so much as opposed to death, but life as more philosophically and psychologically conceived. If life is defined as Eros, the usual psychoanalytic polarity of Thanatos, the implication of this definition is that life is dependent on sharing with others. Ninivaggi and Harris (1976), in a recent study of attitudes in patients with serious cardiovascular disease, concluded that:

> . . . the most outstanding features of this survey are consistent with the theme that meaningful human existence is a function of interpersonal relatedness. . . . This quality of being related in a responsible and caring way to others appears to impart meaning and a sense of personal satisfaction to life. It would appear that interpersonal relatedness is a basic motivating force in formulating attitudes toward living and death in the elderly. (p. 1496)

One of the most fundamental bases of this sharing is in the communication process, which, in turn, depends on the possibilities of shared intersubjectivity. Such possibilities are seriously diminished in dysphasia. This could mean the destruction of Eros, connection or relationship, in the patient's life.

The aim of this discussion has not been to relegate the seriously involved cerebrovascular patient to the category of nonperson. Our aim has been rather to point out the magnitude of the problem for this patient, the family, and staff. The goal of care in the stroke patient is not merely adaptation to living but possibly adaptation to a seriously diminished human life with the attendant feelings of rejection, denial, guilt, frustrated hope, hostility, and despair.

References

Cassirer, E. 1944. *An Essay on Man.* New Haven: Yale University Press.

Ferraro, A. 1959. "Psychoses with Cerebroarteriosclerosis." In S. Arieti, ed., *American Handbook of Psychiatry*, vol. 2:1078–1108. New York: Basic Books.

Ninivaggi, F. and R. Harris. 1976. "Attitudes Toward Living and Death; In Chronic Cardiovascular Disease," *New York State Journal of Medicine*, 76:1496.

Part V
The Life-Threatened Patient

23
To Die from Cancer or from a Heart Attack

Jan van Eys

THERE IS MUCH speculation about the mode of dying that is conceived as appropriate and desirable. The discussion of death has come into the open and is even fashionable. Because of my position as a pediatric oncologist, I am frequently invited to discuss death and dying with various groups. When the problems of dying are discussed, it is obvious from the interaction with the audience that the majority of listeners conjure up a vision of a disease like progressive cancer. However, when one discusses death, the audience begins to imagine a catastrophic heart attack, or another death, equally swift. Clearly, it is not true that cardiovascular disease is always a sudden, irretrievable end; there is protracted dying in cardiovascular disease. Conversely, there are many instances of swift and merciful deaths from cancer. Nevertheless, the observed distinction in reaction is so real and so repetitive, that one is forced to speculate on its origins. This brief paper is such a speculation. There are no true statistical facts on which to base a specific conclusion. Therefore, the following is mainly personal in concept. My personal experience with dying patients has been with children. When seen in the form of congenital malformations, pediatric heart disease is not necessarily viewed differently from malignancies by parents. However, that is not under discussion. The topic is the experience of the living will, rather than the experience of a dying person, or even the experience of an adult responsible for the care of a dying dependent. Much of the imagery is in popular Christian concepts, for only in this context have I had the majority of my observations of adult reactions. Nor have discussions with medical students been different.

There are a number of differences between heart disease and cancer that might be responsible for the fundamentally different response to these two diseases as a conceived terminal event. Sometimes such differences are not based on real distinctions, but rather are imagined by a person who has not experienced either disease. Other concepts are true and give a measure of reality to the differential attitude. These real and imagined reasons are so intertwined that the following discussion will not make a value judgment. In fact, personal reactions and the feelings and reasoning observed in audiences are hardly separable. After all, we have as yet not experienced the Copernican revolution in the science of thanatology. We still allow preexisting concepts to explain phenomena, rather than deriving knowledge from the phenomena themselves. Especially in dying, phenomena are usually explained away, rather than used as clues to reality. This paper will not herald in such a scientific revolution in the psychology of the dying, but the antinomies discussed have helped to interact positively with audiences. In that sense the suggestions, hypotheses if one wants to use this term in this context, have been predictive.

First of all, there is the general idea that one reacts differently with foreknowledge than against the unexpected. In the final analysis, one cannot truly conceptualize being dead. Therefore, in most instances a reminder of dying, the imminence of death, is a very real threat. Cancer, when diagnosed, constitutes such a threat, even when the disease might be treatable, if not curable. The popular fantasy is that a heart attack is quick when it kills, and that the killing will occur with little warning. This may have nothing to do with the reality of the frequently preceding danger signals. Nevertheless, the fantasy is very widespread. In that sense, both cancer and heart disease are associated with death, but only cancer is associated with dying. Death is an unimaginable concept, while dying is imaginable. Sudden death (unassociated with the process of dying) is not expected to truly take place, while cancer is a very realistic possibility, and therefore frightening.

Cancer is an all-or-none battle against the threat to life, while heart disease has an image of being conquerable. Cardiovascular disease is conceived as a process of healing and recurrence, rather than as an ever-present gnawing threat. It is fascinating to note that doctors themselves describe their own cardiovascular disease as an interesting phenomenon, while viewing cancer as a serious threat to life. In a compilation of descriptions of diseases, as they are experienced by doctors themselves, many more instances of cardiovascular disease were related than cancer attacks (Greene, 1971). As a result of this different feeling about cancer and heart disease, there is an entirely different attitude in the approach to the two diseases. The attitude toward cardiovascular disease is a positive one. On the other hand, cancer care is the area in which thanatology has made the greatest inroads. This is now, in fact, one of the burdens of cancer care, since the outlook is not actually that bleak anymore in pediatric oncology (Van Eys, 1976). Nevertheless, this prevailing attitude strengthens the popular image that death from cancer is the norm.

The consequences of having cancer are conceived differently from the consequences of having serious cardiovascular disease. It has already been said that cancer is generally thought to be protracted, while heart attacks are seen as swift. But there is much more to that distinction. Although in both diseases survival, if it occurs, requires the patient's adherence to instructions of physicians, there is a fundamental difference. Time and again, the image of the physician fighting the cancer in the body of the patient is brought up. Teenagers voice this concept frequently. The cancer is inside, destroying the body that is necessary for the spirit to be in the here-and-now. The doctor enters and, in fact, violates the body to do battle. The patient's spirit does not enter in the battle except to allow the doctor to do the fighting. It matters little whether this fight is with surgery, radiation, or chemotherapy. This concept of "battle" probably contributes to the thriving quackery in cancer care. Images of such fights against the cancer border on daemonic struggles. Many patients hedge their bets and follow the advice from medical authorities as well as that from the spiritual healers. On the other hand, after the initial insult is overcome, the patient with heart disease is told about the healing powers of his body and what he can do to promote recovery. The patient retains a sense of self-determination. His own ability to maintain appropriate activity levels, to be sensible about life-style, to stop drinking, smoking, or whatever—all these measures are self-determined. They are followed on advice to be sure, but there is no pill to make the diet salt free, nor is there medication to make the food have less calories. Even disease-directed drugs are apt to be seen as medications to help the failing heart, rather than as drugs to kill the invading cancer. In short, if you do not die from cardiovascular disease, a measure of self-determination is left, allowing the concept of healing and recurrence to soothe much of the fear of a protracted dying process. And even if one fails to follow the doctor's advice, and thereby precipitates the life threat anew, then one still has the self-serving excuse that it was not some higher power that overwhelmed. Even then the image of self-determination is retained.

When all such subconscious or realized rationalizations are rejected, there is still a major distinction between cancer and heart disease. Despite current discussions about brain death, the majority of people still conceive of the heart as the measure of life, not necessarily as the seat of the soul, and therefore not as the equivalent of the person. Rather, it is seen as the index of the body's life, and the body is the vessel of the spirit. The threat to the heart is an all-or-none threat. If the heart fails, then the body is gone, and the spirit may even be thought as liberated. If there is any image of resurrection, fears are allayed since the body is still very much intact, and only a failing heart has to be restored. It must be stressed again that such images are more prevalent among individuals who have not experienced heart disease, and this group is the majority of living people. Cancer, in contrast to heart disease, is far more likely to encroach on far less vital parts. The progressive destruction of the body, without concomitant liberation of the spirit, is very frightening to many. Eventually, death may occur, but it is likely a secondary death, and the actual means by which it occurs is not very clearly conceptualized. The body seems to be destroyed with a heart that is still viable. To be able to incorporate any immortality concept requires greater powers of imagination and rationalization under these circumstances. Even though the separation of body and spirit is widely discussed and mostly acknowledged, the conceptualization of being dead, if it is forced upon one at all, involves living imagines. A brain death is very frightening, because it conjures up an image of a spirit that could not escape the body in time to wait for a reclamation of that body. A brain death seems conceivable only in others by most people. Cancer death is seen as the converse, no real workable body for the spirit to survive in, but a spirit that is not yet liberated.

Sooner or later everyone will encounter death and dying in some close person. Observation of such, still somewhat distant, reality does little to change the concepts of people. Whatever physicians use to fight cancer, it will leave battle scars, while the survivor of the heart attack is, in most instances, visibly intact. As the practice of cardiac surgery for the alleviation of coronary insufficiency increases, this perception may change. Also, as we begin to recognize the genetic predisposition to cancer or cardiovascular disease, we may begin to generate in the general population a personal image of private death, rather than a generalized image of the possible modes of demise. But we are a long way away from that. Although medical knowledge advances very rapidly, the basic concepts and fears of most people are not readily changed.

The question then is whether it matters what the picture is in the minds of those who are thinking about death at all. It is probably not truly important to the progress of thinking how the general public views the difference between heart disease and cancer. That is, truly quantum progress in the evaluation of civilization's thought comes from the direction of the inspired few and not the consensus of the many. Rather, what is important is that the image held by the general public is not entirely foreign to the medical profession. They too had such concepts before they entered the profession of healing. In fact, the choice of the specialty is usually made on some basic but incomplete idea of the realities of the chosen area of medicine. Many physicians accept failure in oncology as expected and therefore react either with anger and challenge to do the impossible, or relaxation and security of doing the best that can be done, without the pressure of requiring success. The cardiologist frequently requires last-ditch efforts because recovery is the expected norm, even if the mortality eventually is very high. Resuscitation is the armamentarium against cardiovascular disease, but is far less frequently practiced on an oncology service. This difference in attitude is significant, because there is consequently less direction toward cure in oncology, especially when contrasted against the optimism of cardiovascular research, which now even accepts the concept of an artificial heart as a realizable goal. Such a device, if truly successful, would in the eyes of the uninformed widen still further the gap between cancer and heart disease.

These ideas should not imply that there is no desperate hope to achieve a cure from cancer. On the contrary, cancer, being the most feared, has in effect been granted priority. But there is a conceptual difference in the goals. In the case of cancer, the disease should be removed in such a way that the patient is freed from the doctor, by making the cancer disappear as a reality, by making it as though it never happened. It is rarely recognized that changing reality will produce utmost despair. For cardiovascular disease, the existence of the disease can be acknowledged. In fact, some small social benefit is accrued from a heart attack. One is thought to have worked too hard, or at least one is allowed to work somewhat slower, but is still regarded as capable of returning to work. Again, this may be far from the reality of a given patient, but the concept persists in the minds of people who have not experienced the illness.

The difference will be erased if oncologists quietly start expecting cures themselves. Not because cures now are the norm (even though we are coming close in pediatric oncology), but because the expected will be achieved some day. When the physician expects to cure, the patients will be more confident. Though this may appear counter to the tenor of a thanatology ideal, it is not actually the case. No matter how accepted death should be, the expectation of the *initial* medical visit is the evaluation of prognosis and how the outcome can be realized. If, indeed, the outcome cannot be changed from death, then medical management should be geared toward helping the patient accordingly. But if cure were achievable, yet death was expected, this would become a self-fulfilling prophesy. To a degree this is beginning to occur in oncology. It would be too far afield to discuss whether such an effort toward cure is worthwhile or whether the cost is prohibitive. That is not germane to the topic at hand. Rather, it is clear that the current attitude from the medical profession, which in itself is derived from popular conceptions, strengthens the differential attitude between death by cardiovascular disease or by malignant disease.

References

Greene, R., ed. 1971. *Sick Doctors*. London: William Heinemann Medical Books.
van Eys, J. 1977. "What Do We Mean by the Truly Cured Child." In J. van Eys, ed., *The Truly Cured Child*, pp. 79–93. Baltimore: University Park Press.

❦ 24

Cardiovascular Disease and Cancer: Comparisons and Contrasts

Roger R. Williams

AN OFFICIAL UNITED STATES government report on the nation's vital statistics for the year 1973 revealed that heart disease was the most common cause of mortality (all ages combined), accounting for 757,075 deaths (38 percent) in the United States (*U.S. National Center for Health Statistics*, 1975). Varying somewhat with definitions of interrelated disease, about 84 to 93 percent of these deaths resulted from coronary heart disease (CHD), 3 to 12 percent from "hypertensive disease," 3 percent from rheumatic heart disease, and an additional 1 percent from congenital heart defects.

This same document indicated that cancer was the second most common cause of mortality, accounting for 351,055 deaths (18 percent) in that same year. In men, lung cancer caused most of the deaths (33 percent), followed by tumors of the large bowel (12 percent) and other digestive sites (15 percent). In women, breast cancer accounted for 20 percent of the cancer deaths, followed by malignancies of large bowel (15 percent), other digestive sites (14 percent) and lung (10 percent). Stroke or cerebrovascular accident (CVA) was third on the mortality list with 214,313 deaths (11 percent) in men and women.

Approximately three-fourths of the deaths from cancer and cardiovascular disease occurred in persons over 55 years of age. Since 1900, a rise in the proportion of the population dying from cardiovascular disease and cancer has been attributed in large part to the prevention of death from infectious disease and, in some part, to new exposures in our modern society.

Geographic Distribution and Etiology

Significant differences in mortality rates from cancers and cardiovascular diseases are observed between areas of the United States (Moriyama et al., 1971; Mason et al., 1975). In some general aspects they are similar for cardiovascular disease and cancers (for example, with high rates in the eastern part of the country and low rates in the mountainous areas of the west). However, more striking differences are seen in international comparisons. Coronary heart disease and large bowel cancer are two of several diseases common in the United States and rare in undeveloped African countries (Burkitt et al., 1974). Even among the developed countries as much as a fourfold difference in mortality rates is observed for coronary disease, strokes, and cancers of the large bowel, lung, stomach, and breast (Mason et al., 1975; Levin et al., 1974). Such large international variations strongly suggest that environment and possibly heredity play major roles in the etiologies of our most common causes of death.

Several environmental risk factors have been defined. Smoking is a major risk factor for coronary disease and stroke (Gordon and Kannel, 1972), as well as for several common cancer sites (*United States Department of Health, Education and Welfare,* 1967, 1971, 1972, 1973, 1974). Factors such as serum cholesterol or dietary fat and fiber intake have also been suggested as playing an etiologic role for both heart disease and cancer (Burkitt et al., 1974; Wynder and Mabuchi, 1972; Haenszel et al., 1973; Kannel et al., 1971), although the data at present are not conclusive.

A strong association with alcohol intake has been found for several major cancer sites (Williams and Horm, 1976). Heredity has been shown to play a substantial role in the etiology of some cancers (Fraumeni, 1975)—that is, colon, leukemias, breast, and lung—and for three major risk factors of coronary disease: hypertension, glucose intolerance, and hyperlipidemia (*National Heart* and Lung Institute, Division of Heart and Vascular Diseases, 1976). Important insights into the interaction of environment with heredity have also been supported by studies of lung cancer with smoking (Kellermann et al., 1973), diabetes with obesity (West and Kalbfleisch, 1971), and hypertension with salt consumption (Fries, 1976).

A broad summary of these epidemiological considerations gives some indications of similar or parallel process contributing to the occurrence of major cancers and cardiovascular disease. In both instances, the patients can find reason to suspect that their own life-style, habits, and environment are largely responsible for their illnesses.

Symptoms and Diagnosis

In contrast to the similarities in the epidemiology of cancer and cardiovascular disease, the constellation of symptoms and diagnostic methodologies is quite different in the two diseases. For most malignancies, symptoms are nonspecific, vague, and gradual in onset. Insidious loss of vigor, appetite, and weight; poorly localized pains, subtle changes in a chronic cough, gradual appearance of blood streaks, constipation, lingering infections, unexplained fevers, and even personality changes can accompany a developing malignancy, although these same symptoms can also accompany a host of less ominous maladies. The initial diagnostic modalities are equally nonspecific and are used to define many disorders in addition to cancer. These include x-rays and scans of all varieties, nonspecific blood tests, stool guaiac, and cultures. With the exception of accessible malignancies such as leukemia or cervical carcinoma, the definitive diagnosis (biopsy) often requires an exploratory operation.

A dramatically different set of symptoms and diagnostic procedures is encountered by the patient with a myocardial infarction or stroke. Chest pains or paralysis are sudden and relatively characteristic symptoms. The specific diagnosis is frequently quite obvious to the patient as well as to the physician. Diagnostic tools are direct, specific, and quite conclusive. They include ECG and myocardial isoenzymes or neurological findings directly referrable to the occlusion of specific cerebral vessels.

Treatment and Survival

With the exception of curative surgery of early tumors, cancer therapy is quite nonspecific and generates a host of undesirable side effects. Radiotherapy and chemotherapy are used for most malignancies and both are well known for their noxious effects on normal tissues as well as tumor masses. Nausea, vomiting, hair loss, hemorrhage, and infections occur all too frequently after repeated treatments. Even surgery performed for palliation or in hope of a "cure" can leave the patient with some sort of "ostomy" or draining wound that refuses to heal. Median survival times for the major cancer sites are six years for breast, two years for large bowel, and less than six months for lung, pancreas, stomach, and esophagus (Axtell et al., 1972).

For myocardial infarction and stroke, the main therapeutic strategy is intensive supportive care in anticipation of spontaneous recuperation. Antiarrhythmics, diuretics, vasopressors, and cardiotonics all have specific indications, titratable endpoints, good expectancy for favorable response, and side effects that are less frequent and less severe than the antineoplastic regimens. In the instance of a patient recovering from a myocardial infarct, few of these drugs would be required for prolonged periods. Anticoagulants which are sometimes used for both stroke and myocardial infarct can induce hemorrhagic manifestations similar to those of cancer patients under therapy. However, in contrast to the bleeding induced by antineoplastics, hemorrhage resulting from heparin or warfarin can be effectively countered by parental pharmacologic antidotes (protamine and vitamin K1). Considering all myocardial infarctions, 16 percent die suddenly and another 16 percent within the first three weeks. For the two-thirds who survive the acute attack, average survival is seven or eight years (Moriyama et al., 1971). For stroke, 20 percent die in the first two days, another 50 percent succumb to the stroke in the next 30 days, and about 20 percent survive five years or more.

The developments in cardiovascular epidemiology and therapeutics have had some apparent success in preventing deaths. After increasing steadily for 25 years, deaths from coronary heart disease have shown a decrease for several years as have deaths from stroke (Levy, 1975). Deaths from cancer are decreasing for cancer of the uterus and stomach and increasing dramatically for lung cancer (Seidman et al., 1976). Although little improvement in cancer mortality rates is visible at present, a relatively new and growing list of environmental risk factors for cancer provides hope for dramatic success in prevention. However, more effective programs must be developed by the general community of health professionals and educators to properly exploit epidemiological discoveries for preventive medicine (Burnum, 1974).

Discussion

Cancer patients, their families, and attending medical staff would seem to have justification for considerable frustration and anxiety generated by vague and gradual prodromal symptoms, multiple nonspecific diagnostic procedures, and oftimes ineffective therapies accompanied by uncomfortable side effects. In contrast, heart patients, their families, and attending medical staff are presented with sudden catastrophic events for which some specific therapeutic measures can provide dramatic relief. A generally better chance of survival would seem to give heart patients a psychological advantage over most cancer patients. However, it is probably not generally appreciated that five-year survival rates are not much different between patients with coronary disease and breast cancer. Survival rates for stroke victims are even poorer.

Through questionnaires and interviews, many of these life-threatened patients and their families become familiar with research efforts to understand and prevent these fatal illnesses. During such encounters, even terminal patients and their families may derive satisfaction from making meaningful contributions toward preventing others from having to share their misfortune.

References

Axtell, L. M., S. J. Cutler, and M. H. Myers. 1972. "End Results in Cancer Report No. 4." DHEW Publication No. (NIH) 73-272. Biometry Branch, NCI, Bethesda, Md.

Burkitt, D. P., A. R. P. Walker, and N. S. Painter. 1974. "Dietary Fiber and Disease," *Journal of the American Medical Association*, 229:1068–74.

Burnum, J. F. 1974. "Outlook for Treating Patients with Self-Destructive Habits," *Annals of Internal Medicine*, 81:387–93.

Fraumeni, J. F. 1975. *Persons at High Risk of Cancer. (Chapters 1. Congenital and Genetic Diseases, and 2. Familial Susceptibility)*. New York: Academic Press.

Fries, E. D. 1976. "Salt, Volume and the Prevention of Hypertension," *Circulation*, 53:589–96.

214   Roger R. Williams

Gordon T., and W. B. Kannel. 1972. "Predisposition to Atherosclerosis in Head, Heart, and Legs: The Framingham Study," *Journal of the American Medical Association*, 221:661–66.
Haenszel, W., J. W. Berg, and M. Segi. 1973. "Large Bowel Cancer in Hawaiian Japanese," *Journal of the National Cancer Institute*, 51:1765–79.
Kannel, W. B., W. P. Castelli, T. Gordon, and P. McNamara. 1971. "Serum Cholesterol, Lipoproteins, and the Risk of Coronary Heart Disease," *Annals of Internal Medicine*, 74:1–12.
Kellerman, G., C. R. Shaw, and M. Luyten-Kellerman. 1973. "Aryl Hydrocarbon Hydoxylase Inducibility and Bronchogenic Carcinoma," *New England Journal of Medicine*, 289:934–36.
Levin, D. L., S. S. Devesa, J. D. Godwin, and D. T. Silverman. 1974. "Cancer Rates and Risks (2nd Edition)." DHEW Publications No. (NIH) 75-691. Biometry Branch, NCI, Bethesda, Md.
Levy, R. I. 1975. "Third Report of the Director of the National Heart and Lung Institute." HDEW Publication No. (NIH) 76-970. NHLBI, Bethesda, Md.
Mason, T. J., F. W. McKay, R. Hoover, W. J. Blot, and J. F. Fraumeni. 1975. "Atlas of Cancer Mortality for U.S. Countries: 1950–1969." DHEW Publication No. (NIH) 75-780. Epidemiology Branch, NCI, Bethesda, Md.
Moriyama, I. M., D. E. Krueger, and J. Stamler. 1971. *Cardiovascular Diseases in the United States*. Cambridge, Mass.: Harvard University Press.
National Heart and Lung Instutute, Division of Heart and Vascular Diseases: Report by the Task Force on Genetic Factors in Atherosclerotic Diseases. 1976. DHEW Publication No. (NIH) 76-922, Bethesda, Md.
Seidman, H., E. Silverberg, and A. I. Holleb. 1976. "Cancer Statistics, 1976: A Comparison of White and Black Populations," *CA-A Cancer Journal for Clinicians*, 26:2–29.
U.S. DHEW, public Health Service: The Health Consequences of Smoking. Reports of the Surgeon General: 1967, 1971, 1972, 1973, 1974. Washington, D.C.: U.S. Government Printing Office.
U.S. National Center for Health Statistics: Vital Statistics of the United States, 1973. 1975. Washington, D.C.: U.S. Government Printing Office.
West, K. M. and J. M. Kalbfleisch. 1971. "Influence of Nutritional Factors on Prevalence of Diabetes," *Diabetes*, 20:99–108.
Williams, R. R. and J. W. Horm. 1976. "Association of Cancer Sites with Consumption of Tobacco and Alcohol and with Socioeconomic Status from the Third National Cancer Survey Interview," *Journal of the National Cancer Institute*.
Wynder, E. L. and K. Macuchi. 1972. "Etiological and Preventive Aspects of Human Cancer," *Preventive Medicine*, 1:300–34.

❀ 25
Role of Death Concern
in Cardiac Illness

W. Doyle Gentry

VERY LITTLE HAS been written regarding the role of death concern in cardiac illness. Rather, clinical investigators have to date concerned themselves with a description of the emotional reactions of patients to this life-threatening event and only recently have begun to study the basis for emotional behavior in the cardiac patient in an attempt to intervene in same. Hackett, Cassem, and Wishnie (1968) first described the affective state of patients suffering from symptoms of acute myocardial infarction (MI) in a coronary care unit. They noted that anxiety was the predominant affect seen in these patients; at least 80 percent of the patients studied evidenced some degree of anxiety as diagnosed by physical indices (restlessness, hyperventilation, excessive perspiration), empathy on the part of the attending physician, third-party evaluations by relatives and nursing staff, and subjective reports by the patients themselves. Gentry, Foster and Haney (1972) similarly reported that the degree of anxiety reported by MI patients on the coronary-care unit was determined by their use of denial as a psychological defense mechanism and also related to their perceived health status. Patients classified as deniers acknowledged less situational anxiety on admission to the cardiac-care unit (CCU) than is typical of normal, nonstressed individuals; while those classified as nondeniers initially reported a level of anxiety comparable to that of psychiatric patients with a primary diagnosis of anxiety reaction. In this study, levels of anxiety were paralleled by patients' ratings of perceived health status. That is, nondeniers initially reported a discrepancy between how healthy they were prior to their current episode of cardiac illness and how healthy (or sick) they were in the CCU, a discrepancy which tended to disappear after five days in intensive care and was associated with lower levels of reported anxiety. Other studies of similar patients have shown that anxiety in MI patients is a function of prior cardiac status (Rosen and Bibring, 1966), social class and severity of illness (Dominian and Dobson, 1969), and in turn can be predictive of subsequent morbidity and mortality in such patients (Hackett et al., 1968; Gentry et al., 1972; Klein et al., 1968).

Only in a more recent study, however, by Gentry and Haney (1975) have investigators begun to look for the basis or cause of the anxiety noted in acute MI patients. In studying 16 patients admitted to a CCU with a clinical diagnosis of acute or probable MI, these authors collected data concerning patient characteristics (for example, age, sex, race, prior cardiac status, severity of illness), prehospital behavior, behavior during the patients' stay on the CCU, and outcome in terms of morbidity, mortality, and functional status 18 months later. In all, the authors studied relationships between 22 different behavioral variables in this single group of patients. Many of the significant findings related to the patients' reported level of *death concern*, which itself was related to certain aspects of prehospital, CCU, and outcome behavior. The findings were as follows.

Prehospital Behavior. Patients who exhibited less delay in seeking medical attention (less than 24 hours) tended to be more concerned about dying and perceived themselves as sicker than did patients who exhibited greater delay (more than 24 hours).

CCU behavior. Patients who reported more concern about imminent death also evidenced: more subjective anxiety in the CCU, a higher level of physiological stress as measured by urinary sodium/potassium values, higher levels of self-reported pain and discomfort, and a greater perception of themselves as critically ill. Interestingly, white MI patients in this study were, as a group, twice as concerned about dying as were nonwhite patients (mean ratings of 3.73 and 1.80 respectively on a 5-point scale of death concern), and thus were characterized by noticeably higher levels of reported pain, anxiety, and physiological stress.

Outcome. At the 18-month follow-up, functional status (that is, how well the patients were able to function in everyday activities) tended to be less in patients who had reported less concern over dying in the CCU than was true of patients who had expressed a high level of death concern earlier on.

What these results suggest to us is that death concern is of crucial importance to the individual experiencing cardiac illness from the moment he or she first suffers the symptoms of acute MI all the way through critical care to eventual recovery and rehabilitation. However, it also seems clear that death concern has both a positive (life-saving) and negative (life-threatening) effect on the patient's response to cardiac illness at different points in the illness process. Initially, fear of dying brought on by a correct attribution of symptoms to a problem with the heart can lead to less delay in getting proper medical attention at an emergency or critical-care facility. Since delay and indecision in responding to MI symptoms are directly related to increased morbidity (congestive heart failure) and mortality, death concern would seem to be an asset to the patient. However, once the patient has secured proper medical attention and, in most cases, been admitted to a coronary-care unit, prolonged or intense death concern can turn into a liability. It clearly is directly related to abnormally high levels of subjective and physiological stress and reported pain and discomfort, which, in turn, gives the patient a poorer prognosis during this critical phase of illness. Patients who fail to be reassured concerning their chances for survival on or shortly after admission to a CCU, both by their physician and the nursing staff, run the risk of being "emotional casualties" of cardiac illness. In short, they may represent self-fulfilling prophecies in that their own concerns and worries about death lead directly to that end, despite courageous attempts by the CCU staff to keep them alive. Finally, it seems obvious to us now that patients' nonphysical functional status following acute MI may, in part, be determined by how concerned they are during and after their stay in the CCU about their own health, well-being, and survival.

Successful outcome and rehabilitation may depend on an individual's ability to focus on restoration of his health as the thing of highest priority, as a consequence of which his will to live will replace his fear of dying. Those patients who deny a fear of dying, or who do not have sufficient medical information to know they should be afraid, and who often report more concern over the cost of hospitalization or their family's health and well-being while in the CCU are less likely to involve themselves in the rehabili-

218   W. Doyle Gentry

tation process actively and thus become less functional over time, independent of the status of their heart. To some degree, this may describe what have traditionally been referred to as "cardiac invalids."

In many cases, the physician, nurses, and relatives of the life-threatened patient in the CCU themselves play down, deny, or ignore the patient's direct or indirect signals of anxiety, which may be based on his or her fears of death. In part, they may do this because of their own personal difficulties in dealing with such concerns in an objective, yet compassionate, manner and, in part, they may fear that dealing with such concerns may in fact make the patient worse. Indeed, some medical personnel and families of patients view the psychologist or psychiatrist called in to help the CCU patient resolve such issues as "potentially dangerous," fearful lest he upset the patient still further with probing, emotionally laden questions. What we suggest here is that these concerns are present in most patients—regardless of what we would like to be the case—and, in fact, one only has to ask the patient about them (for example, Would you rate how concerned you are about dying right now on a 5-point scale?) to get a clear statement of same. These concerns should be anticipated, for example in white patients as opposed to nonwhite patients, and dealt with immediately. Patients with a higher level of formal education, a prior history of cardiac illness and/or admission to a CCU, and younger patients are more likely to be more anxious and require help in coping with such concerns. Where normal reassurance about chances for survival by a physician or nurse do not succeed in lowering the patient's anxiety level, professional consultation from a psychologist or psychiatrist should be initiated. Cassem and Hackett (1971) have shown that where such consultation is available, approximately one-third of all MI patients on a CCU warrant such services.

References

Cassem, N. H. and T. P. Hackett. 1971. "Psychiatric Consultation in a Coronary-care Unit," *Annals of Internal Medicine*, 75:9.

Dominian, J. and M. Dobson. 1969. "Study of Patient's Psychological Attitudes to a Coronary Care Unit," *British Medical Journal*, 4:795.

Gentry, W. D., S. Foster, and T. Haney. 1972. "Denial as a Determinant of Anxiety and Perceived Health Status in the Coronary-care Unit," *Psychosomatic Medicine*, 34:39.

Gentry, W. D. and T. Haney. 1975. "Emotional and Behavioral Reaction to Acute Myocardial Infarction," *Heart and Lung,* 4:738.

Hackett, T. P., N. H. Cassem, and H. A. Wishnie. 1968. "The Coronary-care Unit: An Appraisal of its Psychological Hazards," *New England Journal of Medicine,* 279:1365.

Klein, R. F., V. A. Kliner, D. P. Zipes, et al. 1968. "Transfer from a Coronary-care Unit: Some Adverse Responses," *Archives of Internal Medicine,* 122:104.

Rosen, J. L. and G. L. Bibring. 1966. "Psychological Reactions of Hospitalized Male Patients to a Heart Attack," *Psychosomatic Medicine,* 28:808.

🌿 26
A Cardiac Patient Speaks Out
Jack B. Rostoker

IN 1966, AT AGE 47, I was admitted to hospital with a heart attack. This paper is based on ten years of study, of personal experiences, of discussions with cardiovascular patients, families, medical and paramedical personnel involved with exercise therapy.
This study also includes participation in and observations of, test-
ings and cardiac rehabilitation programs in Canada and the
United States.

    When he enters the hospital, the patient goes through a
cycle of emotions. Many medical and paramedical personnel dealing with cardiac patients can recognize heart disease, but, unfortunately, they cannot recognize the symptoms of another illness
which has to be treated almost immediately, "the Psychological":

Disbelief   —Impossible (it could only happen to someone else);
Anger   —Why me? Why now?;
Fear   —The Unknown;
Depression—What will I be able to do now? (depending on circum-
                stances, family responsibilities, financial situation, age,
                occupation, etc.).

    The doctor must be prepared for many questions. At this
time a decision is made on how much to tell the patient, including medications and therapy. There are many doctors who feel
that this knowledge will cause the patient to worry or that it may
initiate many more questions that could be very time-consuming

to answer, such as, "What is a heart attack?" the technicalities of which the patient would not understand. It may surprise some of these doctors how much a patient will understand if explanations are made in understandable terms, and how he will accept and adjust even to bad news!

Doctors with empathy do not wait for the questions which must come, but encourage them. Once dialogue of this sort has begun, it is not only informative but also helps to establish a relationship of mutual trust and respect. If, on the other hand, the doctor avoids questions, or does not answer them truthfully, there will be distrust and loss of respect.

A vital component of this dialogue in hospital is patient counseling. There may never be a better opportunity for this since the patient is so available and so receptive to suggestions. The purpose of counseling is to stimulate the patient to think because "to wonder is to begin to understand." He will understand the illness: the damage, the time needed for healing, the fact that *it* did not happen overnight. Treatment will mean that there is no instant cure, that it takes time to adjust, and that, like all damaged muscles, the heart needs movement. Seeds are planted to encourage the patient to review his life-style and consider other muscles and systems which may have been affected. With this counseling, the patient will begin to feel hopeful and to visualize himself adjusted, with limited mobility at the start but on the road to full rehabilitation. Overprotection and pampering may create a cardiac cripple or a problem patient. Lack of family understanding can lead to additional overprotectiveness. Therefore, the whole family must also be counseled to understand the anxieties and frustrations of the patient and the treatment that will help him deal with these. Their concerns must be alleviated along with the patient's.

All logic and counseling in the hospital are lost if they are not followed up immediately and reinforced regularly. There is a difference between knowing and doing, especially once the patient leaves the hospital. If properly counseled in hospital, the patient will have learned to realize when he has lost control and when life is running him. He will have to readjust to the "quickie" world: quick bite, quick drink, quick shower, even a "quickie" (sex). Therefore, there is the need for a close follow-up during which time the doctor will be able to assess if the seeds planted require watering or resetting due to "bad weather." The patient now, as before, should always know what is happening, whether he is progressing or regressing. The bond and trust between the doctor and himself is reinforced. In time, self-confidence will arise from the continuous counseling and success in doing.

To become fully rehabilitated, the patient must understand and learn his need for physical activity. The degree of this activity depends on the patient's age and extent of his physical condition and history. He must build himself up once again, including overall muscle tone. He must understand, however, that physical activity is not an instant cure-all, that it requires patience, and that it goes together with diet and rest. He must be aware that physical activity "will be time-consuming," may be boring, and may produce aches in muscles unused for a long time. He must be aware that he can overdo it and become overanxious to prove he is better, therefore becoming too competitive. He must allow the necessary time to warm up and cool down. Together with close follow-up, supervision, counseling, and the setting of realistic goals and objective, the patient will find himself feeling better, healthier, and happier.

Some patients do not participate in or discontinue exercise programs because of family influence, lack of counseling and guidance, informed letter of consent (rare instances of mishaps), fear of testing—"guinea pig" feeling—lack of empathy and personal attention from personnel after awhile, distance to travel, and financial problems.

There are also a few important reasons why the doctors do not recommend their patients for exercise therapy. First, they may still feel that exercise therapy is at the experimental stage and is too aggressive. Secondly, programs have too many patients for proper supervision. Thirdly, if a problem does arise the doctor gets blamed, usually by the family. Finally, but not the least of these, there are legal implications.

Cardiovascular disease suggests that cardiac rehabilitation involves more than a medical approach; it involves psychological and physical ones as well. It would be hard to find any physician who has the time to participate and the experience to be a cardiologist, psychologist, physiologist, dietician, and, in rare cases, a cardiovascular surgeon. With cardiovascular disease growing at the rate it is, might it not be better for a specialized and coordinated cardiovascular medical and paramedical team approach?

❧27
Reflections on Facing Death
Nathan Lefkowitz

THE IDEAS THAT I am going to talk about are close to me. Although I may not have difficulty talking about them, I might have to dig around a bit to get them to the surface. My purpose for presenting these ideas is threefold: first, I have had some interesting experiences with the problem of dying; second, I want to find a way to look at these experiences that will take them out of the realm of one man confronting death; and third, I want to try to see what the general implications of my experiences are and how others would be affected by them. In a sense, I'm trying out ideas.

I don't consider myself to be a person who is dying in the sense of being a terminally ill patient. I don't know how long I have to live. I consider myself to be a middle-aged person who has had a series of encounters with dying and who has had a life-threatening illness; that is, a myocardial infarction. I do expect to die from this condition, but, again, it is only an expectation— whether or not it will happen, I really don't know. I don't expect it to happen today, tomorrow, or the next day, but, as I say, it *is* a general expectation. What we are talking about are people who see themselves encountering death, but who are not in an imminently terminal condition, and who might live with this condition for a long time. I think the thing about it is that death or dying has become a living issue for me (and for others like me) that somehow involves my identity as a person. To use, I think,

Erikson's terminology, this kind of status becomes akin to a developmental path that I have to learn how to resolve; and this developmental path and its resolution have thrown me into an identity crisis which leaves two options open to me. One option is, I can choose to die, not biologically but psychologically and socially, and this is not a very uncommon thing. Invalids from cardiac or other diseases are quite common. Or else, I can choose to live. The kind of person I'm talking about either is in, or has been in, a state of anticipatory mourning about his own death for quite a while. In my case, it has been at least a year and a half, and the critical questions for a person like myself when he is mourning for himself are: "What am I anticipating?" "Am I anticipating my own death?" "Am I anticipating my recovery?" Usually, anticipatory mourning is not thought about in terms of preparing oneself for death but the other way around, preparing for the loss of someone else.

I am raising the question of not looking at mourning as a process with various stages but of looking at the outcome of this process and looking at the two possibilities—the outcome when I anticipate mourning for my death and when I anticipate mourning for a rebirth or a reliving. And what I am looking at more specifically are the factors in this mourning process that determine which of these alternate outcomes I will choose, or which will be chosen for me. Somehow, my prediction is that the way the mourning process works right now predisposes the person to anticipate his own death and to mourn for it. There are many, many reasons why I believe this. I would like to deal with one or two of them; and they have to do with the nature of our culture and with how our culture looks at death.

What I am thinking about in our culture is what I would call the rules for handling the phenomenon of death and the rules for using this phenomenon of death. In our culture, we have rules that we kind of go by and which we use to handle this phenomenon. To illustrate in a mundane way what I mean by these "rules," I propose that in our culture we have rules that tell us what items are proper to handle and under what conditions it is proper to handle them. For example, in our culture we are not supposed to handle feces, under almost any conditions. Yet we can handle somebody else's money or property if we are given permission. There are other rules that tell us whether we should behave passively or actively in handling what we are entitled to handle. Somehow the expression "you can't fight City Hall" is a rule that tells us that we should behave passively in the presence of power, particularly governmental power. Or, as other examples: one is allowed to be active in sexual matters primarily or particularly after marriage; and the male is expected to be more active than the female.

In the political area, we're expected to be active but not so active as to make ourselves into revolutionaries who want to overthrow the system. I think if we look at this notion of rules of handling various phenomena and look at it in terms of dying, our culture has a kind of rule that indicates, suggests, or almost dictates teaching a kind of passivity. We are expected to struggle against death almost until exhaustion sets in; then we are expected to accept death with serenity.

Our culture also has rules for using the phenomena that we are allowed to handle. Again, there are mundane examples to illustrate what I have in mind. Primarily, one is expected to use sex for the purposes of procreation. In terms of death, the individual is not encouraged to use the phenomenon of dying for purposes other than to die. He doesn't have the right to commit suicide and people who take to death-defying behaviors are, in many cases, considered to be mentally ill.

One major area in our society where we are permitted to use the phenomenon of death is connected with the modern state. We can use death against our enemies in war or we can use it to punish people. As far as the individual is concerned, he can use death and dying only under very regulated conditions—when he is a soldier and on the battlefield, face-to-face with the enemy. Other than in that particular circumstance, our culture does not allow people to use death and dying, and I think the idea of the way we handle the phenomenon of death and dying and the uses we make of it, or don't, have severe implications which predispose us to at least make the mourning process a predisposal, to accept death rather than life.

Again, I am interested in this notion of a choosing process. I tried to work out what a model would look like when a person uses mourning or anticipatory mourning to produce death rather than life and what the alternate profits would be when he would choose life over death. I tried to work out some of the major variables. I think when a person takes a passive attitude toward death and he does not use it for social purposes and personal purposes, in a way he begins to almost deny the existence of the phenomenon of dying and he becomes closed as to how this phenomenon works. He lacks the ability to understand the nature of this phenomenon and the properties it has and then he begins to succumb to it. He enters, I think from a social sense, a transitional status of social dying and after that, as part of the mourning process, he enters a situation of acceptance and giving up of himself.

On the other side, I can use mourning as an outcome of life. Rather than the passive, I think I'd take an active attitude toward dying and use it for purposeful goals. This kind of attitude puts the person in a state of denial toward death, setting him into confrontation with it, opening him to the properties of death as a phenomenon just like any other phenomenon in life. Rather than finding himself in the transitional status of social death, he finds himself in a transitional status of rebuilding or reshaping himself, and rather than leading to a state of disintegration, it leads to a state of rebirth. There is literature that stresses the idea of being in a crisis state where there is the potential of destruction or rebirth. Other literature supports the alternative of the mourning process that anticipates rebirth rather than the mourning process that anticipates the death of the self.

Somehow, I feel, we can master the phenomenon of dying by handling it and by using it for our purposes. Somehow, by learning how to handle the phenomenon and using it, we externalize death and make it into an object that is outside of us; and we begin to strip this object of some of the feelings of awe, of mysticism that it has, and that many other objects in our culture had before they were made rational.

What I would like to do is pursue this line of thinking and show how it has applied in my own experience and show how I've handled some of my experiences. I shall select bouts that I've had with death and I'll look at those episodes in terms of the two choices that could have reinforced my sense of dying or reinforced my sense of living. What I experienced in almost all of them was always a field of forces in which both of these were poled as opposites with always the question of a tilt or balance between them. Sometimes the tilt went to the side of dying, but life was still there; sometimes it went way to the sense of life with dying still there.

Before describing the experiences themselves, I want to present a very brief background. I have had three, or maybe four, heart attacks. I had the first heart attack in a subway coming home from a lecture at Columbia, during the rush hour. I was standing, and having great difficulty breathing. It felt like water in my throat—and I was gasping for breath and was very dizzy. I made it home and denied the fact that I had had a heart attack. I went to bed and slept for three whole days, got up, felt good, went back to school, and blamed it on smoking too much.

On election day in 1969, about a month later, I had severe chest pains and since I had stopped smoking, I felt that there was some other cause. I went to the doctor. He said I had had a heart attack. I was hospitalized and went into the CCU. I had the sense of wanting to commit suicide, basically because I had the notion that if my damage was so great as to make me an invalid, I preferred to die. That is a use one makes of death—a choice that I had. I was in the hospital for six weeks.

In January of 1970, about three weeks after I got out of the hospital, I had other heart pains and was hospitalized again. This time it was a false alarm, and I was immersed in self-pity.

About ten months later, in February of 1971, I had a second false alarm. I had the symptoms of a heart attack; however, it turned out that I had jaundice and something wrong with my gall bladder. This was removed, and I was in the hospital about six weeks. I had no thought of death or dying, at that operation. At that point, I found myself ending my state of mourning.

In August of 1971, as I was about to go on vacation, I had a second MI, and it left me with a deep feeling of the premonition of my death—a very severe premonition of it. In September of 1971, about three days before I was to leave the hospital, I had my third MI and I had a feeling of despair, that I was working on my fourth: I vacillated between despair and hope. This experience is still reasonably with me.

All this happened within a period of two years. Before that I was never sick, never conscious of death. I could recall only three recollections of death. One occurred during my Army experience in World War II when I was a combat soldier. The first day in the Army I was put in an Infantry Division. I had a sense of "I won't come out of this alive," although that left me. While cleaning my rifle the night before I went on my first combat mission, I began to cry, had a sense of self-pity, and wrote a letter to my mother, but I tore it up. The third feeling of death was on the assault wave going into this island we were invading. I had a sense of everything around me being unreal, as if I were looking at a movie in which I was one of the actors. I had a sense of detachment for about a half hour and then that disappeared. I had fears of death but never anything more.

The only other feelings of death I had involved my mother's dying. I felt that this was a great gift she was giving to me—the way she died in my presence. I had a sense of a great tragedy, in the classical Greek sense of the word tragedy.

Hence, my general orientation throughout my life up until the time of my heart attacks had been a kind of feeling of unlimited time available to me—a feeling of having a very powerful body whose unlimited energies I could call up at will.

Now I shall discuss some selected experiences in this two-year period with death or with dying and go over them from the point of view of how I responded to them and, perhaps, how they have contributed to my desire to be reborn rather than to mourn my own death.

The first experience took place within the CCU. The impact of having a heart attack did not hit me until I was actually placed in the bed there about two hours after I had been admitted to the hospital. I remember a sense of being completely disinterested in my wife and with my surroundings. I withdrew completely into myself; I had a sense of crawling up into myself, of wrapping myself into a cocoon. My first thought was about how much damage I had, and that if the damage was severe, I would prefer committing suicide. Leading to that was the imagery of my not facing myself as a person with severe damage. But equally important to that were my images of my children (all at that time under fifteen): images like wrestling with my son, of holding my two daughters—and touching them. I didn't want to have my children see me as an invalid. Even now, I don't know if I would have actually committed suicide. But what I do know is that it was a great comforting thought to know that I had this option that things couldn't get so bad that I couldn't cop out if I wanted. I think that that element of control insofar as I exerted it gave me a great deal of strength. It might have even served as a regulator to control the amount of damage I did have.

I wasn't able to get rid of the thought of suicide until I was able to work out, "Supposing I was severely damaged and couldn't do a day's work. What would I do then?" I called up imagery of one of the things I had planned to do when I retire, to tell children's stories. I said, "Aha, I will now have a chance to tell children's stories and make a living at it, and that is something I want to do anyway." When that image came into my mind and I felt it and believed it, I was able to accept the fact that insofar as damages were not crippling, I could accept the heart attack and I didn't have to worry about suicide anymore. So it was the act of coping that made a big difference to me.

The second incident was a more complicated one. It happened about seven or eight days after the first incident. I was taken off the emergency list and transferred from the CCU to the regular medical floor of the hospital. They put me in a room for cardiac patients who had just come out of CCU. It was on the third floor and directly below was an empty lot, where drilling was going on, in preparation for a new mental hospital. Twelve drills were operating at the same time—into stone; and a couple of bulldozers were scraping up the pulverized rocks. The noise was so great that even the head nurse reported that she disliked going into this four-person room because it would give her headaches. The physician of the patient next to me said that when he put the stethoscope to the patient's heart, he could not hear the heartbeat. The patient next to me said that he had gotten out of the CCU the day before I did and the noise was causing him heart pain. I called up a friend of mine and was talking with him when he asked, "What's the noise in the background there?" It was sort of loud.

I became very angry at the noise and told the intern, "Hey, you know, the noise is hurting me." The intern said patronizingly, "No, don't worry about it." I took other action for about two or three days, but nothing really happened so I went "on strike." I refused to eat, I refused to take medication, I refused to have the doctor treat me. It wasn't an act I planned to do. All I had planned to do was take certain actions, like calling up the Board of Health and asking them to send a noise inspector down, talking to the administrator, and things like that. I made three demands of the hospital: (1) that they put an audiometer on the window and measure the decibels of sound and give that to a physiologist and let him decide whether or not it was harmful; (2) that they give the patients earplugs; and (3) that they call in a noise consultant and have him offer suggestions on how to reduce the noise. I think I made seven or eight of those demands and said that I would pay for everything. All were turned down and I was intimidated in many different ways. I stayed on strike for three days until they finally met the demands. The point is that I had the feeling I was being coerced into accepting something that I knew and felt to be harmful to me. I felt that this was wrong. I felt too that I was being stripped of the rights of an adult—the physicians, in effect, would pat me on the head and say, "Don't worry about it little boy," and I looked at the physician and said, "Your treating me is a privilege I grant you, and if I can't trust you, I don't want to have anything to do with you." I think that in the way they were treating me they were trying to induce me to accept something that was harmful to me and to strip me of my status as a human being. I fought that.

The curious thing I found was that the weaker I became physically, the stronger I became mentally, and somehow this behavior helped me maintain myself as a social person and helped me cope with the damage that had been done to my identity as a result of the heart attack. It introduced me to the therapeutic value of protest behavior.

The third incident occurred in the summer, about seven months after that attack. My family came from Vermont; my children were born there. I had done a lot of mountain climbing at Stowe and Camel's Hump, which I guess is about the biggest mountain in Vermont. Somehow this mountain had a mystical meaning to me, so I took my family there. We decided to climb mountains, particularly Camel's Hump. I remember walking up the mountain and getting to the point where my heart started to pound very severely, and I thought of the advice of my physician, "Watch out." My heart is pounding, and if I follow his advice, "Watch out," I have an image of myself as limited in capacity. I didn't like that image and kept worrying. It came to the point where my heart was racing faster and I said to myself, "The hell with it! I'm going to risk it." I pushed myself a little more and got my second wind and kept climbing. I didn't get to the top of Camel's Hump, but I had the sensation of having my heart pound as fast as it had in the past and yet it didn't fall apart. It gave me an exhilarated feeling, that I was back to where I had been before. This was the first time I had the notion that I am now who I was before I had the attack—not completely, but close to that. I felt at that moment that it was worth the risk.

The other incident—the gall bladder operation, was an exploratory laparotomy; they didn't know in the beginning that it was gall bladder; they thought it might be something else because I had jaundice and other complications. Throughout the whole experience, I had no thoughts of death or dying although I went into the operating room. It leads to a very interesting idea, that the thoughts of dying are specific to diseases, that they are learned in connection with specific diseases.

It was June 17, 1970, that I first became aware that I had been mourning and had now ceased to mourn.

In July of 1971, I had the sensation of being caught in this life-death tug and had a sensation that I was on the side of life now. I had a sense of dying to be reborn.

I had my second MI in August of 1971. The strongest feeling I had then was of being abandoned. I had a premonition of death, and I had a premonition of being abandoned. I thought about it and said, "Now why the hell would I feel abandoned?" Then I went back in my own life when I was an infant, and realized that apparently rejection had played an important part in terms of my makeup. This gave me one of the clearer insights I had into the phenomenon of death, that I was able to experience abandonment very deeply. I was able to, as I was experiencing it, pull myself away from my experience and say, "Why am I experiencing this?" Then I was able to kind of backtrack over my life and tried to account for it. It gave me a terrific mastery of the notion of death.

I had a third MI a month and a half after the second, two or three days before I was to be discharged from the hospital. I was in the rehabilitation unit, and the first thought I had was that I didn't want to go back to the medical ward. I always wanted to collect notes on my experiences and write about what a hospital looks like from a patient's point of view. I had a dignity, and I wanted a place where I could do it in dignity. I wanted that room I was in. I insisted that although it didn't have the fancy equipment, I wanted to stay there. That is, I chose the ground on which I wanted to fight, and I think that strengthened me a great deal.

During this time I had been doing a lot of reading about religion, specifically Martin Buber, a man who interested me a great deal. I became concerned about "Do I believe in God or don't I?" Emotionally, I really did want to believe in God, and I asked myself that question in that tense situation. I really did want to believe in God but I can't. There would be more respect for me and for Him if He really exists, and I did believe. This, too, is an act of confrontation, and it gave me a sense of dignity in a situation that was very distressful.

About three days later, I had a dream that I was lying flat on my back in a hotel room and a man came through the door. All I could see of him was from his head to his chest. He had a smile on his face and it was a beckoning smile. At first I thought the man was a thief, and then I looked at him and said, "My God! It's the messenger of Death. He's come to take me." It frightened me very much and I got up; and in that state between waking and sleeping, I said, "I'm frightened, I'm frightened that if I don't go back and talk with that messenger, I'll be trembling for the rest of the days of my life." I went back to sleep and hunted for the messenger of Death. His face was vivid to me then, and it still is. I remember seeking him out. I had a long argument or confrontation with him. The essence of it is: "Look, I'm not ready. When I am ready, then I'll call you." Even now, I have the feeling of him lurking at the edges of my life.

After that came the experience of "I had the third, I'm working on the fourth" and it said why the hell should I get over the third or fourth, depending upon the way you count it, in 22 months? This gave me the idea that, "Well, if I develop some kind of curve, I'll be getting the next one in a few more months." This led me to great despair and a sense of doom. I followed that path for several days, about a week, and I think I found at the end of the path just a dark door—just more gloom and despair. It wasn't a productive way to look at it, nor was that predictive way of looking at it productive. I toyed with the idea in my mind about the connection between science and fate and looking at the physician as a scientist-priest, and that essentially he is both; he has a role pair and not a single role. There are times when you are caught in this kind of bind. I think the way I was able to look at it or get out of it was to recognize that if I phrase it in terms that I'm working on the fourth, it can lead only to doom and despair which are nonproductive. I was looking for a way to create a feeling of some kind of optimism, or some kind of hope. I couldn't take the path of a myth because it gave me the sense of some sort of unreality. When I was caught in the dilemma of either being in a sense unreal or in despair, I opted for despair. I think I prefer being psychologically depressed than psychologically crazy.

I had a bout called a hypoventilation incident, and what it essentially was that the deeper I breathed in, the less air I was taking in. I caught myself gasping for breath and I couldn't breathe. I caught my body quivering and quaking. I found my body in very violent motion, and I said to myself, "So this is how I'm going to die." I had a sense of observing myself in this state. It was odd. I felt a little frightened, but I think I felt comforted that I could look at myself and say, "This is how the end is coming."

There was some connection between what I was doing then and what I was doing when I felt abandoned. At least when I felt abandoned, I had worked out a way of seeing and coping that I then used for this incident.

A physician was called in, and he wasn't able to account for my symptoms. One of the assumptions was that in an MI there are enzymes and chemicals being given off and some of those chemicals might act as a foreign body, coming into your system, causing the attack. The doctors weren't able to find out, and so what happened remained undiagnosed. As a result, I felt that somehow I could put my experiences into a perspective that I chose, and I could look at myself while I am experiencing a very, very frightful thing. I could choose whether to be open to it or to deny it, and somehow openness seemed to give me more strength.

These are only selected experiences and what they've led me to are some observations about the notion of handling and using the phenomenon of death. I think one of the characteristics of handling the matter is whether one denies it or whether one is open to it. Somehow, I felt openness worked for me and it might have been one of the factors that contributed to what I think was my sense of being reborn rather than of dying. I also found that what the specific content of death, what it appears in my experiences—one concept is the fear of being abandoned—is that it is produced by whatever my past experiences had been. It's produced in many, many different ways, and the content is probably different for different people, depending upon whether one confronts death or whether one succumbs to it. Also, it is different if one takes an active stance in relation to the phenomenon.

The other thing I found is that there are pattern-shapers. The house staff of the hospital are in many ways the shapers of the pattern of death. A good example is, I think, when I was in a state of hypoventilation. I guess I was a very horrible sight to look at—a human body bouncing up and down in an uncontrollable fashion. The nurse who was taking care of me never returned. She said she was going to call the doctor. She called him and never came back. When you see a nurse and then you don't see her, it gives you the feeling that something severe is happening. Even the physician, a house guy, would distance himself from me quite a bit. His distancing himself from me also served to shape some of the structure of the pattern.

I think that when one takes a passive stance for handling and using a phenomenon, one isn't allowed to get to know death as a phenomenon that is shapable, rather than as a force which one has to succumb to. In contrast, when one takes an active stand, I think it allows the individual to know the phenomenon of death just as he knows any other phenomenon—sex or what have you— and to take an attitude toward it, and in a lot of ways to shape the phenomenon, to make use of the properties of that phenomenon for social purposes. What I am suggesting is that death can be made into an object and is an object the same way any other natural and social phenomenon can be made to have the properties of an object. When you have a passive handling of the death phenomenon, mourning leads to a giving up of self, and to viewing onself as nothingness, and to a distintegration of self.

Death is awesome, it's mystical, it is something you succumb to. In the passive way of handling it, one enters or one creates for oneself a social position in a sociological sense of social death as a separate and distinct social status. If one takes an active stance in relation to death, one has the sense that "I can handle the phenomenon in such a way as to make it reveal its properties to me and then I can use these properties to understand death and to advance my own psychological social purposes." This kind of active way of handling mourning, I think, leads to a reinterpretation of self, and if not a mastery of death (maybe that's being too ambitious) at least to a feeling that you don't have to succumb to it, that "I know it, I understand it." Death, then, assumes certain properties, and it assumes the properties of an object that is secular rather than sacred. And like any other secular object, it can be mastered and it can be noble. The last thing, I think one enters a social position—rather than a social death—of rebirth.

I'd like to mention some of the properties of death, of dying that I've come to experience. (Maybe properties is the wrong word to use, maybe it's more like the meanings.) One of the properties I found about death—again I'm thinking of the abandonment situation—is that it seems to call forth a return to unresolved conflicts of infancy and youth, a fear of abandonment and a fear of poverty, and many other fears that I had in this state. I could pick out the point in my life when they came about and somehow this phenomenon seemed to call into play the unresolved conflicts I had experienced.

The other property of death is that it leaves one with a damaged or spoiled identity. Death means, "I am what I do not want to be; I am frightened, helpless, vulnerable, dependent."

A third property of death seems to be a summary judgment

of how well I have lived my life. Throughout many of the times, I had a sense of a poorly lived life and a good deal of my mourning had to do with that.

A fourth property of death, at least from the point of view of coping with death, seems to be the property of the need to reaffirm life. I'll give a couple of examples and then get into the point I want to make. Whenever I felt close to dying, it wasn't myself I was most concerned about. The first time I had a dream of dying (this was at the time of my first MI) I had a vision of my son, who was 14 at the time; I felt him unprepared for life. In my dream I saw him unprepared for life and suffering—it was as if I were an onlooker, unable to do anything to alleviate the suffering of someone I loved dearly.

At the third MI, I cried for my youngest daughter (then 12). I felt that somehow she was not prepared for life. I never had this feeling about my middle child (I felt that she was okay). However, I was worried about the fate of my survivors. I was also worried in a great way, more than I recognized, about whether the world would survive, whether civilization would survive. I remember going back to where I grew up (the Lower East Side of New York) and I remember going back to the building where I spent my childhood and sitting on the stoop of the building—by this time there were all Puerto Ricans and blacks living there. I saw a Puerto Rican woman who must have been the age of my mother when we had lived there, and who had a son who must have been my age when I lived there, and the son was carrying a package of groceries up for the mother. I said, "My God! Although it is Puerto Rican now and it was Jewish then, I have faith in these people, they seem to be good." It was a great relief for me—it is not important that I die, because somehow civilization remains. Maybe I am stressing it crudely, but I can pick out four or five incidents where the concept of immortality is not that of the individual but of the race, of civilization, of society.

Another property of death is as an ascribed status that people give you, and I call it in a lot of ways a coffin-status or coffin-category. As people tell me, "Don't go out in the cold," or "Don't work too hard"—things like that—one feels like the unfortunate one, and it is something I don't like. And sometimes that ascribed status can link one onto a status of social death of which invalidism is one property.

The last property of death, and the one that is most meaningful to me, is that death is a spur to solving an identity crisis and to remaking one's own identity. This I have felt strongly.

28

Two Men, Four Episodes
Yvonne M. Parnes

IF CANCER IS considered a killer, coronary incident is viewed as a crippler. Though not mutilating the body image surgically, it alters the mind, imposing sanctions. It is essential from the onset of the coronary to recognize that we cannot divide the patient into mind and body. We must incorporate the science and the art of treating the patient. To cure the body expecting the mind to follow is to ignore suffering.

The similar experiences of two early middle-aged men and their compromise with cardiovascular disease are presented here. To be determined is whether cushioning to prolong life expectancy does indeed encourage one to miss the meaning of life. What is the meaning of life? It is decidedly different things to different people. The search for the magic in life that eludes some may be identified by others as what they have. They may argue that life-threatening disease teaches one to appreciate what is theirs. They may rationalize that in an attempt to broaden themselves they produced the abnormal relationship with their environment resulting in arteriosclerosis. They cannot risk continuing to evolve as they had before their illness. Thomas Hobbes tells us that "men are too fearful of death to give much thought to freedom." Some, invalided, capitulate and become patients.

Not to return to the work one left prior to hospitalization may be a statement affirming previous lack of success, satisfaction, or productivity. Falling back on the security of insurance, resigning to remove challenge or confrontation with chance that being in business means, must be examined as a defection from living. Here is the crutch one may have been looking for—the shelter provided by disease—an umbrella acknowledged by society, endorsed by the medical establishment, and approved! Truly life can still be a gift, not in quality but possibly in quantity, if one organizes one's daily routine to adjust to the sanctions imposed by a coronary episode. Surely, if one lives "properly," getting prescribed amounts of exercise, rest and food, one rationalizes that one has not violated a regimen and will be rewarded with no further attack. If it does occur, accompanying it is increased psychological trauma as to why and how this could have recurred in one who played the game according to the rules.

L. was stricken dramatically on the golf course and was rushed to a CCU where a theatrical wait began. He was not Type A to the eye. Good looking, a charmer, popular in school, he seemed a Peter Pan! His business involved salesmanship and he became proficient in the skills. He mixed well, entertained, provided, procured, and sipped the wine that brought the orders in. If he slept too little, ate and drank too much, played too hard, traveled at a fast pace, it was demanded by competition. He had achieved the status he had been seeking, and consensus of opinion was that hard work and play, coupled with inherited qualities from his mother, who died at 50 from sudden coronary disease, gave him his attack.

After recovering, he gradually resumed the directorship of his company, with policing by his wife, until one year later a second episode pointed to surgery. Following successful surgery, he defected, supplemented by great disability insurance and a wife who agreed to resignation from life because of the status it also afforded her. No longer would he travel without her, so her fears of any lack of stability in the marriage vanished. One may also rationalize that it was not a bad trade: a reconstructed heart, a tax-free monthly income, a husband always there, requiring her care, and security—financial and psychological. Threat of other episodes always concerned her, but day-to-day worries were something she could cope with.

They joined the select group who follow the sun, the "heart condition" crew who live in fear, contemplate risks, and are crippled because the body has healed but the mind cannot recognize it. Gone is *raison d'être* except to survive! What is survival when what is necessary to support life is provided but goals are eliminated? Society fails when it provides greater financial reward to prolong invalidism than to stimulate purpose.

Large firms and financially secure executives usually have the cushion—disability insurance. Tax-free monthly sums are paid when the holder of such a policy is unable to work. Often the determination of when persons recovered from coronary incident may return to work falls into a gray area. With checks arriving monthly is it feasible to attempt to return to work, knowing that illness may strike again? Even those renewed with surgical bypass, giving life to dead vessels, cannot be assured. The productive years may be over and one succumbs because need has been eliminated. Psychologically that may be more crippling than the disease itself.

Logical adjustment on an individual basis should be considered. If a person does work that interferes with a well-ordered life, regular mealtimes, continuous sleep, and adequate rest, could not some readjustment be made to benefit from one's skills without jeopardizing one's well-being? Perpetuating the memory of illness daily serves to warn that venturing outside of the secure environment may spell disaster. Despite two episodes and cardiac surgery, this man has not confronted his mortality, validating the Peter Pan image perceived before his illness.

Conversely, we recognize the fragility of life, and the recipient of the disability checks may have tongue in cheek. He is secure with income, food, and shelter. His medical history assures him of superior health care because he is watched carefully by his physician. He has it made, or does he? One can adjust to being a professional patient. His self-esteem, rather than declining because he is not producing, can be elevated because the attention he receives says, "I am important to my family. They will do anything, go anywhere, to keep me alive." Eventually, he believes it, substituting impetus for passive security. The dimensions of his world become smaller, but safe. When the disability payments stop at 65, social security will take over.

D., an orthodontist, seemed to fade as his father had. It was no surprise that angina-type pain and a visit to the Emergency Room preceded his admission for a heart attack, diagnosed later. He coped for four years, modifying continually. A second episode convinced him of the need to gamble on cardiac catheterization and surgery if possible. He explored every avenue, weighing his options until he found the situation least threatening, most comfortable for him and his family. He describes various giants of car-

diac surgery, practicing mass-production medicine. Deper-
sonalization! One of them was L.'s surgeon and L.'s security
hinged on the fact that his doctor did many cases each day. He
did not mind becoming a number. He thought he was buying experience. "After all, when we get in there, we're all alike."

D. opted for not dividing mind and body. He chose those
who recognized who he was and finally had surgery at a progressive, midwestern medical marvel. His preoperative teaching included the members of his family. L. had had no inkling that this
would happen and states that if he had known, he would have
run. D. was walking on day four post-op and flew home on day
nine. He alludes to nothing but looking ahead, while L. takes one
day at a time, hoping to duplicate the day before. L. is aware of
every bodily change, overly concerned with self, not even allowing for the small quirks of middle age that would be accepted by
anyone else. Again, the Peter Pan syndrome! The scar, running
the length of his chest, may have faded from his body but not
from his mind. It serves as a reminder of what must be avoided at
all cost and is psychologically conditioning. The scar is Pavlov's
bell! Some thrive on routine. It is easier to do the same thing at
the same time every day. It too reduces risk, promising reward
(life) for adherence to "what is best for you." One may feed the
mind with the latest literature, regulate the body, but when in-
centive is withdrawn, only a robot remains, removed from a living
environment.

D.'s recovery was swift, and his wife returned to work as he
planned also to do. She protected her station, because society
accepted her with less question as his wife. Otherwise, she investigated the new status of women, exercised her liberation, and
gave only what was required to continue their arrangement. Perhaps this less than overprotectiveness was just what the patient
needed. He had to go on living, producing, earning (although he
had similar insurance), or he would have been alone. He took his
bypasses as a second chance and improved. He knew of the existence of a third, occluded vessel that could not be revised, but he
felt secure. Life still held enchantment. He was not impeded by
the past nor obviously threatened by the future.

As an orthodontist, was his comprehension of the cardiovascular system more sophisticated than L.'s, the businessman? Or from the initial pre-op clearance, was he convinced that
all he needed to get well was surgical adjustment? He had every-

thing else: a lucrative profession that continued to be challenging and a provocative marital situation. He could not consider anything else because limited living was never his style, and his object in the search was to buy time to continue to be productive, not merely to breathe.

The lack of patient education in hospital is one area to blame. Many institutions have recognized the need to "include the patient in." To understand what has happened to the patient, we must continually explain what we are doing in an attempt to save life, heal the damaged heart muscle, restore the ability to live, and return the patient to familiar environs. The informed patient is less anxious, more cooperative, more willing to participate in rehabilitation. It is necessary to decrease the doctor's omnipotency and achieve rapport so that the patient believes all are working for him. It is conveying that we care! That is why we chose to become partners in the caring professions. Somewhere in the educational process the original initiative is lost, and the most human component needed in treating people is gone. It is not irretrievable.

With all the sophisticated technology we employ to recoup after the coronary incident, the human factor remains perhaps dominant. Fear must be coped with. Dependency on machines is depersonalizing. The patient must understand that caregivers are supervising those machines and are available. It is not enough to reassure that we are watching; it is important to touch.

Does the anxious patient adjust to the presence of the monitor, sound off or on? Fantasy accompanies the medications given, as well as depression in realizing what has happened. Once we can stabilize the patient—and, in the frantic period of accomplishing this, learn to diminish our own anxieties—rehabilitation can begin. This must also be conveyed to the family, continually, in employing them as part of the team.

As with Reach to Recovery, volunteers from the heart clubs should be organized with a set protocol to visit heart patients, families, and cardiac surgical patients. How effective it would be if the volunteer serving coffee in the CCU waiting room were a rehabilitated heart-club member. The time then spent by families, instead of being intensified toward concerns, problems, fears, could be used in anticipation of hope toward recovery and rehabilitation. The time could teach families their role in the care of their loved one, *temporarily* invalided. It could plant the seeds toward believing that an active life is possible. In educating the waiting family, caregivers provide them with the tools to stimulate—not to commiserate with—the patient.

In permitting the CCU waiting room to become a group arena for comparison of symptoms, identification of problems that may never arise—based on stories of others' past experiences—we brew despair. We must initiate hope. We should educate families—and the patient—by lecture, audiovisual materials on the nature of coronary disease, and instructions on how the heart heals to return to normal patterns of living. The hospital fails too often to make proper use of the time spent in such waiting rooms.

Most patients do not have the option of security that disability insurance can offer. It then becomes part of the care plan to provide for rehabilitation as thoroughly as intensive care planning is provided for. This will begin in the hospital. The goals to be evaluated by the medical team evolve from adjustments in lifestyle to eliminate old habits which produce the coronary threats inherent in an affluent society. Substituted must be new routines that will become habit, as in preventative medicine. Medical care should encourage patients to be reviewed in advance of disease, so that screening procedures can identify risks, in order for steps to be taken as a way to avoid massive occurrences. As research identifies the causes of the syndrome leading to such insults, we can refine our system of health care so that those falling into high-risk categories can be better protected. The availability of such protection should be equitable, for it is the preservation of the future.

29

Commemoration Wishes

Nathan Lefkowitz

I FEEL THAT I'm down the homestretch. Not that death is waiting for me but that I'm in a critical zone in which I could turn to life or to death. Last night I had several ventricular irregularities which I interpret as a bad omen. It may be the precursor of an arrhythmia of the heart attack or it may make an open-heart surgery more risky. Yesterday morning I was told that I would be going up to the medical floor. This morning I was told that they still want to observe me. I felt like making a bowel movement. The aide put me on a commode. While I sat on it, he said that I should not have been on it but should be kept on complete bed rest. Another ominous sign—complete bed rest. I had some shortness of breath on the commode and some tingling in the chest area. I don't know if these are signs of anxiety or signs of angina.

The aide asked me if I were going to have open-heart surgery and asked if the surgeon had been in yet. I asked, "What have you heard?" and it took him aback, as if secret information had been leaked. He said, "I heard your arteries are in bad shape." He shaved me this morning, which pleased me, for now I can make a presentable appearance to Sarah Lynn, my older daughter.

I will have to talk to the children this morning about my plans for burial, should I die. I told my brother Irving and sister, Edith, that I would like to be buried at the cemetery with Mom and Dad. I will tell the children that I want a plain, simple coffin and a prayer by an Orthodox rabbi but no eulogy. I cannot see a rabbi who knows nothing of me summarize my life for me. Perhaps in the days of old when the rabbi was a teacher and was close to his congregation, he could eulogize the dead one. But today that is only a ritual.

My wish is to have my immediate family, made up of my wife and three children, my two brothers and my sister, Edith, and their children gather in a circle around the coffin, be it open or closed. Each should speak his or her piece about me and their relationship to me. Let them not eulogize me, but let them speak of the encounters we have had together and the imprints upon each other. Let this not be something to be said once in one or two sentences. On the contrary, let each speak when moved—say their say. Let there be silence; and let the second person who is moved speak his piece. Let this procedure be repeated until the summary of my life has been accomplished to each one's satisfaction. Let the tone of the meeting be one of the living experience, where people feel the tragedy of death and the beauty of life. Let them think of the concept of tragedy in the Greek sense rather than the American modern sense. More accurately, let them think of it in the Hebraic sense, in the sense of the prophets. Let them be guided by the words of Isaiah. As I remember this prophet said, "And we shall conquer death."

Let dying and death bring out the highest of spirituality in each member of my family. Let them stamp out pity toward themselves or toward me. Let them stamp out notions of injustice by God toward themselves or toward me. Let them stamp out the idea that my life has been cut short and is incomplete. Let them be guided by the thought that I have lived my life as a search, whose aim in the end has been to understand how humans can build a consciousness that helps them construct a reality that is inhabitable by humans—that which manifests love and justice and truth. Let them realize that I came to the end of my search, but that I am merely passing on the baton to others, who will continue it in either my form or any other form that is meaningful to them.

Yes, I would have liked to have simulated or culminated in more than the general ideas which are locked within me. Yes, I would have liked the opportunity to communicate the wisdom I have arrived at. But yes, I thank God and thank my fellowmen and my families for their aid in promoting my search. I feel content because the essence of life is doing, is becoming, rather than completing or being completed. God is one who creates rather than one who has created. If all He had done was to create once and for all, He would have died at birth. In the human world, man creates and recreates. When I say my life has been devoted to searching, I mean to learning how humans can create a human reality that they find to be livable.

Finally, let my dying be a gift—a gift that spurs each of you individually and together to seek out that which you individually and together wish to make *your* life's quest. Do not duplicate mine. Not because it has been unworthy or unfruitful, but because each of us has to find our own quest. To duplicate mine would merely be to try in vain to perpetuate my life in a form in which it can no longer be lived. Do not fear, it will be lived in another form beyond what we are able to conceive of. In conclusion, on my tombstone, put the inscription, "A searcher for a livable human reality."

I am making these preparations, not because I think I'm going to die, but because I am in sadness, and death is a possibility—a reasonable possibility. I am stronger now spiritually than I have ever been and will end that way. Tears roll from my eyes as I speak, and sadness oozes from me. Yet, I feel released by speaking and comforted by speaking these thoughts. It is my way of gathering my psychological and spiritual resources to climb the mountain I will be facing in the next few days or few weeks, or however long it takes. My family: please rest assured that I will fight and fight harder for life, but yet I will surrender to death in the midst of battle. If my life depends upon my will, all will go well.

As a last thought and as a precaution, let there be no argument or cause for argument over any of the wishes I have described above about the ceremony. If some favor an open coffin and others do not, let there not be an open coffin. I care not if I am commemorated before or after I am put into the ground. Should one person have strong feelings on any of these, then let that one thing be eliminated. (I have in mind the open or shut coffin, or having the coffin open while family members are talking about me.) In addition, if the rabbi must make a eulogy as part of the ceremony, let it be a simple one that would not violate my tastes.

EDITORS' NOTE: *Dr. Lefkowitz died in Israel in January 1978 during the course of a month-long visit, his first trip there. Before he became ill, he attended a Martin Buber Festival and traveled by himself through the country—fully aware that death might be imminent. His wife, son, and daughters were with him when he died in a hospital and arranged to have his final wishes carried out—one was that he be buried in Israel.*

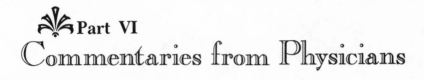

Part VI

Commentaries from Physicians

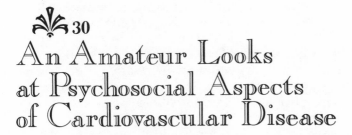

30
An Amateur Looks at Psychosocial Aspects of Cardiovascular Disease

Irvine H. Page

YOU ARE ENTITLED to my credentials. I am not a psychologist, psychiatrist, sociologist, or philosopher. I have been actively engaged in medicine for over 50 years, have seen countless patients with cardiovascular disease, have been editor of the Coronary Club Bulletin for four years, have answered myriad unsolicited letters from the public, and had a myocardial infarction all my own nine years ago.

Hypertension and coronary disease often rank with bronchopneumonia as the old, or debilitated, person's deliverer. Death from hypertension usually results from stroke or myocardial infarction, and coronary disease regularly causes myocardial infarction. Death in this manner is not always easy but it is to be preferred to that from acts of violence and terrorism.

Provided death is not hindered, when it is inevitable, by meddlesome medical care or ethics innocent of compassion and common sense, death from cardiovascular disease usually is a tranquil process.

Since I know nothing of the psychological mechanisms involved, I can only relate my own experiences gained from patients, their families, the public, and interviews with myself.

I am convinced that many people do not really fear death, they only regret that it must occur. Personally, I am more curious about the unknown than afraid of it. If there is nothing after death, I shall never know it—and if there is, I do not shun it. On a number of occasions I have been told by patients of their premonition of death and then have seen it occur. There was no fear involved.

What most younger people do not realize is that as one ages, the competitive spirit is replaced by noncompetitive serenity. Unlike patients with cancer, those with heart disease are seldom faced with a foreseeable time of death. Hope is engendered in the cardiac patient by the possibility that a more hygienic regimen will prolong life. In some circumstances, surgical operations may be life-saving. Then too, modern antihypertensive drug therapy has been very successful. In short, there is a great deal that can be done for these patients if they are willing to participate faithfully and intelligently in the prescribed treatment.

The purpose of the Coronary Club Incorporated, for example, is to provide guidance and understanding derived from firsthand information and experience to those who want to avoid cardiovascular disease or to live with it.

The families of cardiac patients must also learn to participate in the therapy. I have for many years required my patients to take and record their own blood pressures. If low-salt, low-cholesterol diets are prescribed, then everyone in the family can learn to enjoy them, especially since they may well benefit by them. The motivation to regular exercise and rest also will be greatly strengthened by family participation.

There need be no secrets in the diagnosis of cardiovascular disease, its treatment, or its prevention. Patients should be encouraged to voice their fears (of dying suddenly in a strange place or while driving an automobile). They should also be encouraged to ask for expert advice when in doubt, because fortunately this is readily available.

I realize I have said nothing new, but I hope it gives a quick view of the problem as physicians see it. The effort to be human is the only psychosocial aspect I try to fulfill.

❀ 31
Responsibility of the Physician in the Preservation of Life

Franklin H. Epstein

BECAUSE HOSPITAL INTENSIVE care units are in some ways the epitome of modern medical technology, they are often the focus of the questions that doctors and nurses must ask themselves from time to time about the very reason for their existence. Anguished relatives wait in the wings, expecting and fearing that death will come and sometimes disappointed that it does not. In an attempt to relieve what are felt as unbearable pressures, physicians in charge of such units are tempted to assert their sole right to determine when life has lost its meaning for their patients, and to decide when care can be given over, the plug pulled. It was easier thirty or forty years ago in the days of therapeutic nihilism. Then, for many more patients than at present, the matter seemed to be out of our hands. There were fewer decisions to be made and a gentle manner and firm, wise countenance did wonders for the doctor and the family, if not for the patient. "Pneumonia," said Dr. William Osler, "is the friend of the aged." Antibiotics were yet to come, blood transfusions were given in homeopathic amounts, and mechanical respiratory assistance was almost unheard of. It was easy to let an old man die and even to believe that it was God's will that he go quickly.

But it is harder for us. We have become, some feel, too successful in rescuing life. For some perverse reason, God has made respirators and antibiotics available, and we don't know whether Osler (or God) would call them friends of the aged or not. Liberal clergymen talk easily of "the right to die" with all the fervor of a Rousseau declaiming the natural rights of man. And on this subject every reporter and perhaps every lawyer has recently become a philosopher.

I should like to detail briefly some of the special considerations that will be appreciated best by doctors and nurses, why my own years in the care of desperately, often hopelessly, ill patients have led me to espouse the rule: When efficacious treatment is at hand, try as hard as you can. The doctor's duty is to his patient, to relieve his suffering and preserve his life.

1. *Pain can be relieved.* With proper care and modern techniques, physical pain can be assuaged in almost every instance. If necessary to relieve pain, a patient can be put to sleep or made drowsy for most of the day. Excruciating pain is almost never present in dying patients and when it is, it can be controlled. There is a clear distinction between putting a person to sleep and taking his life.

2. *"Dignity in death."* Talk about a "dignified death" usually comes from onlookers, not from the patient. Most patients want to live, need to have some hope of staying the inevitable end, and need to feel that their doctor is helping to keep hope alive. Dignity lies in their fight for life and in their struggle to maintain contact with humanity. Kindness, personal attention, and good nursing help to preserve a patient's dignity. Euthanasia for old people whose bodily functions and control are failing relieves primarily the distress of the relatives, not that of the patient.

3. *The doctor is not omniscient.* Doctors are fallible. Their wisdom tends to be greatly exaggerated by the popular press and too often by doctors themselves. Patients have an enormous need to feel that their doctors can prognosticate with great accuracy, but the kindest, best-intentioned doctor is often wrong. Moreover, a doctor's prognosis tends to be weighted toward pessimism, because patients who do badly claim most of his time and attention and remain in his memory longer than those who do well.

Doctors in charge of intensive care units have a special problem to overcome in that their training and experience is often heavily weighted toward the care of acute emergency illness rather than that of chronically ill patients. When an old man with chronic cardiopulmonary disease and acute bronchitis is placed on a respirator, the expectations of the nurses and doctors may be attuned to the usual prompt recovery of a young postoperative patient with respiratory failure rather than to the slow convalescence of a chronic pulmonary cripple.

It is tragic to see life support withdrawn because of a mixture of impatience and ignorance. Equally tragic is the assumption that an incurable but indolent illness is causing new symptoms, when in fact a coincidental curable disease is at fault. The best way to ensure that a cure is not overlooked is to make it very hard for the doctor to give up.

4. *The doctor is an interested party.* Psychological pressures on the doctor caring for terminally ill patients conspire against his impartiality. The doctor suffers when the patient doesn't get well and his suffering ends when the patient dies. It is hard to appreciate how difficult it is to attempt to support a dying patient day after day with condolence and hope; how frustrating to contemplate months of decline, of weary and anxious relatives, of *nothing working.* Doctors and nurses know the overwhelming sense of relief that comes when on hurrying to the patient's room, steeling oneself to face the ordeal of a patient's not getting better, you learn that death has arrived, unexpectedly, an hour earlier. The sense of relief can be so intense that it is hard to remember that the patient cannot share it.

5. *The doctor's contract.* Our obligation to assuage the pain of our patients is sometimes discussed as if it involved an equal obligation to minimize suffering of relatives, friends, and other onlookers. In fact, much of the "suffering" of terminally ill patients from nasal oxygen tubes and intravenous drips exists only in the imagination of shocked relatives who are sickened and frightened by unfamiliar procedures and apparatus. The doctor must remember that he has only one client—the patient. He is the advocate of the patient—not of the family, nor the welfare agency, nor the kindly clergyman, squeamish at the sight of tracheostomy.

6. *Useless treatments.* If we are indeed obligated to do everything we can to preserve our patients' lives, then we have a special and balancing obligation to evaluate our expensive methods of treatment in impartial, prospective studies, so that resources will not

be unnecessarily squandered. It should be clear that when life is irretrievable, useless treatments should not be employed. But ad hoc judgments about the "quality of life" should be discouraged as a major factor in such decisions.

In the best hospitals, the principle that human life itself has dignity and worth will inform all of the actions in every department. To maintain that attitude is the unique responsibility of the medical profession. In the last analysis, that attitude may be as important for society as any miracle that modern technical medicine can perform. Death always comes at last, despite our best efforts. But the little we can do carries a message to our patients and to the world: Human beings are important. Humanity is to be preserved.

32

Death

George E. Burch

DEATH, AN INEVITABLE event for all living things, has not received the attention of scientists and physicians that it warrants. The biologic phenomenon itself has been studied extremely little, regardless of its cause. This is an astonishing fact. Such a universal biologic phenomenon deserves much greater attention. Death among patients with heart disease, as with almost all diseases, can be: slow and chronic, rapid or subacute, or sudden or acute. These are all different clinical states. All three have quite different effects upon the dying person, as well as upon family and associates and friends. The effects involve emotional, financial, business, domestic, marital, political, and future security for the family—as well as family readjustments and many other innumerable factors of varying importance. Death of an important member of the family is a tremendous and catastrophic event for any family. The family's reaction to an illness of one of its members must always be seriously and properly considered by the physician.

Death is a simple and apparently not unpleasant phenomenon (Burch et al., 1968). It is the process of dying that offers more difficulties to all concerned. It is at this time that the physician's role is most important. The "art" of medicine, bedside manner and attitude, and its interaction with bereaved, emotionally disturbed, and concerned people becomes extremely important. The visits to the bedside and with the patient's family and friends become most important when the disease is incurable and irreversible, and hopelessness becomes a part of the emotional consideration. The visits to the bedside must be frequent and pleasant and must reflect optimism to the patient and some hope, yet honesty, to the family. The physician should prepare the family for the worst, with willingness to help and support the family in many little ways. At this time, little things count enormously. The situation and behavior differ for patients who have been under the doctor's care for many months or years from the situation and behavior for patients seen by the physician during their last illness for the first time. These differences are readily evident. In the first instance, the patient and family are usually known fairly well by the physician, whereas, in the latter instance, the patient and family are strangers to the physician in the midst of one of humanity's most serious problems. The management of the dying patient and family requires proper and satisfactory background, childhood, early adulthood, and attitude toward people of the physician himself—experience with people under *all* circumstances, both happy and sad ones. Some people do not have the personality required to be a compassionate doctor—this is readily obvious during the premedical training period. The selection of undergraduate students for medicine is based primarily upon grades, tests, and computerized psychiatric evaluations, but personality and personal character traits are relegated to the background.

Doctors Treat People with Disease States

A physician must know the signs of impending death. The earlier he recognizes the approach of death, the better he can manage the associated problems. Dying can be an extremely gradual event or a sudden catastrophic one. The family appreciates a knowledge of its approach and often responds hysterically when it occurs suddenly or without advance knowledge. Here again the physician is the pivotal person. He must be prepared and able to answer questions truthfully, and not be reluctant to permit or invite consultant physicians of the family's choosing or upon request. It is even better to initiate the family's interest in a consultation. This has a tremendous and soothing influence on the family and even on the patient. When a patient dies and the family has doubts as to whether all available medical and scientific techniques and *reasonable* effort and agents have been brought to bear, the family often tends to suffer from self-incrimination. After all, the loss is bad enough, but emotional disturances should be held to a minimum in degree and duration following the death of a loved one.

Thanatology has been neglected. This is an important and extensive subject. Like birth, it involves all people. The phenomenon of death as a biologic entity needs more study, as do the associated economic, social, family, and physiologic problems. Many people, including the dying, are too often unnecessarily disturbed, with members of the family even being emotionally crippled for the remainder of their lives, becoming disturbing to those about them or dependent upon them.

Small children left behind without a loving mother are most pathetic. Even here the physician can be helpful in guiding the children and their father. The responsibility of the physician to the patient and his family is extensive and almost never ending. The performance of physicians seems to be best in rural areas, where the physician and his patients and their families know each other intimately and the physicians are less callous. The richest and greatest satisfaction and rewards from the practice of medicine are realized under conditions of helping a dying patient and family. If the attitude of the physician is one of compassion and helpfulness, these rewards can be experienced in large cities as well as in rural areas.

Death is not the final event for the family—it is often just the beginning.

Reference

Burch, G. E., N. P. DePasquale, and J. H. Phillips, 1968. "What Death Is Like," *American Heart Journal*, 76:438.

Part VII
Psychosocial Aspects of Bereavement

🎋 33
Understanding Your Grief

Arthur C. Carr

THE GRIEF YOU are feeling is a universal experience occurring as a natural reaction to the death of a loved person. Your response to this loss is likely to arouse many emotions, feelings, and reactions which will be unique to you, both in intensity and kind. You may also undergo many experiences which are predictable and part of all "grief reactions," shared by others who have endured a loss similar to your own.

At the time when your loss is most recent, in the "winter" of your grief, you may feel that your present feelings will be unchanging ones. Believe that "this, too, shall pass," although it may be difficult for you to accept such apparently easy comfort at the moment. Various people, however, find sustenance in a variety of thoughts: some in their religious convictions; some in the knowledge that death is inevitable; some in the comfort that comes from having shared a meaningful life with a loved person; some in memory, and some in hope.

Before your current mourning has run its course, you may experience a gamut of complicated and even contradictory feelings, which it may be well for you to anticipate. You should know that possibly, even in deepest grief, it is not unusual for a person to experience transient feelings of relief for a death that occurred at the particular time it did; irrational feelings of anger over seemingly having been abandoned by the dead person; thoughts of the gains and rewards possibly accruing from the death; or many other "unacceptable" feelings, which seem inappropriate to the depth of your feeling and the magnitude of your loss. These are a natural result of a basic condition of all human relationships and, if they occur, these are not unique to you.

Variations in how we respond are not unusual. Complicating your reaction to your recent loss may be any experience you have had with loss earlier in life. If your feelings now appear out of proportion to the present event, it may be that you are reacting in terms of earlier losses in life. On the other hand, if your feelings do not seem proportionate to your present loss, you may be temporarily postponing feelings which are, at the moment, too difficult or painful to handle. Or, it may be that the loss followed only after a long illness and that in anticipating the outcome you already expended your grief in what is known as "anticipatory grief."

The effects of grief are such that some authorities characterize the condition as an actual illness marked by the disruption of normal bodily and sensory reactions. Loss of appetite, insomnia, feelings of "numbness," fatigue and irritability, diminishing of sexual interests, susceptibility to physical and emotional illnesses—all these may occur and support the contention that a grieving person is in a physically vulnerable state. In the early stages of grief, a bereaved person may develop physical symptoms similar to those which the deceased had; such reactions can be interpreted as attempts to identify with the dead person or to perpetuate his memory. In contrast, there may be transient periods when you "forget" your loved one has died, and you find yourself acting as if the event had not occurred. Even more vividly, you may have sensory impressions which seemingly can be explained only as coming from the dead person. Without understanding and preparation, such apparently unusual experiences might cause unnecessary anxiety and fear. Should such signs or symptoms of grief persist, however, it would be wise to seek professional counsel.

Because of the unusual pressures on your physical makeup during a grief reaction, it would be wise to delay any elective surgical or dental procedures for a period of at least eight weeks after your loss. While you should strive to carry out all necessary obligations and responsibilities during this period, prudence dictates postponement of any major financial or personal decisions until such time as you have more fully worked out the effects of your loss.

Your reactions to others in the weeks ahead may be highly variable. At times you may want to be alone. Friends who sense this, and who are actively respecting your wishes for privacy, may act in a way that actually seems thoughtless or rejecting. It may require extra effort to understand *them* and *their* feelings of inadequacy at being unable to help you with, or participate in, your grief. Indeed, their efforts to help may often fail. For example, while trying to be sympathetic and helpful to you, they may insist on how bereaved *they* feel, as if to say that *they* are the ones who need comfort! Well-meaning people can sometimes appear very unthinking and inept in their interactions with bereaved friends.

If there are young children in your family, this may be an especially difficult time for you and them. While there are no prescribed rules and no easy way for dealing with this situation, it is generally better if children are told in simple terms what has happened, and if they are allowed—in some way appropriate to their age—to share the experience and express their feelings at this time.

About pain, the philosopher Gibran wrote, "Your pain is the breaking of the shell that encloses your understanding." In your present loss and grief, such an outlook promises that even suffering may provide a sustaining growth experience. As with other, earlier life privations, you may find that change itself stimulates unsuspected areas of growth. Your own capacity to adjust will reveal many new strengths within you. Some individuals are even able to channel their grief creatively, reaching out to help others with similar life problems.

🌿 34
Methodological Problems in Assessing the Relationship Between Acuteness of Death and the Bereavement Outcome

Paula J. Clayton, Ramon H. Parilla, Jr., and Michael D. Bieri

ONE OF THE most controversial issues in bereavement research today is the relationship between the length of the terminal illness and the adjustment of the survivor. Contrary to common sense, but consistent with the results of the majority of well-designed bereavement studies, sudden deaths do not produce more disturbed survivors. Maddison and Viola (1968), Bornstein et al. (1973), Clayton et al., (1973), Schwab et al. (1975), and Gerber et al. (1975) found that sudden deaths did not predict poor outcome. In fact, Schwab reported that survivors of longer illnesses were more likely to show negative effects in the bereavement period than survivors of acute illnesses. And Gerber et al. reported that although survivors whose spouses had chronic fatal illnesses experienced more—but not significantly more—ill effects than survivors of acute illnesses, there were significant differences in the adjustment of those who survived short and long chronic illnesses. Those survivors whose spouses' illnesses were of more than six months duration experienced more deleterious effects in bereavement than those who survived shorter chronic illnesses. Only Parkes (1975) has shown a positive correlation between sudden deaths and poor outcome. Because this issue is crucial in relation to intervention efforts, the authors will use data from a recent study of young bereaved to illustrate some of the problems involved in research concerning this issue. It is not the intent of this paper to settle the issue, but merely to review the problems in the area.

We have interviewed a group of white, recently widowed men and women, under the age of 45, one and thirteen months after their spouses' deaths. We attempted to collect a consecutive series of young bereaved from the St. Louis City and County area. We also have collected an age- and sex-matched group of controls from the voter registry. Out of a possible 94 subjects, 62 consented to be interviewed, an acceptance rate of 66 percent. Those who refused the interview were similar in age and sex to those who accepted. The causes of the spouses' deaths of the refusers were also similar, with the majority being deaths from cancer and cardiovascular diseases, but a significant minority being accidents, suicides, alcoholism-related deaths and unexpected postoperative deaths. For the purposes of this paper, our population will be limited to 14 survivors of cardiovascular deaths (10 women and 4 men) and 22 survivors of cancer deaths (7 women and 15 men). From this it can be seen that the survivors of cardiovascular deaths were more often women, and survivors of the cancer deaths more often men. (A chi-square with a Yates correction of 3.914 is significant at the .05 level.) The average age of the survivors of the cardiovascular deaths was 39.8 years (38.9 years for women and 42.0 years for men), and of survivors of cancer deaths was 38.0 years (34.4 years for women and 39.7 years for men). Survivors of cardiovascular deaths are not significantly older than the survivors of cancer deaths. The women survivors from the cancer group are significantly younger than their male counterparts and just miss being significantly younger than the women survivors of cardiovascular deaths (student t-test). Applying the Otis Dudley Duncan socioeconomic index (a prestige rating from 0 to 100, based on years of education and income) to the man of the family's last job, the two groups were similar (53 for cardiovascular and 47 for cancer) and well above the national average (37.7). Finally, 42 percent of the deaths from cardiovascular diseases compared to 86 percent of the deaths from cancer occurred in the hospital. This difference is significant at the $< .01$ level using the Fisher exact probability test. The cardiovascular deaths occurred in the home in 36 percent of the cases, at work in 7 percent of the cases, and on the street in 14 percent of the cases.

Reviewing the articles on reactions to sudden deaths, there seem to be four areas that contribute to the controversy and confound the results: the age of the survivor, the definition of sudden death, the definition of "disturbance" in the survivor, and the sex of the survivor.

Those familiar with the literature of bereavement research would recognize that the differences between the first five papers mentioned above and Parkes' paper was the age of the survivor. Parkes's widows and widowers were under 45; Maddison's were between 45 and 60; and all of the other authors dealt with the elderly populations. Because Parkes's population of the young showed a positive correlation between acute illness and outcome, it was concluded by some that as a person ages, deaths among friends and relatives act as rehearsals for deaths of closer people, so that when a significant other dies, the response seen is more muted. Thus, after a subject reaches a certain critical age, no death could be considered "untimely." That explanation might be plausible if it were just that the reaction of the elderly to an acute death was no different from their reaction to a death after a long illness. However, Gerber and his group have clearly shown that survivors of longer terminal illnesses show more signs of distress in the year following bereavement than those with shorter terminal illnesses. The age of the survivor, thus, affects outcome, with both acute deaths in young survivors and long terminal illnesses in older survivors causing difficult bereavement outcomes.

More crucial to the methodological problem is the definition of "sudden death." In our studies, we have let the subject define the length of the terminal illness of the deceased by asking, "How long was your husband ill?" "When did the illness begin to interrupt his life?" or "When did it become a continuous downhill course that you knew would end in death?" Then, we arbitrarily defined "sudden deaths" as illnesses of five days duration or less and compared them to illnesses of longer duration. The following case histories illustrate the problem inherent in this definition.

Mrs. R. was a 37-year-old white woman, mother of five, whom we saw 23 days after the death of her 43-year-old spouse. She reported that he had died of a myocardial infarct, but that he had been sick for one year and eight months. He had been retired for that period of time, but previously had been the manager of a service station and had made an adequate income. He was a diabetic who took Orinase, but had been in good health until 20 months previously when he experienced acute chest pain and was admitted to the hospital with a diagnosis of myocardial infarct. He stayed approximately six weeks. During this time he lost weight and no longer needed to take an antidiabetic drug; however, he was discharged from the hospital on Coumadin, Diuril and Aldomet for high blood pressure, and Librium. He did well for approximately 12 months until he had a recurrence of chest pain which lasted 2½ to 3 hours. He was not admitted to the hospital. Two months before his death, he had two more light spells of chest pain. The month of his death, he saw his physician, and was told he was doing fine, that his blood pressure was normal, and that he was to return in eight weeks. On the day of his death, he was the co-chairman of a street picnic. He arose early and went down to help set up the stalls. His wife talked to him at 10:30 AM. She was called shortly thereafter, told that he had developed severe chest pains and passed out. He was taken to the hospital where he died four hours later. Even though the death was sudden and unexpected, she insisted that she had anticipated it for 20 months, and it was something she lived with continuously.

In contrast, Mrs. M. was a 35-year-old white woman, mother of three, whose 41-year-old husband died of a myocardial infarct and pulmonary emboli. We saw her 25 days after his death. She reported that his death was sudden, unanticipated and she felt that it was less than a five day illness. The deceased had been a produce manager for a supermarket until he became disabled three and a half years before his death. Approximately five years before, the patient had had chest and arm pain and was taken to a hospital, but was told it was indigestion and sent home. Then three and a half years before his death, he had the same symptoms, only more severe. Again, he was taken to the hospital and after an EKG, he was to be sent home, but "an enzyme in his blood" was elevated; he was retained and told that he had had a myocardial infarct. The length of that hospitalization was three weeks. The patient was also told at the time that he had varicose veins. Approximately six months after the first myocardial infarct he had a vein-stripping operation. Then six months after that he had a second myocardial infarct and was in the hospital again for three weeks. After his second myocardial infarct, he continued to have some shortness of breath and chest pain, which the wife attributed to his heavy smoking. During the last year of his life, these pains became worse. However, two weeks before his death he went on a vacation trip with neighbors. While on the trip, he began feeling quite ill and returned home after two days. Because the pains persisted, he went to the hospital and was again admitted. In the hospital she was told he had had another myocardial infarct, and an embolus was identified in his lungs. He became weaker and weaker and died on the fifth hospital day.

According to our method of classification, the first lady would be classified as a survivor of a chronic illness and the second a survivor of an acute illness, although the courses seem similar and, if anything, the course of the second patient seems more chronic than the course of the first.

Parkes felt that because a sudden death, occurring during the course of a chronic illness that was not expected to be fatal, could be just as traumatic as a death from a brief illness, the illnesses should be defined according to what he called "short" and "long" preparation. A person was defined as having short preparation for the death if she had less than two-weeks warning that the spouse's condition was likely to prove fatal and/or less than three-days warning that death was imminent. Because of Parkes's work, we redefined our illnesses in all of our patients accordingly and thus classified both of the previous subjects as having short preparation. In another study Glick, Weiss, and Parkes (1974) divided their widows into three groups, the first being the short-preparation group similar to the one mentioned above but now called a "no anticipation group." Women were placed in this category if their spouses died in an accident, of a myocardial infarct with no previous illness, or of an illness which initially was not understood to be fatal. The second category was "an uncertain category" where the respondent should have anticipated the spouse's death on the basis of the information but did not. In this group, they classified four women whose husbands had suffered one or more heart attacks before being fatally stricken, and one woman whose alcoholic husband had been told that if he continued to drink he would die. The third category, which needs no explanation, was those whose spouses died of "anticipated deaths." The uncertain group in the authors' comparisons looked more like those who did not anticipate the deaths.

Gerber's definition is still different. "Acute illness death" was defined as a death occurring without warning and prior knowledge of the condition or a death after a medical condition of less than *two months* duration with the absence of multiple attacks and hospitalization. A "chronic illness death" was any condition, cancer or cardiovascular, of two or more months duration, truly life-threatening by medical standards and supported by multiple attacks and hospitalization.

Of our 14 cardiovascular deaths, 7 had had previous myocardial infarcts. Depending on the definition used, these 7 survivors would be classified differently in each of the different studies. One survivor considered that her husband's illness was of six-month duration, and she would be called, according to anyone's system, a survivor of a "chronic illness death." The two women described earlier had husbands who were on disability because of their previous myocardial infarcts. They could be classified either way in any system. The other four with myocardial infarcts were spouses who had returned to work and were functioning in a normal way up until the times of their deaths, so they could most easily be called "sudden death." Reclassifying according to Parkes's first dual subdivision led us to put 13 of the 14 cardiovascular survivors in the "no anticipation group." All of the 7 would be called "uncertain" in his and his colleagues' three-part classification.

The measures of "disturbance" in the survivor are also difficult. In our work, we have used the presence or absence of a depressive-symptom complex to quantify the degree of disturbance in the survivor. Thus, we compare the percent of men and women who were depressed at one month or one year in the acute versus the chronic illness groups. Those subjects whose spouses died after chronic illnesses were more likely to have depressive symptoms at one month, but by one year there were no differences between the two groups.

Parkes's definition of disturbances is vague in his one-month data and at one year similar to ours. At two to four years it is also difficult to judge. He uses discriminate function analysis to define outcomes. He speaks about the fact that a one-month preparation did not prevent early grief or grieving, but that somehow those who survived after an acute illness had "less capacity to cope." At the end of 13 months, 74 percent of the short-preparation group, and only 42 percent of the long-preparation group had a depressive-symptom complex. These differences are significant ($p < .05$). At the end of a two- to four-year period, he found that the short-preparation group had more problems with "role functioning," and "financial affairs," and had a "less favorable attitude toward the future." In the book by Glick, Weiss, and Parkes, using the three groups as defined previously, the authors state that those

who anticipated their husbands' deaths had "moved toward remarriage" and those who had not had more clearly moved in "an
other direction toward reorganization." They go on to state that
most of the widows whose husbands died without warning, like
the other widows, established new sexual relations of some importance, and organized their lives around these relationships,
but did not want to remarry, even in two cases where they had
had a child by the boyfriend. The authors felt that these widows
were fearful of marriage and that they felt they could avoid further catastrophe by avoiding marriage. Again, outcome measures,
measure outcome. Is it really marriage that should be valued here
as a "good outcome," or should it not be the ability to establish a
close, confiding relationship?

Gerber's measures of disturbance are clear-cut. He counted
the number of physician visits, the number of times the subjects
reported feeling ill without consulting the physician, and the
amount of psychotropic medicine that the bereaved consumed,
and compared these outcomes in the acute and chronic illnesses.
He found, as reported, that survivors of very long terminal illnesses, particularly widowers, had significantly increased physician visits, days of illness, and increased amounts of intake of
psychotropic drugs.

Sex, acuteness of the death, and outcome may also be related. If one of the measures of outcome is remarriage, then outcome must be evaluated separately by sex. Clearly, the data show
that women are less likely after becoming widowed to remarry
within the first five years than are men. So if—as in our group of
survivors of cardiovascular deaths—there is an excess of women,
there will be less dating, sexual intercourse, and remarriage in
the year following the death of the spouse than in our survivors of
cancer deaths. Gerber has also shown among the older bereaved
that being a widower is related to poor outcome in those who survive long, chronic illnesses.

Despite all these qualifications, from our data on survivors of
cardiovascular deaths (judged according to Parkes' criteria to have
short preparation illnesses in 13 out of 14 cases compared to 3 out
of 22 of the survivors of cancer deaths), it may be that in young
bereaved acute illness is related to poor outcome. At one month,
64 percent of the survivors of cardiovascular deaths compared to
32 percent of the survivors of cancer deaths had a depressive-
symptom complex. This barely fails to reach chi-square significance. At one year, only 8 percent of the survivors of car-

Clayton, Parilla, and Bieri

diovascular deaths and 15 percent of the survivors of cancer deaths had a depressive-symptom complex. These figures are strikingly low compared to those reported by Parkes earlier in the paper. In contrast, however, at one month, the acute-illness survivors had significantly more physician visits (57 percent versus 18 percent, $p < .025$ by Fisher exact probability) and took more tranquilizers (43 percent versus 23 percent) although the differences here were not significant. At one year, they continued to have more physician visits with 85 percent of the survivors of the cardiovascular deaths having seen a physician compared to only 60 percent of the cancer death survivors. This difference is not significant. And, they continued to use more tranquilizers, this time at a significant level (46 percent versus 10 percent; significant by the Fisher exact probability test at the .02 level). Whether these differences are due to the length of the preparation or the differences in the sexes of the two groups will only become clear when the control-group data are analyzed. It also must be remembered that the numbers in these two groups are small and larger N's would certainly provide more clear-cut data.

In conclusion, bereavement research will yield more useful and reproducible information as we become methodologically more sound. Gerber's clear definitions and outcome measures in his aged bereaved should serve as a model in future research in this field, although it could be argued that severe psychological distress or poor social and work adjustment may be missed by these outcome measures. We have repeated evidence that, in fact, these two measures do not sort together (Clayton et al., 1972; Bornstein et al., 1973). Those with a whole host of depressive symptoms are no more likely to see a physician than those with no or minimal depressive symptoms. Obviously, the most comprehensive study would combine both measures.

References

Bornstein, P. E., P. J. Clayton, J. A. Halikas et al. 1973. "The Depression of Widowhood After Thirteen Months," *British Journal of Psychiatry*, 122 (570):561–66.

Clayton, P. J., J. A. Halikas, W. L. Maurice. 1972. "The Depesssion of Widowhood," *British Journal of Psychiatry*, 120(554):71–77.

Clayton, P. J., J. A. Halikas, W. L. Maurice et al. 1973. "Anticipatory Grief and Widowhood," *British Journal of Psychiatry*, 122(566):47–51.

Gerber, I., R. Rusalem, N. Hannon et al. 1975. "Anticipatory Grief and Aged Widows and Widowers," *Journal of Gerontology*, 30(2):225–29.

Glick, I. O., R. S. Weiss, C. M. Parkes. 1974. *The First Year of Bereavement.* New York: Wiley.

Maddison, D. and A. Viola. 1968. "The Health of Widows in the Year Following Bereavement," *Journal of Psychosomatic Research,* 12:297–306.

Parkes, C. M. 1975. "Unexpected and Untimely Bereavement: A Statistical Study of Young Boston Widows and Widowers." In B. Schoenberg et al., eds. *Bereavement: Its Psychosocial Aspects,* pp. 119–38. New York: Columbia University Press.

Schwab, J. J., J. M. Chalmers, S. J. Conroy et al. 1975. Studies in Grief: A Preliminary Report." In B. Schoenberg et al., eds., *Bereavement: Its Psychosocial Aspects,* pp. 78–87. New York: Columbia University Press.

❧35
Survivors of Cardiovascular and Cancer Deaths

Paula J. Clayton, Ramon H. Parilla, Jr., and Michael D. Bieri

THIS IS A companion paper to the preceding contribution. We shall compare the bereavement symptoms and adjustment of survivors of cardiovascular deaths and cancer deaths. We shall consider that these two groups represent short and long preparation deaths respectively. We shall then discuss the results in comparison to Parkes's similarly aged widowed (Parkes, 1970; Parkes and Brown, 1972; Parkes, 1972; Glick et al., 1974; Parkes, 1975).

As already stated, this is a consecutive group of young (under 45) widowed men and women seen two times in the first year of mourning. The number of subjects is small (cardiovascular, 14; cancer, 22; follow-up, 13, and 20 respectively), so that only the most extreme differences could be statistically significant. Therefore, "trends" will be noted. There are also significantly more women whose spouses died of cardiovascular disease and more men whose wives died of cancer. Because the majority of the subjects come from the suburban county they had good educations, good jobs, and high socioeconomic indexes. They were, for the most part, Catholic and Protestant although some professed no religion, and only one-half considered themselves "religious."

This study supported, in part, by USPHS Grants MH-13002 and MH-05804.

Thirteen of the 14 subjects who survived a cardiovascular death compared to 3 of the 22 survivors of cancer deaths were considered connected with short preparation illnesses ($p < .001$ by chi-square with Yates correction). The cancer death victims had an average length of illness of 5.2 months, with the range being from 0 to 540 days.

Marriages were long and happy. Survivors of cardiovascular deaths had 4.07 children per family, and the cancer death survivors had 2.09 children per family. The children in both groups were all ages. This difference could be due to the fact that the survivors of cardiovascular deaths are healthy women, compared to the cancer victims, who are slightly younger women stricken in their reproductive years. There were no young infants in the cardiovascular group, so that at least the immediate reproductive rate was no different. In fact, the youngest child in the cardiovascular group was 3 years old. Or perhaps men who die from cardiovascular disease for some reason have more children. This should be investigated further, as it could be a factor to be considered in post-bereavement counseling. There were no significant religious differences in the two groups to account for the difference.

There were no differences in the subjects' characterizations of their marriages. Most of them felt they were closer than other couples they had known, and no differences in sexual problems in the marriage between the two groups. Despite this, as table 1 shows, the cardiovascular survivors reported more problems in every area of marriage, and significantly more often had two or more problems within the marriage. In particular, drinking was noted by five survivors of cardiovascular deaths compared to two cancer survivors. This barely fails to reach significance by the Fisher exact probability test. There are several explanations for

Table 35.1 Problems in Marriage as Reported at First Interview

Symptoms	Cardiovascular Survivors (N = 14) (%)	Cancer Survivors (N = 22) (%)
Money	36	23
Children	14	5
Drinking or drugs	36	9
Sex or infidelity	14	0
Any problem	57	36
Two or more problems	43[a]	5

[a] $p < .01$ by Fisher Exact Probability.

these findings. It could be that men who die of cardiovascular diseases actually are heavier drinkers and have more problem-riddled marriages; because there are more women survivors in the cardiovascular group, they may be more sensitive to drinking and other problems, and more likely to report any kind of problem; a long preparation for death could allow the survivor to come to grips with the problems of a marriage, and to put them aside so that by the time the spouse dies, these problems are poorly remembered or at least poorly reported. There were no differences in the two groups in the problems they talked about in the immediate bereavement period or in the kinds of help they received. Although we recorded people in the environment as being helpful, not helpful, disappointing, and a hindrance, we did not look at those variables for these two groups.

Table 2 shows the psychological symptoms in the two groups in the first month of bereavement. As can be seen, most of the symptoms are only slightly more common in the short-prepara-

Table 35.2 Psychological Symptoms in the First Month of Bereavement

Symptoms	Cardiovascular Survivors (N = 14) (%)	Cancer Survivors (N = 22) (%)
Crying	86	73
Depressed mood	71	59
Insomnia	64	68
Loss of interest	64	41
Anorexia	50	50
Weight loss	50	23
Restless	50	45
Difficulty making up mind	50	24
Numbness	43	23
Difficulty concentrating	43	27
Slowed thinking	43	41
Guilty	43	37
Someone to blame	43	32
Poor memory	38	36
Wish dead	36	27
Irritability	36	23
Fatigue	36	36
Reverse diurnal variation	36	18
Diurnal variation	29	18
Feels angry	21	18
Hopeless	14	18
Worthless	7	0
Thoughts of suicide	8	16
World unreal	0	9
Body unreal	0	0
Depressive-symptom complex	64	32

tion subjects. Only three comparisons are of such increased frequency in the cardiovascular survivors to be nearly significant. These are weight loss, difficulty making up their minds, and occurrence of the depressive-symptom complex. The weight loss is severe in the cardiovascular group, with most of them having lost more than 10 pounds within the first month. "Blame" in the short-preparation subjects was directed at various people—the deceased, the physician, the in-laws, and others—whereas all the cancer victims blamed the physician. This may be a point worth noting for the health-care professions.

We asked our subjects a list of physical symptoms that Maddison and Viola (1968) found to be prominent in the bereavement period. All the physical symptoms that they noted were rare and equal in both groups. There was no one in the first month who said that he or she had general poor health. Table 3 shows the medical attention the two groups sought. There was no difference in the drinking habits reported by the two groups in the first month. The cardiovascular survivors used more hypnotics and more tranquilizers, and in the latter case it barely fails to reach significance. Interestingly, 36 percent of the long-preparation group (cancer survivors), compared to 7 percent of the short-preparation group, reported that they had no physician. This barely fails to reach significance by the Fisher exact probability test. In keeping with this, the cardiovascular survivors had significantly more often seen or called a physician in the first month.

Table 4 shows the symptoms the subjects reported at one year. All symptoms have diminished and seem to be even more equally distributed in the two groups. However, the psychological depressive symptoms, depressed mood, feeling guilty, worthless, a burden, nothing to look forward to, hopeless, wish-

Table 35.3 Physician Visits and Drug Use in the First Month of Bereavement

Symptoms	Cardiovascular Survivors (N = 14) (%)	Cancer Survivors (N = 22) (%)
Increased alcohol consumption	7	10
Used hypnotics	29	14
Used tranquilizers	50	23
Had no physician	7	36
Saw or called physician	64[a]	23
Saw physician	57[b]	18

[a] $p < .05$ by chi-square.
[b] $p < .025$ by Fisher exact probability.

Table 35.4 Psychological Symptoms at One Year of Bereavement

Symptoms	Cardiovascular Survivors (N =13) (%)	Cancer Survivors (N =20) (%)
Crying	46	25
Depressed mood	38	35
Insomnia	46	35
Loss of interest	38	40
Anorexia	23	20
Weight loss	8	30
Restless	54	45
Difficulty making up mind	23	15
Numbness	23	10
Difficulty concentrating	23	20
Slowed thinking	8	20
Guilty	8	35
Poor memory	8	25
Wish dead	0	15
Irritability	38	40
Fatigue	31	35
Reverse diurnal variation	46[a]	5
Diurnal variation	8	5
Hopeless	15	15
Worthless	0	5
Thoughts of suicide	0	10
World unreal	0	0
Body unreal	8	5
Burden	0	5
Nothing to look forward to	15	20
Fear lose mind	8	10
Depressive-symptom complex	8	15

[a] $p < .01$ by Fisher exact probability.

ing for death, and thinking of suicide are as common, or more common, at one year in the survivors of the cancer deaths. The depressive-symptom complex is also slightly more frequent in the cancer survivors. Reversed diurnal variation, feeling worse when the spouse should come home, or in the evening, is significantly more prominent in the cardiovascular group.

Physical symptoms had increased slightly, but not a great deal, and again they were equal in the two groups. Many of the physical symptoms were reported only by one or two people. No physical symptoms were reported by 23 percent of the cardiovascular survivors and 25 percent of the cancer survivors; 62 percent and 40 percent, respectively, had one; and 15 percent and 35 percent, respectively, had more than one. Two of the cancer survivors reported "general poor health," and none of the cardiovascular survivors did so. (Remember this is a young group

Table 35.5 Physician Visits and Drug Use in the First Year of Bereavement

Symptoms	Cardiovascular Survivors (N = 13) (%)	Cancer Survivors (N = 20) (%)
Drinking increased	23	10[a]
Used hypnotics	31	20
Used tranquilizers	46[b]	10
Used either	54	30
Saw physician	85	60
Saw psychiatrist	8	0
Other counselor	0	5
Hospital, surgical	8	10
Hospital, medical	8	0
Hospital, psychiatric	0	0

[a] An additional 20% increased their drinking early in bereavement, but had decreased it by one year.
[b] $p < .025$.

of people with relatively few physical symptoms.) Table 5 gives the physician visits and drug use in the first year of bereavement. As can be seen, about one-fourth of the people increased their drinking. A significant number of the cardiovascular survivors were using tranquilizers, and most of the cardiovascular survivors had seen a physician. Only 60 percent of the cancer survivors had seen a physician. The one woman who saw a psychiatrist had seen him before her husband's illness. One woman went to see a minister for counseling in the bereavement period. Then, despite the doctoring and use of medicines, there was minimal use of psychological support and there were minimal hospitalizations. Sixty-nine percent of the cardiovascular group and 65 percent of the cancer group reported that they felt better than at the last interview, and most of them felt the improvement occurred between three and six months after the death.

Table 6 gives the subjects' social and sexual adjustment. Al-

Table 35.6 Social and Sexual Adjustment at One Year

Future Plans	Cardiovascular Survivors (N = 13) (%)	Cancer Survivors (N = 20) (%)
Remarry		
Female	0 (N = 9)	0 (N = 7)
Male	0 (N = 4)	31 (N = 13)
Not remarry	31	37
Dated	31	60
Intercourse	23	55

though there are no statistically significant differences, the differences noted are due to the fact that the survivors of cardiovascular deaths are largely women, and the other group is composed mainly of men. There are no women in the study with any plans to remarry. We have found in previous studies that this is due mainly to the fact that the pool of available men is small for women, perhaps not quite so limited at this young age, but still limited.

Table 7 gives the actions of the survivor in regards to the spouse and also in regards to mourning. This table is included mainly to give the reader some idea of the frequency of these thoughts, feelings, and actions. The only differences that approach significance are that the survivors of cardiovascular deaths have more regrets and feel that they would have done things differently both in relationship to the marriage and the illness. And, the survivors of cancer report more often that their period of mourning is over. This all seems consistent with the idea that a longer preparation for death gives the survivor an opportunity to come to terms with the difficulties in the marriage.

Table 8 gives the replies to questions Parkes found distinguished his bereaved from controls at one year. There are minimal differences, none of which is significant.

Table 35.7 Actions of Survivors Concerning Spouse and Mourning

Actions	Cardiovascular Survivors (N = 13) (%)	Cancer Survivors (N = 20) (%)
Think of spouse daily	77	60
Sense he is around	46	30
Guides decisions	15	25
Feel presence	46	30
Do things to remind self	46	30
Avoid things	23	40
Excessive mementos	8	5
Kept clothes at home (packed)	23	10
Acts as still alive	38	10
Difficulty accepting the death	31	15
Angry	38	40
Do crazy things	0	10
Blame someone	23	35
Regrets	69	40
Done things differently	69	40
Rash decision	0	15
Child sleeps in bed with parent	38	30
No grave visits	23	10
Mourning is over	31	60
Severe anniversary reaction	15	0

Table 35.8 Feelings Inquired About at the End of the First Year

Feelings	Cardiovascular Survivors (N =13) (%)	Cancer Survivors (N =20) (%)
"I feel somewhat apart and remote even among friends"	31	25
"During the past year my memory has seemed to be all right"	100	85
"It's safer not to fall in love"	54	32
"Most of the time I don't care what others think of me"	42	45
"When I go out, I usually prefer to go by myself"	8	20
"I worry more than I used to"	38	35
"I am the kind of person who takes things hard"	18	47

Parkes (1975) reported striking differences between his short- and long-preparation young bereaved. His findings were based on a group of 60 Boston widows and widowers under the age of 45 seen three to four weeks, six to eight weeks, thirteen months, and two to four years after the deaths of their spouses. His study population differed from ours in several ways. Both of his groups had an equal percentage of men—29 and 28—similar to the 29 percent in our short-preparation group (survivors of cardiovascular deaths), but strikingly different from the percent of men (59) who survived their wives' cancer deaths. Our groups were only white whereas his were black and white (33 percent of his short-preparation group was black). His short-preparation group was also from social classes five and six in approximately 50 percent of his cases. Our groups were of similar social class and above the national average. Finally, his short-preparation group were the survivors of various types of sudden and unexpected deaths, whereas ours were only survivors of cardiovascular deaths.

At one month, he showed that more of his short-preparation group reported disbelief, guilt, resentment, and would welcome death. There were no differences in any symptoms in our groups at one month including numbness, guilt, feeling angry about the death, and wishing for death itself. The percent of people who report positive responses to the various questions is similar in his long-preparation group to our long-preparation group (both cancer death survivors), but our short-preparation group report reduced numbers of distressing symptoms. Still, using the depressive-symptom complex and visiting a physician as an index of disturbance, our findings also point to the short-preparation group as being more disturbed.

No visits, one visit, and/or less than five visits to the grave are similar at one year in our two groups. We did not record when the first visit occurred. Parkes found that significantly fewer of the short-preparation group had visited the grave by six to eight weeks, which he interpreted as being a denial that the death had occurred or an avoidance mechanism.

By one year, we again did not replicate Parkes's findings of symptom differences including the occurrence of a depressive-symptom complex in our two groups. Parkes reported 74 percent of his short-preparation group were experiencing this depressive-symptom complex compared to only 7 percent of his long-preparation group. Our findings are markedly different, with only 8 percent of our short-preparation group and 15 percent of our long-preparation group reporting enough symptoms to qualify for the symptom complex. In reviewing the records of our 14 cardiovascular-death survivors it was my impression that a number of the respondents had symptoms, but few admitted to being depressed enough to qualify for a positive scoring on the symptom, "depressed mood." Without this symptom or a synonym, these people could not be classified as having "the depressive-symptom complex." This is corroborated by the fact that 69 percent of the cardiovascular survivors had one or more depressive physical symptoms (anorexia, weight loss, fatigue, and so on) and only 55 percent of the cancer survivors did. At one year, our two groups had almost equal numbers of people who reported loneliness as the worst problem (54 percent compared to 50 percent), whereas Parkes reported significant differences at two to four years between the two groups on that symptom, as well as others.

However, at one year, our short-preparation group was taking more tranquilizers than the longer-preparation group. There was a trend toward having more physician visits and a trend for them to wish they had done things differently and to have regrets about the death and not to feel that their period of mourning was over. In general, however, the psychological and physical symptoms were extremely similar in the two groups by one year.

In summary, we would agree with Parkes that these young survivors are more troubled and have more difficulty in the first year of bereavement than similarly studied older bereaved. Taking the use of medicine and physician visits, there is some indication that those in the short-preparation group do less well than those who have a longer preparation for death. We did not feel, however, as Parkes did in referring to the short-preparation group that "somehow the lack of preparation for a massive loss has prevented a normal process of unlearning from taking place. Instead of repeated frustration of the search, leading to its gradual abandonment, it seems almost as if grieving has become a normal part of life." He felt these subjects used excessive avoidance mechanisms. We found (as noted in table 7) more overt avoidance in the cancer survivors, although slightly less avoidance of the grave. As a contradiction to this finding, in his London widows followed prospectively (Parkes, 1970), more of the short-illness survivors "treasured reminders" of their spouses (slightly more of ours did also, table 7).

Except for the first case that follows, we did not find any other short-preparation survivor who could be labeled a "pathologic mourner." Instead, as the case of the cancer survivor indicates, it seemed to us that there were small percentages of each group who do poorly for reasons that are still poorly understood. In looking at the data from the entire sample, which is not presented here, one additional factor in postbereavement adjustment seems to be the survivors' prebereavement psychological makeup. Our cases will illustrate this. We found that subjects who had experienced a depressive-symptom cluster, whether it was primary or secondary to some other psychiatric illness, such as hysteria (chronic hypochondriasis), anxiety neurosis, or alcoholism, were more likely to do poorly in the bereavement period than those without such a cluster.

Because our groups are selected only as cardiovascular or cancer victim survivors, this study will be replicated with the total sample divided into short- and long-preparation groups to confirm the findings reported here.

The following are case histories reviewed for the paper. The first and second are cardiovascular death survivors and the third a cancer death survivor. The first is one of the most disturbed women seen by this investigator. The second is the last woman in the study and a more typical response. The third case is a cancer death survivor who did not do well.

Mrs. C. was a 42-year-old, married, white, female, mother of five with children ranging from 4 to 20, whose husband died suddenly at home of a myocardial infarct. She had no prior warning of illness. On the evening before his death, he had chest pain and discomfort. The next day he went to work, but felt bad, so he saw a physician at a downtown clinic where apparently no treatment was given. He returned to work, continued to feel ill and went home. She found him dead when she returned from a shopping expedition.

Both she and her husband had college educations and her husband had a good job. She had not worked although she was trained to be a teacher. At the beginning of the interview she said, "I plan to start teaching next year" (approximately nine months in the future), "but I don't think I will like it."

When she was seen for the first time she had all the symptoms of depression with terrible sleep, no appetite, a 16-pound weight loss, irritability, and loss of interest in reading and her children's schoolwork. She felt restless the first few nights and wanted to be left alone. She felt hopeless and had trouble making decisions. She felt guilty about not finding him in time, and worthless and no good. She felt she had nothing to look forward to. She wished she were dead, but denied suicidal thoughts "because of the children." She had a strong sense of his presence in that she felt she was being guided by him. She also felt at times that the house was like a cocoon and she was surrounded by him. She complained of unreality feelings—as if she were standing outside watching herself. She felt numb and she had some palpitations. She also felt angry, bitter, and that God and the clinic were to blame for her husband's death.

In her past history, it was difficult to decide if she had been psychiatrically ill. She had never seen a psychiatrist. She answered no to the question, "Have you ever felt that you were a nervous person or have you had a nervous breakdown," but qualified it by saying, "my friends may think I am weird." She had had symptoms associated with depression in the past, but they had never clustered into a syndrome. She had frequently lost her appetite in response to stress, such as college exams, and she had had periodic sleeping difficulty. One year she lost 60 pounds on a diet and did this again with a pregnancy. She admitted to being irritable occasionally for several days at a time, and to having trouble making decisions. She also had had some anxiety attacks with apprehension, shortness of breath, choking sensations and fear. However, they occurred so infrequently that we were not convinced that she had an anxiety neurosis. She also had headaches, but no other physical symptoms. She had taken a hypnotic and sodium butisol t.i.d. for several years and had been on vitamins and energizers—amphetamines—for weight loss in the past. When we reviewed her record we called her undiagnosed, ? no psychiatric illness.

She and her husband had had a long and happy marriage and she had no complaints. When asked if she had ever considered separation or divorce, she replied that they joked about the fact that whoever got divorced would get the children. She had not seen a physician, but she had called a physician and asked him to send her additional hypnotics and tranquilizers. He renewed the prescription she had in the past.

She was seen by us approximately one year later. The physician seeing her described her as "emotionally bitter." One of the first questions was, "How do you feel compared to the last time?" She answered, "not sure," but then added, "I feel fine, just like before." She continued to have low mood, sleeping problems, loss of appetite (she lost 50 pounds in the first three months), fatigue, irritability, and loss of interest chiefly in herself and her house. She cried often and felt she had nothing to look forward to, and that life was hopeless. She denied thinking of suicide. She said bitterly, "No one gives a damn, even the kids." She had thought about running away, but then qualified it by saying that she wasn't serious. She was aware that she should be making active plans for her future, but just could not bring herself to do this. She made many derogatory remarks about the children. She said life was better now that one of her children had gone off to college. When we asked her about her children's activities she said that she was struggling to get things done, but that it was a burden, because before, at least, she could share some of these activities with her husband and now she had to handle them all herself.

Physically she admitted to even more anxiety symptoms, stating spontaneously, "I would have sworn I had four or five heart attacks in the last several weeks," describing sternal chest pain and some palpitations. She again admitted that she had had this kind of symptom before, but generally with exposure to cold and not at other times. She complained of abdominal pain which occurred at 7:00 to 8:00 in the evening "after a battle with the children." She also complained that she just "could not get warm." She disliked the responsibility of the children and felt this was her worst problem. She felt "tied down" by them.

She was financially well off, although she realized that she should be thinking about going to work. She was looking less and less concerned with her personal appearance.

She said that she thought about her husband constantly. She did not do anything to deliberately remind herself of him, saying, "I don't need to." She put off getting a driver's license for six months, but finally did get it with difficulty. She still had most of her husband's clothes. She felt she had to push herself and everything she did was done "as if her husband were alive," meaning that she needed this kind of encouragement to keep herself going. She still felt angry about the death and that God and the physician were to blame. When asked if she would have done anything differently, she said she would have gotten him to his regular physician sooner and requested that he do the "stress test" (she must have talked to someone about this). In answering the questions that Parkes thinks are important she had positive answers to "it is safer not to fall in love," "most of the time I don't care what others think of me," and "I worry more than I used to." She said that friends had brought up the idea of remarriage, but she did not think she would remarry "because of all the kids." She had gone to couple parties, but had not really dated and had not had sexual intercourse. Despite this, however, when asked "How do you feel you are functioning?" she answered "Well." She had not been to a physician since her husband's death, but was still continuing to take Placidyl and Butisol.

On the second interview we did the family history of psychiatric illness and this was entirely negative.

This woman seems to have a picture consistent with the kinds of reactions that Dr. Parkes reports in young widows and widowers. In view of her past tranquilizer use and the history of anxiety attacks, although infrequent, we feel it is possible that she has anxiety neurosis. There is an indication in the literature that anxiety neurotics are "stress responders."

In contrast, Mrs. Z. was a 43-year-old, white woman, mother of two, a high school graduate who had never worked. She was married 21 years. Her husband was a 43-year-old engineer who died suddenly of a myocardial infarct. He was stricken at home, but was pronounced dead at the hospital. When seen for the first time, she said that she had been to a physician in the past few months because of headaches. He had discovered that she had high blood pressure and diabetes. She was currently taking medicine for both. The symptoms she admitted to within the first month were irritability, feeling restless, having difficulty concentrating, and thinking less clearly, and having a poor memory, but she denied being depressed and characterized herself as "cranky." She denied all other physical or psychological symptoms.

She, too, reported the marriage had been a good one. She said that about seven years previously she had lost interest in sex for about six months, but that it had come back spontaneously and they had had no other problems. She felt that they were as close, if not closer than other couples they had known. She was impressed with all the solace and comfort and help she had gotten from people. They had moved to St. Louis not too long before and she felt that this was the best place for her to be and she was very glad to be here. She took comfort in the fact that he had had a quick death. She felt that he could have lingered in a long illness and this would have been very bad for him and for everyone. And, she also took comfort in the fact that he was home a lot, that he was handy around the house, and had left a lot of things for her to remember him by. And, that they had had a lovely Caribbean cruise the summer before his death. Her only question was concerning the heritability of cardiac disease. She was concerned about her 18-year-old son and whether she should in some way be doing something to prevent him from having an early death, like feeding him a different diet, or something of this order.

When we saw her at a year, she said that she felt the same. When we asked her about her mood, she described it as "jealous, feeling sorry for myself," which was a reference to her own loneliness. She admitted to feeling worse in the evenings and to having some restlessness, but the other symptoms of which she had complained previously had cleared three to six months after his death. She did feel that she had lost interest in clubs and social activities which was consistent with her feeling lonely, neglected, excluded, and out of place. She had not gone to work. Her son had left for college, so she was living at home with her one daughter. She felt that she was cooking less and doing less housework, but that she was as concerned about her personal appearance and the other things in her life as she had been before her husband's death. Although she was a very light drinker before her husband's death, she said she was having about three drinks a day on the follow-up, but had no alcohol-related problems. She still thought about him every day around the time he should arrive home from work and did sense his presence, but she did nothing to remind herself of him or to avoid reminders. She had given away her husband's clothes early in the bereavement and kept only a memento. She had difficulty accepting the fact that he was dead, but did not feel angry or that anyone was to blame, nor did she have any regrets. She had done nothing odd, crazy, or unusual in the bereavement period. The only question in the series of questions that we took from Dr. Parkes's work that she answered positively to was, "I worry more than I used to." She was an active churchgoer and had continued in this. She said that people had brought up the idea of remarriage, but she did not think she would and did not give any reason. She had not dated and had not had sexual intercourse. She had a very adequate income. She had continued to see her physician for the same reason she had in the past, blood pressure problems and borderline diabetes. She had seen him about eight times and she felt that this was not related to the death. She had had no hospitalizations and was taking no medicines other than those prescribed—no tranquilizers. In her family history it is interesting that her mother was recorded as being a heavy drinker. The interviewer felt that she had done well and showed no symptoms of pathologic mourning.

Mrs. B. was 43, a mother of two. She was married for 21 years. Her husband had died at age 42 of stomach cancer with metastases. She realized six weeks before that death was imminent. About one year before his death, he had felt an uncomfortable sensation in his chest, as if food did not go down well. He went to a physician who did an upper gastrointestinal series, but it revealed no ulcer and no cancer. The next month he was still not feeling well, returned to his physician who still could not find the cause of his ill health. Despite additional physician and clinic visits, it was not until June, seven months later, that he saw another physician who put him in the hospital with the feeling he probably had some kind of tumor. On July 5, he had exploratory surgery and a cancer of the stomach with metastases was discovered. After surgery he returned to work and worked approximately two months despite continued symptoms and radiation therapy. He finally was forced to go into the hospital again because he was too weak to eat. He could not breathe properly. The last few days he slowly slipped into coma and died.

The subject herself, when first seen, had all the symptoms of depression—feeling low, sleeping trouble, appetite and weight loss, feeling tired, irritable, guilty about the husband's terminal illness, and occasionally wishing she were dead, thinking why didn't God take her. She admitted to being nervous, and that little things worried her. She had a huge array of physical symptoms most of which had been present long before her husband's death—headache, blurred vision, dizziness, nausea, vomiting, abdominal pain, constipation, diarrhea, urinary frequency, dysmenorrhea, skin rashes (psoriasis), crippling arthritis, and a numb feeling in her right leg with weakness. Her current medicines were thyroid, Indocin, Donnatal, Placidyl, Vistaril and Valium. She had eight previous hospitalizations beginning in 1944 with (1) an appendectomy (age 14), (2) "a dropped kidney," (3) a uterine suspension, (4) a heavy bleeding spell for which she needed a D & C, (5) a work-up because of a "kink in her right kidney," (6) tests for stomach trouble for which Donnatal was prescribed, (7) another time for a cystoscope, and (8) a psychiatric hospitalization for "nervousness and a compazine reaction." She did not clarify this last admission very much and it was difficult to tell exactly what did occur. She was only hospitalized six days. She had been scheduled for a hysterectomy before her husband's death, but she postponed this.

She did feel the physicians were to blame for her husband's death.

On mental status she was not tearful and did not appear depressed. She described herself as always wanting to be in control and felt that her brief stay in the psychiatric hospital had been helpful because she now was not bothered if she felt jittery, anxious, etc. for brief periods of time. She was reassured with this hospitalization about her mental health and she found this comforting. She felt that her stay had helped her not to let her emotions get the best of her, helped her to understand her emotions and to allow them to exist, and to learn to assert herself.

She felt she had had a happy marriage and there were absolutely no problems. Everyone had been helpful in the bereavement period.

Between her interviews we received some of her medical records (no hospitalizations). She, indeed, had had numerous visits to the physician for various reasons, for example, "tires easily," physical—normal. Since 1965, she had been on various antianxiety drugs and hypnotics, such as, Placidyl, Librium, Vistaril, and Donnatal. In 1961, her physician noted "no more refills until patient comes in for a visit." She was not seen by that particular physician anymore. She was then followed for about four years by another physician who gave her Donnatal, Valium, Indocin, thyroid, and Placidyl. He stated that she was being treated for "osteoarthritis of the spine, obesity, hypothyroidism, and chronic nervous tension." He had referred her to a gynecologist who wrote "she came in because she wanted a recommendation in regard to a hysterectomy." She had a uterus that was enlarged to 2½ to 3 times the normal size, but had minimal other symptoms except abdominal pain.

When interviewed a second time by telephone she had moved east to be with her siblings and parents, and also because her son had decided to go to school there. She moved seven months after her husband's death and wished she had not moved. She said she felt better, but still admitted to depressed mood, crying, feeling irritable, restless and fatigued. She had lost 45 pounds since the death of her husband, and had insomnia. She also felt guilty, had nothing to look forward to, and wished she were dead, and sometimes worried about losing her mind. She continued to have multiple physical symptoms and admitted to general poor health. She listed numerous problems since the death. She still felt angry about the death, and that both she and the initial physician who saw her husband were to blame. She had not had a bad reaction to the anniversary of the death. She had just been sad for one day. Her in-laws and minister had told her they thought she should remarry, but she said, "No, she didn't think she would" and then said, "It is possible, but I just can't think of it now." She had not gone to any parties, dated or had sexual intercourse. She thought she should be taking some college courses so that she would not be a burden as she grew older, but had not done so. She had had multiple physician visits and she had had her hysterectomy six weeks after her husband's death.

This woman might be considered by us a Briquet's Syndrome or an hysteric. At other places she would be called a patient with chronic hypochondriasis. However, since we had no hospital records, the physician who saw her also raised the possibility that she had some collagen disease, although this seems unlikely. She made some major changes in her life which she regretted. Her postbereavement course, however, was felt to be more consistent with her psychiatric problems than with the death of her spouse. She did not impress the interviewer, at either time, as "bitter" which may be the most pointed observation of the woman who did so poorly.

References

Glick, I. O., R. S. Weiss, and C. M. Parkes. 1974. *The First Year of Bereavement*. New York: Wiley.

Maddison, D. and A. Viola. 1968. "The Health of Widows in the Year Following Bereavement," *Journal of Psychosomatic Research*, 12:297–306.

Parkes, C. M. 1972. *Bereavement: Studies of Grief in Adult Life*. New York: International Universities Press.

Parkes, C. M. 1970. "The First Year of Bereavement: A Longitudinal Study of the Reaction of London Widows to the Death of Their Husbands," *Psychiatry*, 33(4):444–67.

Parkes, C. M. 1975. "Unexpected and Untimely Bereavement: A Statistical Study of Young Boston Widows and Widowers." In B. Schoenberg, et al., eds., *Bereavement: Its Psychosocial Aspects*, pp. 119–38. New York: Columbia University Press.

Parkes, C. M. and R. J. Brown. 1972. "Health After Bereavement: A Controlled Study of Young Boston Widows and Widowers," *Psychosomatic Medicine*, 34(5):449–61.

❧36
Living with Cardiovascular Disease: A Widow's Perspective

M. L. S. Vachon, K. Freedman, J. Rogers, W. A. L. Lyall, A. Formo, and S. J. J. Freeman

IN THEIR BOOK, *The First Year of Bereavement*, Glick, Weiss and Parkes document some of the problems which develop when a spouse dies suddenly from heart disease. Few authors, however, have attempted to detail systematically what happens when the first heart attack or stroke does not lead immediately to death but, instead, to an extended period of uncertainty.

This paper is a retrospective account of living with heart disease taken from interviews with widows, many of whom were questioned one to two months after the death. These recently widowed women are part of a larger longitudinal study of women whose husbands were 67 years of age and under at the time of death.* Of the 168 widows involved in the study, 61, or 38 percent, had husbands who had a history of cardiac or cardiovascular problems prior to their deaths from the same. Most of the data presented in the present paper will be anecdotal in nature.

Despite the nature and extent of previous warnings, most widows of heart disease victims report that the death occurred

This study "A Preventative Intervention for the Newly Bereaved" was funded as a Demonstration Model Grant by the Ontario Ministry of Health (DM 158).

unexpectedly. This apparent lack of preparation would seem to be due to the operation of at least two factors: when a husband has survived a series of heart attacks or strokes, one comes to think of him as being inherently strong and invulnerable; and the final heart attack or stroke has often been preceded by a period of time characterized by feelings of tremendous peace and well-being.

To illustrate:

> Mrs. A. went to work as usual that morning, leaving her husband at home where he was recovering from his sixth heart attack. He had been busy over the past few days, purchasing both a new boat and a completely new wardrobe for himself.
>
> Mr. A. called his wife at 4:00 that afternoon to report to her that he was feeling better than he had ever felt in his life and that he thought he would go for a drive with their daughter. At 4:15 P.M. the daughter called Mrs. A. to tell her that her husband had had another heart attack.
>
> On her way to the hospital, Mrs. A. mentally rearranged her busy schedule so that she would have time, over the next few weeks, to visit her husband in the hospital.
>
> When she arrived in the Emergency Room, Mrs. A. was informed that her husband had just died. She reacted with stunned disbelief and a sense that this could not really be true. Hospital staff provided no assistance at this time. Mrs. A. was left to drive home alone and to notify other relatives of her husband's death.

In instances where repeated attacks have occurred, there often develops a routinized pattern of coping with both times of crisis and the periods of relief that follow. While experience is teaching family members that heart attacks can be survived, and when patient needs demand continual care, the possibility that death may occur at some vague time in the future can only be of secondary importance. This emphasis on immediate issues suggests that women whose husbands die of heart disease will tend to differ from survivors of other long-term illnesses with respect to their utilization of any resources that may be available to the families of terminal patients. The question also arises of whether or not the concept of anticipatory grieving is at all useful in understanding what takes place at this time.

Many of the women in our study spoke of the difficulty they experienced in living with their husbands' reaction to the diagnosis of heart disease. Responses varied tremendously, but most men at some time expressed feelings of denial, fear, anger, and depression. Some, like Dr. D., kept their heart disease a secret from their wives, refused to see a physician, and carried a busier workload than ever. Others were faced with unemployment or early retirement as a result of their illness. Long hours at home often led to increasing agitation and, ultimately, to difficulties in interacting with other family members. Anger would be displaced onto others. In one situation, the husband threatened his wife and children with a gun saying, "If I'm going to die with this, I'll see all of you go first."

Such behavior is obviously a sign of mental illness, but one of the real problems many of the women experienced was gaining the cooperation of family physicians in treating such disorders or others resulting from the stress of leading severely restricted lives. No one wants to institutionalize a man to protect him and his family only to have the man die from the upset associated with threat of hospitalization. All of the women concerned had no difficulty in anticipating the guilt they would feel should he die under such circumstances. So, at the cost of destroying family life, they "hang on."

Children, especially adolescents, have tremendous difficulty during this time. Often their homes have assumed prisonlike qualities where their friends are no longer welcome, voices must be hushed, and parents cannot be disturbed. Pleasant family occasions become times of tremendous unexpressed fear, because even the emotions stimulated at such times can lead to that fatal attack.

> Mr. P. had three sons marry in a period of four years. His first heart attack occurred on the drive home from his oldest son's wedding. The second, preceded his next son's wedding by one week. The wedding party went to the intensive care unit for pictures, having been told the day before that Mr. P. would not leave the hospital alive. He left the hospital only to develop cancer two months later.
>
> When his third son married, Mr. P. had been dead for one month.

Children get caught in an approach-avoidance conflict wherein they cannot stand to be at home witnessing the tension and anxiety, constantly wondering if father will die in the middle of one of the emotional flareups that frequently occur. On the other hand, they cannot stand to be away from home for fear father might die without their knowing it. An attempt may be made to master such anxiety with behaviors such as leaving home, acting out, sexual promiscuity, and drinking.

Although most of the men in the study knew that their disease would eventually prove fatal, few discussed this with other family members, including their wives. The man who began to school his wife in practical matters following his first heart attack was a rarity in this study. For the most part, husbands and wives dealt individually with their own particular concerns for the future.

The threat of dying, however, could arise in a manipulative fashion from either side in an attempt to control the behavior of one's spouse. Such threats were verbalized by husbands, for instance, wishing to make unilateral decisions about finances, vacations, and so on. Wives, on the other hand, often expressed their fears as tools to get the patient to follow physicians' orders. For example, one wife whose husband suffered from hypertension constantly nagged him to look after his health or "suffer the consequences." Fears stated in such a manner are left to hang in the air, never elaborated upon, and never discussed in a mutually illuminating manner.

Interchanges dealing with health care frequently lead to arguments and angry outbursts. This same woman who continually cautioned her husband provoked him on one of these occasions to shout, "I hope I don't live to go through this again." When he died a short time later, the wife was filled with guilt at the thought that she had "nagged him to death." Another wife who had nagged her husband frequently about his health felt remorse for another reason. She wished that she had not so severely curtailed all of the activities he had enjoyed so much, since, in fact, he had only a short time to live.

Both of these anecdotes serve to illustrate the emotional tightrope wives of heart-disease victims walk in their dual role as wife/caretaker. The pressure placed upon women in getting their husbands to comply with doctor's orders cannot be overemphasized. Wives prepare special low sodium, low cholesterol diets which husbands refuse to eat; they hide cigarettes and liquor and nag about overwork. This type of supervision tends to lead to increased tension and the feeling of being caught in a vicious cycle. If a husband does not change his life-style he might die, but, by forcing the issue, the wife might "kill" him. Usually, the women interviewed felt that the maintenance of this precarious balance was their sole responsibility. Immediately after the deaths of their husbands, they were plagued by feelings of guilt about the quality of care they gave—"If only I had done more";

"If only I had done less"; "If only I had paid attention to all of the symptoms."

Another major problem which develops concerns the question of sexual relations. Although many couples are told that they may resume a normal sexual life, much anxiety is generated in worrying that the husband will die in the middle of lovemaking. The conflict engendered in one widow whose husband died in such a manner resulted in an unresolved grief reaction lasting for several years. Conflict created at the thought of contributing to one's husband's death is further magnified by the fear of what others might think if, indeed, such a situation did occur. Will one be criticized for indulging in "base desires" at such a time, or will one be reprimanded for denying pleasure to a man who may not live to see tomorrow? The impact of preoccupation with such concerns on one's sexual life is obvious.

So far, this paper has concentrated on those widows whose spouses have had heart attacks. The problems experienced following cardiovascular accidents are somewhat different. In many of these instances, husbands are invalided for months, or even years, before their deaths. The wife's entire life, in such cases, has been focused around either continuous care for him at home or daily visiting with him in hospital. These women frequently experience a social death long before their husbands actually die. Family and friends drop away during the lengthy illness, leading the wife to harbor extreme resentment, which may surface at any time during the illness or initial stages of widowhood. The cessation of normal patterns of interaction so early on in the process makes loneliness a very real problem for women in these circumstances. It is doubtful if very many of them will be able to regenerate a social life similar in any respect to the one eroded by time and bad feelings.

The manner in which women cope with long-term illness varies tremendously among individuals.

Mrs. A. nursed her husband, paralyzed by a stroke, at home for ten years because he was afraid of hospitals. During that time they spent all of their savings, went into debt and lost their home. Throughout this period, they lied to relatives about the life they were leading, since they had come to Canada to build a better life.

Mrs. A. kept herself busy during her husband's illness by taking numerous home nursing courses to better care for him.

The husband of another woman lost considerable weight in the one and one-half years following his stroke. Each pound he lost, she put on, almost in an attempt to personally compensate for his dramatic reduction in size. Looking back at this time, once the death had finally occurred, she described it as a period of tremendous physical and psychological strain, far harder on her than her grief as a new widow. This woman sleeps a great deal now, in contrast to the many nights she would remain awake in order to care for her husband when he was still alive.

Another widow experienced the opposite reaction. Her husband was on the verge of death for many years. She sought to escape the situation, in which her husband and their lives together were radically altered, by staying in bed as much as possible, getting up only when it was absolutely necessary. Now that her husband has died, this woman finds it difficult to remain at home and suffers from severe insomnia.

These are but a few examples illustrating the range of behaviors that may accompany long-term care of a spouse with heart disease and the initial stages of widowhood. In order to look at these reactions more systematically, one might develop a continuum based on the two indexes of type/amount of care required and the extent to which there is a disruption of normal activities. At one pole would be the widows who regarded their husband's illness as tremendously stressful and a great drain upon their personal resources. This group constitutes 35 percent of women in our study whose husbands had chronic cardiovascular disease. They now describe themselves as feeling both exhausted and still tense, following their husbands' deaths.

One of the women in this category had a husband who was continuously in and out of hospital for two years. During his periods at home, she could never leave him for more than fifteen minutes at any one time. One day, following his death, she stood waiting for a cashier at the grocery store. When she realized how long the line was, and how slowly it moved, she experienced a rush of panic, dropped her groceries, and hurried home. She was halfway there before she realized that she no longer had to rush, her husband did not require her care now.

It is women such as this one, who, after the death, initially have great difficulty in coping with the large amount of time that is now available. No amount of planned activity seems to provide a substitute for the many hours spent in the routine, but constant, care of one's husband. Finding a meaningful, time-consuming substitute can become a major problem for widows used to being needed and suffering from an excess of nervous energy.

At the other end of our continuum, one could place those women who approximate one particular widow, who had so routinized her husband's care that it was simply seen as part of her housework. She did not think of him as ill but merely as having a "condition" that required routine care but was in no way disruptive to regular family functioning. Following his death, she feels no particular stress.

When husbands finally die, the women who have lived through the strokes feel a sense of loss, mixed with one of relief that the suffering for all concerned is now over. Many have difficulty starting to build a new life for themselves, because social contacts and skills have deteriorated during the lingering illness. In addition, there is often anger at those who have disappointed and dropped away, and guilt over tasks grudgingly done. Some anger is also frequently directed at physicians for their lack of honesty with respect to symptom watching, drug reactions, and eventual outcome.

In conclusion, living with the threat of death from heart disease can create tremendous stress in a family situation. Reactions may vary but usually include denial, anger, fear, depression, and a flight into overactivity. Unlike the case with the wives of cancer patients, there is often no anticipatory grieving in heart disease, because the husband may appear quite well between heart attacks or may seem to have stabilized following a stroke. Nevertheless, there is a constant, unexpressed fear of death which precludes the enjoyment of life and usually results in constant anxiety, particularly whenever the spouses are separated.

Death, when it comes, is usually seen as quite unexpected. Guilt and remorse frequently follow, but there is also a sense of relief that the suffering is over at last for the entire family. Resuming a new life is difficult but, given time, most of these women adjust quite well.

Reference

Glick, I., R. S. Weiss and C. M. Parkes. 1974. *The First Year of Bereavement.* New York: Wiley.

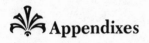**Appendixes**

ꙮ Appendix A
The Facts of Cardiovascular Disease

Aaron B. Shaffer and Gerald Glick

THE MODES OF cardiovascular death are limited. These are cardiovascular failure, shock, cardiac arrest, and stroke (local destruction of brain tissue). The first three of these can be regarded as constituting a continuum of mechanisms of circulatory failure distinguished by their durations and rates of progression. Cardiovascular failure may run a course of years; shock, of hours or days; and cardiac arrest, of seconds or minutes. An individual dying a cardiovascular death frequently traverses all three. Furthermore, shock is a common terminal event of noncardiovascular diseases such as septicemia and cancer. The attitude of the physician, and his approach to these problems, should be determined by the clinical setting in which they occur, a concept that is stressed throughout this chapter.

It should also be borne in mind that since the function of the circulation is to sustain all the tissues of the body, and since the circulation may be inadequate in this function for periods ranging up to years before death, secondary organ degeneration, mainly involving the lung and liver, and to a lesser extent the kidney, is a feature of advanced cardiovascular disease and contributes to its morbidity and mortality.

Aneurysms

A localized thinning and ballooning of a blood vessel wall is termed an aneurysm. Aneurysms most often involve arteries and present a danger because they carry the risk of rupture. Aneurysms of major importance are those of the aorta and cerebral arteries. Aortic aneurysms are most often atherosclerotic in origin. These are usually found in older persons, and tend to develop gradually. Dissecting aneurysms may occur in younger as well as older individuals, often in association with systemic hypertension or the Marfan syndrome, and tend to be sudden in onset. Mycotic aneurysms may occur in the aorta or elsewhere, usually in association with overwhelming sepsis. Berry aneurysms occur at certain sites of predilection in the cerebral arterial system. These are congenital in origin and are a common cause of stroke in young people.

Gross rupture of an aneurysm at any of these sites is usually rapidly fatal; death may appear to be instantaneous or survival may be for only a few minutes. Death is due to massive internal hemorrhage or extensive brain damage. The basic treatment of aneurysm revolves around prevention of rupture. Frequently, clinical signs or symptoms or radiologic findings will suggest that rupture is likely or impending (evidence of enlargement of the aneurysmal sac or evidence of a slow leak). Complete diagnostic studies and operative intervention when feasible can frequently bring about cure of the disease.

As noted above, gross rupture of an aortic aneurysm leads to almost immediate death from hemorrhagic shock and damage to contiguous organs. Once rupture occurs, heroic measures such as massive transfusion or emergency operation are rarely effective. The same ominous prognosis attends external rupture of a dissecting aortic aneurysm.

Other acute features of dissecting aneurysm that affect morbidity and mortality are involvement in the dissection process of peripheral branches of the aorta (such as vessels to brain or kidney), involvement of a coronary artery producing acute myocardial infarction, possibly with resultant ventricular fibrillation, rupture of the aneurysm into the pericardial sac producing acute pericardial tamponade, and involvement of the aortic valve producing aortic regurgitation, which if severe may culminate in left ventricular failure. Acute measures that may support life in these circumstances include electrical defibrillation, pericardiocentesis, and treatment of acute congestive heart failure. Other important emergency measures include intravenous administration of agents such as trimethaphan (Arfonad) and propranolol (Inderal) to keep arterial pressure at relatively low levels, and to reduce the velocity of ejection of blood from the heart with the object of minimizing the possibility of further dissection or rupture. Aortography and emergency operation (if the pathologic anatomy is suitable), including aortic valve replacement when necessary, may prevent additional manifestations of the dissection and correct some of them. At times, conservative management with drugs alone may bring about apparent cure for long periods of time. Signs that a patient is approaching the terminal phases of this disease include the development of stroke and progressive congestive heart failure not responsive to medical management, which leads to intractable pulmonary edema and a shocklike syndrome.

In the case of rupture of a cerebral arterial aneurysm, death may be instantaneous, or a complete spontaneous recovery may ensue. The manifestations of ruptured berry aneurysm in the surviving patient are those of subarachnoid hemorrhage or stroke. Signs of increased intracranial pressure are usually present. A cautious spinal tap will give a measure of intracranial pressure and will show whether blood is present in the spinal fluid. Heroic measures include cerebral angiography, and subsequent ligation of one internal carotid artery, or a direct operative approach to the aneurysm itself if this procedure is feasible. The supportive measures are those used in the treatment of stroke, including attention to respiratory function (nasal suction, oxygen, use of respirators, changing the position of the patient), adequate hydration and nutritional intake (intravenous fluids, feeding through a nasogastric tube), urethral catheter in order to monitor urinary output, support of the circulation (measures to prevent pulmonary embolization and sometimes to lower arterial pressure), and appropriate nursing care (patient hygiene and sanitation, prevention of bed sores). Signs that the patient is medically terminal are as in other instances of stroke. Signs of death, notably complete unresponsiveness, respiratory paralysis, and pupillary findings, are also those of stroke.

Consultations that may be useful in the above instances are medical, neurological, general surgical, cardiovascular surgical, and neurosurgical. If death occurs in the hospital, donor suitability for potential transplantation of various organs will depend on the age of the patient, previous general state of health, and the level of organ damage resulting from the underlying acute or chronic disease.

Arrhythmia, and Cardiac Arrest

Arrhythmias interfere with cardiac function by causing the heart to beat either too fast or too slowly to meet the circulatory needs of the body. Some arrhythmias cause loss of the normal sequence of atrial and ventricular contraction which also interferes, usually to a lesser degree, with cardiac function.

Ectopic tachycardias may be well tolerated or lead to congestive heart failure or to a shocklike state. Unless the severity of the' underlying heart disease does not permit, such arrhythmias are readily amenable to such measures as drug therapy, cardioversion by external electrical shock, rate overdrive through the use of artificial pacemakers, or, in extremely unusual cases, experimental operations aimed at altering the anatomy of the conduction system of the heart. If a patient is terminal in this setting, it is usually because severe underlying heart disease is associated, or the arrhythmia has culminated in cardiac arrest (see below).

Drastic slowing of the heart rate, as in many instances of complete heart block, brings about a clinical syndrome suggestive of congestive heart failure, and may cause clouding of the sensorium in addition. Such severe bradycardias may culminate in cardiac arrest and death if complete failure of ventricular pacemakers occurs, or, as is frequent, the course is punctuated by episodes of ventricular tachycardia or ventricular fibrillation (complete cessation of organized ventricular contraction). Either train of events may give rise to so-called Stokes-Adams attacks (acute periods of unconsciousness with or without convulsions), that may revert spontaneously within a few seconds or that may constitute actual cardiac arrest leading to almost immediate death in the absence of emergency treatment. The manifestations of complete heart block, including Stokes-Adams attacks and cardiac arrest, can usually be treated or prevented by insertion of an electrode catheter into the heart, which allows either temporary or permanent artificial pacing. Sometimes only temporary artificial pacing is necessary, as in some instances of reversible complete heart block complicating acute myocardial infarction. In other instances, artificial pacing may be totally ineffective because of myocardial damage. Thus, arrhythmias per se rarely cause death unless they culminate in intractable shock, intractable heart failure, or cardiac arrest.

Cardiac arrest is, effectively, complete cessation of the circulation. Unconsciousness and frequently convulsions occur within ten seconds as the cerebral circulation comes to a standstill, and if the state persists untreated for longer than three or four minutes, permanent brain damage will probably result, despite subsequent cardiac resuscitation.

Since dying always culminates in cardiac arrest, much consideration has been given to identifying categories of patients that should be resuscitated. Surely a patient with an acknowledged terminal illness, such as widespread carcinoma, should not be subject to resuscitation nor should it be attempted in patients who have had untreated cardiac arrest for longer than several minutes. Otherwise, any individual is a candidate for resuscitation in whom cardiac arrest is unexpected. In addition, patients in a coronary surveillance unit, in whom such episodes are expected, are ideal candidates for resuscitation, since they frequently resume a benign course if tided over the acute episode.

Teams organized for the emergency treatment of cardiac arrest, consisting of house staff, nurses, anesthesiologists, and so on, exist in all hospitals. The most important steps for successful resuscitation are the securing of an airway, initiating some form of mouth-to-mouth artificial respiration, instituting external cardiac massage, providing intravenous therapy (to correct metabolic acidosis and for the administration of appropriate drugs), and electrocardiographic diagnosis to determine whether ventricular fibrillation or cardiac standstill is the underlying abnormality, followed by defibrillation with external countershock or by emergency insertion of a cardiac pacemaker as indicated. The remaining treatment is that of the underlying disease, if any.

Treatment is, of course, intensive until the circulation is restored or death supervenes. Cessation of all vital activities and dilated, unreactive pupils are accepted as signs of death. Should the circulation be restored but the patient remain unconscious, intravenous hypertonic glucose or dexamethasone may be used as a therapeutic trial to treat cerebral edema that may possibly be present. Supportive therapy such as use of respirators, support of renal function, appropriate nursing care, and so forth, are then indicated for some days, although the possibility of recovery decreases as time goes on. Death is diagnosed from eventual failure of the circulation, pupillary changes, loss of all reflexes and a flat electroencephalogram reflecting absent neuronal activity.

Atherosclerosis (including stroke)

Atherosclerosis is a generalized disease of the arterial wall. Its underlying cause is unknown, although a hereditary basis has been suggested. Atherosclerosis also has a known relationship to systemic hypertension, diabetes mellitus, some hyperlipidemias, cigarette smoking, dietary patterns, and certain obscure metabolic disorders. Most of its manifestations are due to thickening of blood vessel walls with consequent encroachment on the lumen and interference with the blood supply to various organs. Involvement of the aorta in this process may lead to the development of aortic aneurysms. Manifestations of atherosclerosis are far more common in, but not restricted to, older persons. Atherosclerosis has certain sites of predilection which tend to group its manifestations into fairly well defined clinical syndromes. These sites include the coronary vessels with resulting angina pectoris, myocardial infarction, or congestive heart failure; the arteries of the brain (cerebrovascular disease) with resulting stroke due to cerebral artery thrombosis as the most common manifestation; and the small vessels of the kidney with resulting hypertension and possible renal failure. Mesenteric artery occlusion leading to bowel necrosis and signs of mechanical intestinal obstruction is less common. Involvement of the arteries of the lower extremities producing intermittent claudication and often gangrene, although relatively common, is less immediately life-threatening.

About 80 percent of cases of stroke (cerebrovascular accident) are due to thrombosis related to cerebral arteriosclerosis, about 10 percent are due to cerebral hemorrhage related to berry aneurysms or systemic hypertension, and about 10 percent are due to cerebral arterial emboli related to underlying rheumatic heart disease or coronary artery disease. It can be deduced from the foregoing that stroke is largely a disease of older people and that coronary artery disease is likely to be associated in a high percentage of cases. The acute nature of stroke on the basis of thrombosis or embolism is due to dependence of the brain on a second-to-second oxygen supply. Interruption of the blood supply to a region of the brain causes ischemia within a few seconds and in-

Appendix A   311

farction within minutes. Cerebral hemorrhage, which may be subarachnoid, intracerebral, or both, produces its effects mainly by physical injury and compression of the brain substance.

The manifestations resulting from a compromised cerebral circulation vary widely. Regions of infarction are frequently an incidental finding at autopsy; symptoms may be fleeting or short-lived as in the commonly occurring transient ischemic attacks. Manifestations of established stroke depend on the location and extent of damage. Recovery, if it occurs, may be rapid and complete, or slow and variable. Appropriate physiotherapy may play an important role in reducing residual impairment. A considerable mortality attends the first episode of stroke. Prognosis depends upon the age of the patient, the extent of neurological deficit, the presence or absence of associated heart disease, and the chances of recurrence. Severely disabled individuals with a relatively unclouded sensorium require careful medical management throughout their lives. Such management is aimed at the avoidance of renal, respiratory, nutritional, and cutaneous complications. Loss of consciousness or a course characterized by progressive impairment of consciousness and of other vital functions, such as coughing and swallowing, carries a poor prognosis.

Transient unconsciousness can be associated with intracranial hemorrhage. In the case of a large hemorrhage, rapidly progressive loss of consciousness often ensues, leading to coma and early death. Delirium and lethargy are also indications of severe brain damage. In these circumstances, the patient may appear functionally decorticate or decerebrate. Hemorrhage involving the brain stem leads to rapidly developing quadriplegia, unconsciousness, pinpoint pupils, and death. Generally, the prognosis in cerebral hemorrhage is poor. In the case of hemorrhage due to aneurysm, recurrence is likely. Unremitting coma indicates a poor prognosis, mortality approaching 100 percent in cases of coma related to intracerebral hemorrhage due to hypertension.

Coma, then, characterizes the medically terminal patient who has experienced a stroke, especially in the setting of cerebral hemorrhage. A similar grave prognosis attaches to the patient who undergoes a gradual deterioration of the sensorium after the acute episode, particularly if it is associated with deterioration of other vital functions, notably respiration and circulation. On the other hand, transient lethargy or coma associated with the onset of a stroke does not necessarily preclude a benign outcome.

Radical therapy, such as emergency operation after cerebral

angiography is rarely of avail once deep coma is present. Palliation is aimed at otherwise maintaining the functional integrity of the individual, and buying time for spontaneous improvement in cerebral function, which, however, becomes less likely as the days go by. Many interrelated measures are included under the heading of palliation. Adequate respiratory function may require oxygen, tracheobronchial suction, use of assisted respiration, tracheotomy, serial blood-gas measurements, and systematic changes in the position of the patient. Measures aimed at preserving the circulation may include, in addition to some of the above, the use of elastic stockings to prevent venous stasis, sometimes anticoagulant therapy, cardiotonic drugs, and artificial pacemakers.

Maintenance of nutrition and fluid and electrolyte balance usually requires intravenous therapy, nasogastric tube feeding, and an indwelling urinary catheter for monitoring urinary output. Intensive nursing care is needed to provide necessary personal sanitation and to prevent decubitus ulcers from developing. Prophylactic antibiotics are not used, but specific therapy for respiratory or urinary tract infections may be indicated.

It is clear that support of the patient's bodily functions and prevention of complications may keep the patient in an alive or seemingly alive state indefinitely. Two distinct questions arise in deciding the disposition of such patients: When can intensive therapy be discontinued on the basis that survival is impossible, so that the patient may be allowed to die in dignity? How is actual death diagnosed in a comatose patient in whom vital functions are artificially maintained? The answer to the first question depends on the underlying diagnosis, the prognosis as known, the duration of coma, the evidence of continuing dissolution of function, and the complex psychosocial factors involved in physician-patient-family interrelationships. The criteria used to answer the second question must of course take into account the life-support systems that are being employed. Although universal agreement does not as yet exist, the present tendency is to define the occurrence of death as follows: deep coma with total unresponsiveness, no spontaneous movements, no active breathing on turning off the respirator for short periods provided that immediately before turning it off the arterial oxygen tension was normal and room air had been breathed, complete areflexia which involves total abolition of central nervous system activity including fixed, dilated pupils, absent superficial and deep reflexes, and a flat electroencephalogram, including absence of electroencephalographic responses to noise or painful stimuli. The duration of time necessary for these signs to be present before pronouncing death still remains controversial and ranges between 30 minutes and 24 hours.

Criteria on which to base the potential for transplantability of organs include the age of the patient, duration of illness, associated illnesses, state of function of these organs at the time of death, actual mode of death, and freedom from infection.

Atherosclerotic Heart Disease

Atherosclerotic heart disease (coronary artery disease, ischemic heart disease) is one of the major causes of morbidity and mortality in the Western world, particularly involving middle-aged and older people. This disease has a wide spectrum of manifestations, including sudden death or cardiac arrest without warning in previously asymptomatic individuals. Atherosclerotic coronary artery disease is of course the most common cause of chest pain on exertion (angina pectoris). Its two most potentially fatal manifestations are acute myocardial infarction and congestive heart failure. Death from myocardial infarction is usually the result of either cardiogenic shock, for which no suitable routine management is available at present, or cardiac arrest stemming from abnormal rhythms or heart block, which most coronary care units are now equipped to anticipate and treat appropriately. For further information see: Arrhythmia and Cardiac Arrest, Atherosclerosis, Cardiovascular Failure, Myocardial Infarction, Shock.

Congestive Heart Failure

See Cardiovascular Failure.

Congenital Anomalies

Congenital cardiovascular disease embraces a broad spectrum of conditions varying from those that are incompatible with extrauterine life to those that do not interfere in any way with a normal lifespan. The highest rate of serious morbidity and mortality are in the early weeks and months of life when the more severe and

complex anomalies will manifest themselves. Cardiac catheterization and palliative or corrective operations, frequently on an
emergency basis, are feasible even in the early hours of life.
When death occurs it is usually due to hypoxia or congestive
heart failure, with cardiac arrest frequently supervening. Operative mortality has also been high in this age group. Important
psychosocial relationships entering into the management of infants with severe congenital heart disease include the parents' attitudes toward the baby and the level of their confidence in its
care.

Mortality from congenital heart disease is relatively uncommon during later childhood and young adulthood, and involves
those with severe, but not rapidly lethal, lesions and those who
have undergone operations that permit survival past infancy. Sudden death due to congenital aortic stenosis may occur in this age
group, particularly in symptomatic patients.

Certain common types of congenital heart disease, such as
atrial septal defect, are usually quite well tolerated into adult life.
Congestive heart failure presenting in adult life in patients with
congenital heart disease is usually readily amenable to operative
correction and should not be a cause of death. Acute and potentially fatal complications of coarctation of the aorta include dissecting aneurysm and stroke. Certain congenital lesions, including
ventricular septal defect, patent ductus arteriosus, and coarctation
of the aorta, are subject to infectious endocarditis or endarteritis.
Death in patients with tetralogy of Fallot or hemodynamically
similar lesions results from hypoxia or from the remote complications of palliative operations.

Obstructive pulmonary vascular disease associated with large
septal defects or aortico-pulmonary communications (Eisen-
menger syndrome), is one of the most common causes of disability and death due to congenital heart disease in adult life and is
not routinely amenable to operative treatment. This syndrome
may give rise to physical disability at any time but is frequently
compatible with a near-normal life-style until about 40 years of
age. Dyspnea, fatigue, and cyanosis are the main clinical features.
Polycythemia is usually present. Hemoptysis is a poor prognostic
sign. Sudden death after age 40 is frequent, presumably as a
result of cardiac arrest; congestive heart failure associated with
pulmonary artery thrombosis is the other major cause of death.
Treatment is symptomatic and palliative. Such measures as use of
cardiotonic agents and diuretics, as well as phlebotomy for severe

polycythemia, and chronic anticoagulant therapy, frequently relieve symptoms, but their effects on the natural history of this disease are unclear.

See also Aneurysms, Arrhythmia and Cardiac Arrest, Cardiovascular Failure, Endocarditis.

Endocarditis (excluding rheumatic)

Bacterial or infectious (nonrheumatic) endocarditis mainly affects the heart valves and is loosely divided into two overlapping types, acute and subacute. Acute bacterial endocarditis is usually the result of overwhelming sepsis and may affect normal heart valves. The manifestations of generalized sepsis frequently mask those of heart involvement. In this setting, bacterial endocarditis is almost always fatal, or death is due to overwhelming infection, septic shock, or renal failure.

Subacute bacterial endocarditis is usually the result of a transient bacteremia becoming engrafted upon a valve that has been damaged by rheumatic fever or upon a congenitally malformed valve or other structure of the heart (e.g., a bicuspid aortic valve). In recent years, subacute bacterial endocarditis involving prosthetic heart valves or involving normal valves, usually the tricuspid, on the basis of drug abuse by the intravenous route, has also become a very significant problem.

Subacute bacterial endocarditis must be suspected when a chronic infectious process occurs in association with a cardiac murmur. The definitive laboratory diagnosis hinges on obtaining positive blood cultures. Medical management is based on treating the infection with high doses of appropriate antibiotics for four to six weeks.

Three major factors contribute to morbidity and mortality in subacute bacterial endocarditis. One of these is the infection itself. A second is partial or complete destruction of heart valves leading to mitral or aortic insufficiency, which, with occasional direct involvement of the myocardium itself in the infectious process, can lead to acutely developing heart failure. Third is embolism, which may result from sterile fragments or from infected material that may have broken away from the involved valve. When the left side of the heart is involved the cerebral, coronary, mesenteric, and renal arteries are prone to embolism with the consequent production of stroke, myocardial infarction, mesenteric insufficiency, bowel necrosis, or, infrequently, renal failure. Right-sided involvement leads to infected pulmonary emboli. The downhill course following acute heart failure may be rapid. Emergency cardiac catheterization and operative intervention with replacement of the diseased valve by a prosthesis frequently bring about recovery.

Hypertensive Disease

Systemic hypertension is a common disease whose morbid manifestations tend to appear in older people. The etiology of hypertension is unknown in the vast majority of cases ("essential hypertension"), or it may be associated with chronic renal parenchymal disease. Rarely (as in various adrenal tumors, coarctation of the aorta, renovascular disease, or unilateral renal parenchymal disease) is hypertension amenable to operative therapy that may be curative.

Hypertension denotes simply elevation of systolic and diastolic blood pressure. The main complications of high blood pressure involve the heart, kidney, and brain. These complications develop acutely or chronically, and it is now evident that these complications can be forestalled by appropriate medical therapy aimed at lowering the blood pressure to normotensive levels.

Hypertension accelerates the progression of atherosclerosis and thus augments the incidence, morbidity, and mortality of myocardial infarction stemming from coronary artery disease. By the same token, systemic hypertension predisposes to stroke on the basis of cerebral atherosclerosis leading to cerebral artery thrombosis and cerebral infarction. Also, hypertension is the most common underlying cause of massive intracerebral hemorrhage. Renal insufficiency may develop insidiously in the course of longstanding hypertension and is a frequent cause of death. Strain on the left ventricle leads to chronic congestive heart failure or acute left heart failure (acute pulmonary edema).

Two ill-defined, somewhat overlapping, but clinically recognized syndromes—malignant or accelerated hypertension, and hypertensive encephalopathy—may suddenly aggravate the previously stable course of essential hypertension or hypertension of known etiology. Both are amenable to therapy, and to some extent are preventable. They are, however, potentially fatal and indicate a poor prognosis. Hypertensive encephalopathy, which appears to involve vascular spasm of the cerebral vessels over and above anatomic damage to these vessels, is characterized by headache, focal and diffuse neurologic findings, abnormal retinal findings, and possibly convulsions or coma. Accelerated hypertension is marked by a sudden sharp further rise in arterial pressure associated with cardiac and retinal manifestations, and acceleration of renal failure.

Another rare type of hypertensive heart disease is primary pulmonary hypertension, which leads to strain and failure of the right side of the heart. This is a rapidly progressive disease of middle life, mainly involving women. It is due to the insidious development of obstructive pulmonary vascular disease. As the name implies, the etiology is unknown, and although treatment is unsatisfactory, anticoagulation and certain antihypertensive medications have been advocated. Other treatment is as described for obstructive pulmonary vascular disease.

Myocardial Infarction

Myocardial infarction is one of the most common causes of morbidity and mortality in middle and older age groups, especially men, although by no means is it restricted to this age and sex. The underlying cause is usually atherosclerotic coronary artery disease. Much less commonly, myocardial infarction may result from coronary emboli originating from the vegetations produced by bacterial endocarditis, or from fibrin clots in the left atrium in patients with mitral stenosis, or by involvement of a coronary artery in the course of a dissecting aneurysm of the aorta. Rare diseases of the arterial wall may also cause myocardial infarction. As noted above, incidence, morbidity, and mortality are heightened by coexisting high blood pressure.

The manifestations of myocardial infarction are many, and it is probable that the natural history of the disease will be altered significantly by coronary artery bypass procedures and related surgical developments. Acute myocardial infarction may or may not be preceded by a history of angina pectoris.

The clinical course of acute myocardial infarction, characterized by chest pain and electrocardiographic changes, is frequently benign with rapid recovery, the only residuum being the increased statistical possibility of future episodes. On the other hand, recovery from myocardial infarction may be incomplete and attended by chronic illness, such as development or worsening of angina pectoris, or development of chronic congestive heart failure.

Death from myocardial infarction also takes a variety of forms. At one end of the spectrum is the occurrence of sudden death in previously asymptomatic individuals, presumably as a result of ventricular fibrillation. Under these circumstances the typical pathologic picture of myocardial infarction does not have time to develop. Depending on the definition one chooses for sudden death, up to 50 percent of individuals suffering an acute myocardial infarction will fall into this category, and will, therefore, never reach the hospital. Other, less fulminant, causes of death are the following:

1) Tachy- or bradyarrhythmias that progress to cardiac arrest. In an intensive care unit, these arrhythmias can generally be treated or prevented by such measures as drug therapy, temporary insertion of artificial pacemakers, or electrical countershock. At times, however, these measures are insufficient, and protracted tachyarrhythmias may prove ultimately fatal as cardiac arrest, shock, or heart failure supervene. Recently, operative removal of the infarcted area has been found successful in the treatment of some otherwise refractory chronic arrhythmias.

2) Cardiogenic shock, which is characterized by a marked fall in arterial blood pressure, cool, pale and sweaty skin, oliguria, and clouded sensorium. This syndrome occurs when 40 percent or more of the heart muscle is involved in the infarction process. Established cardiogenic shock carries a mortality of 80 percent to 100 percent. This mortality has not been diminished significantly by the development of modern coronary-care units, which is in marked contrast to the beneficial effects these units have had on the incidence of death from arrhythmias. Heroic measures presently being developed and assessed include assisted circulation by intra-aortic balloon counterpulsation and emergency coronary-artery bypass operations.

3) Ventricular rupture, which results from softening of the ventricular wall. This complication is nearly always fatal, usually occurs in the first week, and is most common in hypertensive individuals.

4) Heart failure which takes the form of acute pulmonary edema or chronic progressive congestive heart failure. Acute pulmonary edema may develop suddenly because of widespread damage to the left ventricular wall, formation of a ventricular sep-

tal defect as a result of rupture of the septum, or development of torrential mitral regurgitation on the basis of papillary muscle dysfunction or rupture. These complications are frequently fatal. In the acute stages, routine medical management may be of some avail; if failure persists, surgery to bypass the coronary artery obstructions, repair the ventricular septum, or replace the mitral valve, may be necessary.

Chronic congestive heart failure may develop after recovery from the acute infarct, or may occur later, especially if there is aneurysm formation, that is, ballooning of the left ventricular wall. Sometimes it is necessary to remove the aneurysm by operation, either with or without additional procedures such as coronary-artery bypass or mitral valve replacement. Frequently, such operations yield extremely gratifying results. Diffuse dysfunction of the left ventricular wall that is due to coronary artery disease, with or without multiple myocardial infarctions, is a cause of congestive heart failure and is at present subject only to palliative medical therapy.

Pulmonary Edema

The most common causes of acute pulmonary edema are acute left ventricular failure and other acute circulatory failure states characterized by sharp rises in left atrial or pulmonary venous pressure. Pulmonary edema due to noncirculatory causes such as respiratory irritants, high altitude disease, or that related to cerebral lesions, head injury or drug abuse, will not be considered here.

The usual causes of acute left ventricular failure leading to pulmonary edema are coronary artery disease with myocardial infarction, systemic hypertension, and aortic stenosis. Less commonly, acute pulmonary edema results from aortic regurgitation or mitral regurgitation, especially when these conditions come on abruptly as in subacute bacterial endocarditis or myocardial infarction. The most common circulatory cause unrelated to left ventricular failure per se is mitral stenosis. Other such causes include rare types of left atrial or pulmonary venous obstruction (e.g., left atrial myxoma). Uremic acute pulmonary edema, an entity whose mechanism is complex, sometimes occurs in patients with chronic renal failure. In the marginally compensated heart, trachyarrhythmias, undue exertion, or fluid overload may precipitate pulmonary edema.

In a patient who may have had few previous complaints, the sudden onset of dyspnea, tachycardia, pallor, cold perspiration, orthopnea, cyanosis, bubbling rales, and frothy sputum is a terrifying event. However, depending on the underlying cause, acute pulmonary edema is frequently self-limited or responds rapidly to medical measures including intravenous morphine, oxygen, tracheobronchial suction, sitting position, rotating tourniquets, and diuretics and digitalis. In the relatively uncommon event that these measures, or measures aimed at combating precipitating causes such as infection, hypertension, tachyarrhythmias, or hypervolemia, are not successful, then more vigorous efforts aimed at palliation, such as intermittent positive pressure breathing, assisted ventilation, correction of metabolic acidosis, and use of antifoaming agents must be employed. In selected patients, more radical steps such as assisted circulation or appropriate cardiac operations should be considered. In most instances, pulmonary edema resolves itself in a matter of hours, culminating either in recovery or death. Poor prognostic signs, besides evidence of failure of response to medical management, include: progressive hypoxemia and respiratory acidosis, hypotension, depressed sensorium, and development of cardiac arrhythmias.

Pulmonary Embolism

Pulmonary embolism, or lodging of solid material within the pulmonary arterial system, is a condition that is encountered commonly. Thrombi or blood clots which form in the veins of the lower extremities or the pelvis are the usual sources. Much less commonly, pulmonary emboli originate from the lesions of subacute bacterial endocarditis of the right side of the heart, as is seen most commonly in drug addicts. The latter, and other types of emboli such as tumor emboli from the right side of the heart, fat emboli, air emboli, amniotic-fluid emboli, and emboli of foreign material as may result in the course of drug abuse, will not be considered further here.

A small but definite incidence of pulmonary embolism occurs in apparently healthy young people. This incidence has been increased somewhat by the use of birth control pills. Pulmonary embolism is most common in older persons whose blood circulation has been slowed by heart disease, or who have been immobilized by illness or operation.

Massive pulmonary embolism may cause death within seconds or minutes. Smaller pulmonary emboli are manifested by chest pain, tachypnea, sinus tachycardia and, frequently, changes in electrocardiographic contour. Evidence of pulmonary embolization may be apparent on chest roentgenograms, but such findings are usually subtle. Proof of diagnosis depends on studies of blood gases, radioactive lung scans, or pulmonary arteriography. If pulmonary infarction (death of lung tissue) occurs as a result of an embolus, pleuritic chest pain and hemoptysis develop, and characteristic findings are seen in the chest roentgenogram. Larger pulmonary emboli also produce evidence of circulatory collapse, notably hypotension or shock, and jugular venous distension indicating right heart failure. A rarer manifestation of pulmonary-embolic disease is the syndrome of multiple small pulmonary emboli giving rise to a syndrome resembling progressive congestive heart failure that is intractable to usual medical therapy.

Therapy of established pulmonary embolism is for the most part palliative and centers around support of right ventricular function and maintenance of arterial pressure in the face of acute obstruction to right ventricular outflow. The most important medical therapy is prophylactic and takes the form of anticoagulant therapy in order to prevent further embolization. In addition, some evidence suggests that such therapy has a direct effect on the lung to promote survival and recovery. Insertion of an inferior vena caval umbrella, a minor surgical procedure, along with anticoagulant therapy, appears to be the most effective means of preventing further emboli. There is evidence that thrombotic pulmonary emboli may lyse spontaneously over the course of days, weeks, or months. Hastening of dissolution of clots by fibrinolytic therapy remains an experimental procedure.

All pertinent preventive measures having been applied, immediate prognosis is good in most cases of pulmonary embolism, or depends upon any underlying disease state. In some instances, as in pulmonary embolism with shock, the embolism itself is life-threatening on a mechanical basis and emergency pulmonary arteriography and embolectomy may be life-saving. Such patients may survive one to several days but the prognosis is bad even with operation.

Rheumatic Heart Disease

Rheumatic heart disease as seen in the adult usually stems from acute rheumatic fever occurring in childhood or early adolescence and is due to involvement of heart valves in the acute process.

Rheumatic heart disease usually becomes manifest symptomatically at around age 40, after a latent period that may exceed twenty years. In as many as 50 percent of cases of rheumatic valvular heart disease, however, a definite clinical history of acute rheumatic fever cannot be obtained. Also, not all individuals with acute rheumatic fever develop valvular heart disease, and in some the latter condition is asymptomatic throughout life.

The etiology of rheumatic heart disease is unknown except that it is believed to have an immune basis and is related to antecedent streptococcal infection. Prompt treatment of streptococcal infections and antibiotic prophylaxis for acute or recurrent rheumatic fever remain as important community problems at the present time.

The typical clinical picture of acute rheumatic fever is well known and includes a history of antecedent streptococcal infection—notably sore throat, fever, polyarthritis, chorea, subcutaneous nodules, and erythema marginatum. Acute rheumatic fever produces a pancarditis of variable clinical severity. Endocarditis may cause a transient murmur and pericarditis may cause a friction rub, but neither are clinically important, except as indicators of the severity of the attack. Myocarditis produces functional murmurs, gallop sounds, electrocardiographic changes, and possibly cardiomegaly. Myocardial involvement may progress to the point of congestive heart failure, which is usually amenable to routine medical management and the use of salicylates and steroids. However, when death occurs in acute rheumatic fever it is due to progressive heart failure that is unresponsive to these measures. (See also Cardiovascular Failure.)

Rheumatic valvular heart disease is a consequence of the slow healing process that follows acute rheumatic endocarditis. The mitral valve is most often involved (usually mitral stenosis) and women are more frequently affected. Isolated mitral regurgitation is rarely due to rheumatic heart disease. The aortic valve is the next most commonly involved (aortic stenosis or aortic regurgitation) and this involvement occurs predominantly in men. Both these valves are frequently damaged by the rheumatic process in the same individual; in fact, isolated aortic valve disease is rarely rheumatic. The tricuspid valve is virtually never the sole site of valvular damage, and its involvement may be organic (i.e., the result of the rheumatic process) or functional. Organic damage can lead to either tricuspid stenosis or regurgitation; functional regurgitation results from right ventricular failure that is secondary to long-standing pulmonary hypertension. Rheumatic damage to the pulmonary valve is extremely rare and never isolated.

The natural history of rheumatic valvular heart disease depends on the valve most severely involved and the number of valves involved. Its clinical course has been altered considerably by operations aimed at correcting or replacing the damaged valves. Since tricuspid valve disease is rarely isolated, and since the hemodynamically significant abnormalities generally reside in the aortic and mitral valves, involvement of these two alone will be discussed further.

The symptoms of mitral stenosis include exercise intolerance, orthopnea, and paroxysmal nocturnal dyspnea. These symptoms tend to progress, pulmonary hypertension develops, right ventricular failure ensues, and, if appropriate therapy is not initiated, death supervenes. Chronic atrial fibrillation is frequently present. Long-standing mitral stenosis may lead to severe obstructive disease of the pulmonary vascular bed, which increases morbidity and operative mortality. The elevated pulmonary vascular resistance, however, usually regresses after successful mitral valve surgery.

Acute manifestations of mitral stenosis, punctuating the clinical course and contributing to morbidity and mortality, include: (1) acute pulmonary edema, which may be the first clinical presentation of mitral stenosis and is rarely fatal; (2) hemoptysis, which has been known to cause death when profuse, and is treatable in such circumstances by emergency operation; and (3) systemic embolization, which is a particularly frightening complication. Clots may pass from the left atrium in otherwise asymptomatic individuals, and may be the cause of death when a cerebral artery is involved, leading to stroke, or a coronary artery is involved, leading to myocardial infarction.

Operative intervention is indicated when definite progression of symptoms occurs despite optimum medical management (which includes the use of digitalis and diuretics, salt restriction, exercise restriction, etc.) or when an embolic episode takes place. Although it is now apparent that mitral commissurotomy and mitral valve replacement have relieved symptoms and prolonged life, potential complications associated with these corrective operations still exist. Mitral restenosis is common in the case of mitral commissurotomy, and the relatively rare complications of a prosthetic mitral valve include bacterial endocarditis, embolic phenomena, and mechanical dysfunction of the valve itself culminating in a syndrome of congestive heart failure. Reoperation has a place in the treatment of some of these complications. Also, since anticoagulant therapy is a frequent requirement in patients with prosthetic mitral valves, the long-term risks of anticoagulation per se are an additional hazard.

Both aortic stenosis and regurgitation of considerable severity may run an asymptomatic course for many years. The initial symptom is usually exercise intolerance, which may progress to chronic congestive heart failure, punctuated by episodes of acute pulmonary edema. However, acute pulmonary edema may occur also in otherwise asymptomatic individuals. The appearance of heart failure is a poor prognostic sign, indicating survival for an average of two years; at the present time, the onset of failure is an urgent indication for aortic valve replacement. Angina pectoris is a common symptom of aortic stenosis, and in this setting, coexisting coronary artery disease may also be present. The development of angina is an ominous event and requires prompt diagnostic workup and operation. Similarly, syncopal episodes are an urgent indication for operation. Subacute bacterial endocarditis is an important complication and occurs in patients with aortic stenosis or aortic regurgitation. Sudden death is the most dramatic complication of aortic stenosis and occurs in both symptomatic and asymptomatic individuals.

Venous Thrombosis

The importance of venous thrombosis as an ultimate cause of death resides mainly in such thrombi being a source of pulmonary emboli. The most frequent sites of involvement are the veins of the legs and pelvis. The incidence of thrombosis appears to be higher in women taking contraceptive pills. Less common sites of thrombosis are the large venous sinuses of the brain, usually on the basis of underlying infection; these are potentially fatal. Migratory thrombophlebitis is important as a clinical manifestation of underlying carcinoma, particularly of the pancreas. Massive venous thrombosis may accompany disseminated intravascular coagulation syndromes (i.e., rapid utilization of serum fibrinogen and platelets with resulting hemorrhagic tendencies). This is a rare but important feature of various severe acute and chronic diseases, including premature separation of the placenta, septic abortion, amniotic fluid embolism, metastatic carcinoma of the prostate, and, at one time, was a complication of extracorporeal circulation. If treatment with fresh blood and heparin is instituted promptly, the prognosis becomes that of the underlying disease process.

Cardiovascular Failure

Cardiovascular or heart failure is a common cause of morbidity and mortality. It is a syndrome characterized by low cardiac output and venous congestion—pulmonary, systemic, or both. The causes of this syndrome are legion.

Normally, the heart is finely attuned to the circulatory demands of the body. It is subject to an input load, the end-diastolic volume, and it ejects against an output or pressure load that is approximated by the arterial blood pressure. The amount of blood ejected is determined by the force and duration of the myocardial contraction. Heart failure exists when myocardial contractile function is inadequate with reference to the input load or bodily requirements. Because of compensatory mechanisms in the heart itself and in the peripheral vascular bed, early myocardial failure is frequently asymptomatic, so the exact time of onset of failure cannot be determined. Eventually, acute or chronic and progressive symptoms develop as a result of low cardiac output, venous congestion, or both. The venous congestion is due usually to high ventricular end-diastolic pressures that are transmitted back to the atria and veins.

A great deal of attention has been given to semantic problems of defining and subclassifying cardiovascular failure. One such subclassification, useful because of its therapeutic implications, uses the term "heart failure" or "myocardial failure" for instances in which the syndrome is due to myocardial dysfunction and retains the term "circulatory failure" when the heart muscle itself is not directly involved in the disease process. For example, venous congestion due to entities such as tricuspid stenosis or pericardial tamponade would be classified as circulatory failure, as would congestive syndromes that may at times be produced by tachy- or bradyarrhythmias. In these entities, therapeutic measures aimed at improving the heart muscle's contractile function are not indicated. On the other hand, prompt therapy is necessary when heart failure results from diseases that involve the myocardium either directly, or indirectly through excessive pressure or volume loads. On this basis the causes of heart failure can be divided into three groups: (1) diseases of the heart muscle itself, such as arteriosclerotic coronary artery disease, various types of myocarditis or cardiomyopathy, and various rare infiltrative processes such as amyloidosis and hemochromatosis; (2) entities that interfere with the pumping action of the heart, such as mitral stenosis, aortic stenosis, pulmonic stenosis, systemic or pulmonary hypertension and pulmonary emboli. In these entities, the pressure work that the left or right ventricle must perform in order to maintain forward flow is much increased and the strain eventually results in myocardial failure; (3) entities that subject the ventricles to excessive volume loads, for the most part unrelated to bodily requirements. Included in this group are hypervolemia, as may occur in acute glomerulonephritis, mitral and aortic regurgitation, the common types of congenital cardiovascular disease giving rise to large left-to-right shunts, such as atrial and ventricular septal defects, and situations in which a drastic reduction in peripheral vascular resistance exists as in hyperthyroidism, systemic arteriovenous fistula, beriberi, Paget's disease, and patent ductus arteriosus. High flow loads are seen also in patients with anemia and in some patients with pulmonary parenchymal disease. In all of these conditions, one or both ventricles is subject to an increased input load which may result in high ventricular diastolic pressures and venous congestion even as ventricular stroke output remains high. Eventually, the strain imposed by the high input load brings about actual myocardial failure and the ventricular output becomes normal or reduced.

Venous congestion due to severe prolonged heart failure leads to anatomic and functional changes in certain of the organs of the body that in turn contribute to morbidity and mortality. Such changes are most evident in the lung, which undergoes fibrosis, and the liver, which undergoes cell necrosis and fibrosis in a pattern known as cardiac cirrhosis. Through mechanisms that are not fully understood, the failing heart influences the kidney to retain salt and water, which accounts in part for the peripheral edema and pulmonary congestion that are part of this syndrome. Renal function is, however, not otherwise compromised until late in the course of heart failure, when the combination of severe failure and attempts at its correction by the use of diuretics bring about various electrolyte abnormalities and transient or progressive renal insufficiency.

The symptoms and signs of circulatory failure depend on the underlying etiology, whether involvement is of one or both ventricles, and on the rate of progression of the circulatory or myocardial dysfunction. Many conditions that eventually cause heart failure may be asymptomatic for years. The main symptom resulting from reduced cardiac output per se is exercise intolerance, taking the form of excessive fatigue or dyspnea on exertion. In addition, left heart failure produces pulmonary venous congestion, which contributes further to the dyspnea on exertion. The high pulmonary venous pressure leads to pulmonary interstitial edema, which increases the work of breathing, and to pulmonary or alveolar edema, which interferes with respiratory gas exchange and gives rise to characteristic physical findings. Further symptoms of pulmonary venous congestion are orthopnea and paroxysmal nocturnal dyspnea in which shortness of breath occurs at rest while the patient is lying down. Acute left ventricular failure gives rise to acute pulmonary edema as described above. Elevated left heart pressures, as seen in patients with left ventricular failure or mitral stenosis, are the most common causes of right ventricular failure, which is secondary to the raised pulmonary arterial pressure. Isolated right ventricular failure, as for example in patients with pulmonic stenosis, is much less common than left heart failure. In addition to exercise intolerance, right ventricular failure causes jugular venous distension, hepatomegaly sometimes associated with right upper quadrant pain, peripheral edema, anorexia, and sometimes ascites.

Treatment of congestive circulatory failure is aimed directly at the cause, and may include such measures as pericardiocentesis, artificial pacemakers, and the use of antiarrhythmic drugs or electrical countershock. Treatment of heart failure is both supportive of the compromised myocardium and directed to the underlying cause. Supportive measures include digitalis preparations to improve the contractile state of the myocardium, appropriate physical and emotional rest, measures such as salt restriction and diuretics to ameliorate water retention, and the use of oxygen and assisted ventilation when necessary. Medical measures directed to an underlying cause include correction of anemia or hypoxemia and treatment of associated diseases such as infection, thyrotoxicosis, beriberi, etc., as well as other measures mentioned above for the treatment of acute pulmonary edema.

Surgical intervention has altered the natural history of many conditions causing heart failure. In the case of diseases that affect the myocardium itself, coronary artery disease is the most amenable to operation in selected cases. Such operations include coronary artery bypass, infarctectomy, aneurysmectomy, closure of acquired ventricular septal defects resulting from an acute myocardial infarction, mitral valve replacement or, in rare cases, direct closure of a ruptured ventricular wall. Apart from procedures on the myocardium itself, operations have been most effective in correcting mechanical defects. Such operations include closure of septal defects, correction of other hemodynamic abnormalities such as pulmonic stenosis and patent ductus arteriosus, palliative valve surgery or valve replacement for the treatment of mitral or aortic stenosis or regurgitation, etc. Although cardiac operations can be life-saving in emergency circumstances, they are best carried out at a stage in the disease when damage to the myocardium and other organs is minor or reversible.

Congestive heart failure is potentially fatal, although, as noted above, it is increasingly amenable to cure. Furthermore, by the use of routine supportive measures, life may be sustained at a productive level for many years. Heart failure causes death when specific treatment of the underlying cause is impossible and supportive measures become ineffective. A slowly progressive downhill course of congestive heart failure is characterized by a loss of body muscle mass because of low cardiac output and poor nutrition. The latter is related to gastrointestinal dysfunction which may be drug induced or may result from mesenteric venous congestion. In any case, the appearance of cardiac cachexia that is due to a combination of tissue wasting and peripheral edema is quite characteristic. Exercise intolerance will increase to the point that the patient is restricted to a bed and chair existence, and he will frequently be dyspneic at rest. As a result of very low cardiac output, the patient will have blue- or purple-tinged lips, or may be overtly cyanotic—so-called peripheral cyanosis. Jaundice on the basis of cardiac cirrhosis may also be present. In those circumstances and with no further effective therapy available, the patient may be regarded as terminal. At this stage, hyponatremia and azotemia may supervene.

The objective of treatment at this time is to keep the patient as comfortable as possible. Hospitalization may not be absolutely necessary during this period. The patient will be restricted to bed or chair, and should probably have a nearby commode. He should wear elastic stockings to prevent venous stasis in the legs and thereby minimize the chances for phlebothrombosis and pulmonary embolus; at times anticoagulant therapy may be indicated. He may require oxygen or assisted ventilation. Because of fatigue and gastrointestinal upsets, he may be limited to small feedings. Normal contacts should be maintained except that visits likely to bring about unnecessary emotional responses should be avoided. Life-supporting measures such as pacemakers may be used as required, but heroic therapy such as cardiac massage, artificial respiration, and defibrillation have little place in such cases. Assisted circulation may be tried for a time, but because of secondary organ degeneration, patients in terminal heart failure are usually not amenable to heart transplant. Death is heralded by a fall in arterial pressure with progression to a shocklike state and clouding of the sensorium, culminating in coma or cardiac arrest. Death is diagnosed from complete unresponsiveness and cessation of respiration and all reflexes.

Shock

Shock is a life-threatening clinical syndrome of multiple etiologies. The hallmark of the shock state is a low arterial blood pressure. Survival depends on the underlying cause, the depth of shock, and the speed with which effective treatment is initiated. Clinically, shock is characterized by inadequate organ perfusion due to circulatory collapse, which is due, in turn, to inadequate circulating blood volume in relation to blood vessel capacity, or to profound weakness of the heart as a pump.

The causes of shock may be classified into three broad groups. The first group consists of direct insults to the cardiovascular system. The most common entity in this group, and indeed one of the most common of all types of shock, is cardiogenic shock, which develops when 40 percent or more of the left ventricular myocardium is involved in an acute myocardial infarction. It is notoriously resistant to medical management and the mortality in fully developed cases is 80 to 100 percent. Recently, radical approaches to this problem have been employed successfully, but these must still be regarded as experimental. Massive pulmonary embolization is another cause of circulatory collapse and shock. In extreme cases pulmonary embolectomy has been performed and with some success. Acute pericardial tamponade is another cause of shock which, however, is often readily amenable to therapy if the cause is recognized. The second group brings about profound hypovolemia with consequent failure of venous return. The prototype of this group is acute, severe hemorrhage, with bleeding either externally or into a body cavity as in ruptured aortic aneurysm. Marked loss of plasma as a result of extensive burns or peritonitis is another basis for hypovolemia. Severe dehydration and electrolyte imbalance, as may occur in protracted vomiting, diarrhea, intestinal obstruction, or diabetic acidosis, may also result in shock. The keystone of treatment of these conditions is correction of the underlying cause and prompt restoration of the circulating blood volume. The third group is characterized by vasomotor paralysis and collapse as occurs with high fever or during anaphylaxis. Septic or endotoxic shock as seen in gram negative septicemia is in this group.

Shock may be regarded as reversible or irreversible. The ultimate outcome depends mainly on the duration of the shocklike state, which in turn depends on the underlying cause and response to treatment. If this state is prolonged unduly, inadequate organ perfusion will lead to disturbances of cell metabolism and cell death that will bring about the death of the patient even though other aspects of the shock state are treated adequately and appropriately.

Warm skin, bounding pulses, and a relatively low blood pressure in an acutely ill patient may indicate incipient septic shock. However, this picture will eventually give way to the fully developed shock state, which is much the same regardless of etiology. The patient will then have a pale, cool, moist skin with a grayish or bluish tinge, and will be oliguric or anuric. His sensorium will be clouded as manifested by restlessness, apathy, or coma. The pulse will be rapid and thready. Arterial pressure may be difficult to obtain, but the systolic pressure will usually be in the range of 90 mm Hg or less, although this figure must be interpreted in the light of the patient's preexisting blood pressure, since a hypertensive patient may be in shock at a higher pressure. One of the abovementioned causes of shock will usually be evident clinically.

The medical treatment of cardiogenic shock involves pressor agents in order to raise the arterial pressure to levels that will insure adequate coronary artery perfusion. Recent work indicates that drugs such as phentolamine or nitroprusside that decrease peripheral vascular resistance, and thereby decrease the ventricular workload may also be helpful. If ventricular filling pressures are low, volume replacement is indicated. The potential usefulness of digitalis, isoproterenol or other inotropic agents in the setting of cardiogenic shock is uncertain. The response to treatment is best assessed on the basis of serial left atrial pressure and cardiac output measurements. Other, more radical modes of therapy that are not always available, include intro-aortic balloon counterpulsation, with emergency coronary arteriography and subsequent coronary artery bypass or infarctectomy.

General measures in the treatment of hypovolemic shock include bed rest and lowering of the head and elevation of the legs. More definitive measures include rapid replacement of blood, plasma, or water with electrolytes as appropriate, as well as treatment of the underlying cause. Pressor agents alone are of little value. Appropriate cultures and antibiotics, along with supportive therapy, form the basis of treatment for septic shock. Steroid therapy may have a place here.

Since shock may enter an irreversible phase if treatment is delayed, inadequate, or not possible, an important basis of prognosis is the duration of the shock state. Thus, failure of clinical response to appropriate therapy carries a bad prognosis. Other signs of irreversibility include failure to restore the arterial pressure or urine volume. The same is true of changes in the sensorium progressing to unconsciousness or coma. Terminally, cardiac arrhythmias may develop, culminating in cardiac arrest.

It should be recalled that shock, like cardiac arrest, may be a terminal event in many diseases. Thus, heroic measures are best limited to those instances in which shock is due to an acute, potentially treatable insult. Resuscitative or radical forms of therapy are not indicated if shock is part of the terminal state of a chronic, incurable disease. Palliative measures that should be instituted in the course of shock include maintenance of nutrition, chemotherapy as indicated, appropriate nursing care, use of oxygen, and an indwelling urinary catheter for hygienic purposes and for monitoring urinary output. Patients should be kept comfortable and at physical and emotional rest as far as is possible. Since the course of shock is rapid, it is probably best to keep the patient's family aware and informed of the gravity of the situation. Life supporting measures such as dialysis and assisted respiration and heroic measures such as cardiac massage, electrical defibrillation, and assisted circulation may have a place depending on the individual situation.

Unless shock is of extremely short duration, these patients are not usually suitable donors for organ transplantation because of severe secondary organ degeneration.

❧ Appendix B
The California "Right To Die" Law

THIS BILL WOULD expressly authorize the withholding or withdrawal of extraordinary life-sustaining procedures, as defined, from adult patients afflicted with a terminal condition, as defined, where the patient has executed a declaration in the form and manner prescribed by the bill at least 72 hours in advance. This bill would relieve physicians and health facilities from civil liability, and would relieve physicians from criminal prosecution or charges of unprofessional conduct, for withholding or withdrawing extraordinary life-sustaining procedures in accordance with the provisions of the bill. It would be provided that such a withholding or withdrawal of extraordinary life-sustaining procedures shall not constitute a suicide nor impair or invalidate life insurance, and the bill would specify that the making of such a declaration shall not restrict, inhibit, or impair the sale, procurement, or issuance of life insurance or modify existing life insurance.

The bill would make it a misdemeanor to do certain acts relative to the forgery or falsification of such a declaration, effecting a false revocation thereof, or concealing it, or withholding personal knowledge of a revocation with intent to cause withdrawal or withholding of extraordinary life-sustaining procedures contrary to the declarant's intent.

This bill would also provide that neither appropriation is made nor obligation created for the reimbursement of any local agency for any costs incurred by it pursuant to the bill.

Vote: majority—Appropriation: no. Fiscal committee: no. State-mandated local program: yes.

An act to add Chapter 3.9 (commencing with Section 7185) to Part 1 of Division 7 of the Health and Safety Code, relating to medical care.

The people of the State of California to enact as follows:

SECTION 1. Chapter 3.9 (commencing with Section 7185) is added to Part 1 of Division 7 of the Health and Safety Code, to read:

Chapter 3.9 Natural Death Act

7185. This act shall be known and may be cited as the Natural Death Act.

7186. The Legislature finds that adult persons have the fundamental right to control the decisions relating to the rendering of their own medical care, including the decision to have extraordinary life-sustaining procedures withheld or withdrawn in instances of a terminal condition.

The Legislature further finds that modern medical technology has made possible the artificial prolongation of human life beyond natural limits.

The Legislature further finds that such prolongation of life for persons with a terminal condition may cause loss of patient dignity, unnecessary pain and suffering, and an unreasonable emotional and financial hardship on the patient's family, while providing nothing medically necessary or beneficial to the patient.

The Legislature further finds that there exists considerable uncertainty in the medical and legal professions as to the legality of terminating the use or application of extraordinary life-sustaining procedures where the patient has voluntarily and in sound mind evidenced a desire that such procedures be withheld or withdrawn.

In recognition of the dignity and privacy which patients have a right to expect, the Legislature hereby declares that the laws of the State of California shall recognize the right of an adult person to make a declaration instructing his physician to withhold or withdraw extraordinary life-sustaining procedures in the event of a terminal condition.

7187. The following definitions shall govern the construction of this chapter:

(a) "Declaration" means a written document voluntarily executed by the declarant in accordance with the requirements of Section 7188, directing the withholding or withdrawal of extraordinary life-sustaining procedures in the event the declarant is diagnosed as a qualified patient by reason of a terminal condition.

(b) "Extraordinary life-sustaining procedure" means any medical procedure which utilizes mechanical or other artificial means to sustain, restore, or supplant a vital function, without which the patient would die and which is not a usual or ordinary course of continuing treatment. "Extraordinary life-sustaining procedure" includes artificial assistance to respiration.

(c) "Physician" means a physician and surgeon licensed by the Board of Medical Quality Assurance or the Board of Osteopathic Examiners.

(d) "Qualified patient" means a patient diagnosed and certified in writing to be afflicted with a terminal condition by two physicians who have personally examined the patient.

(e) "Terminal condition" means an incurable condition caused by injury, disease, or illness, which but for the application of extraordinary life-sustaining procedures would, with reasonable medical certainty, produce death, and where the application of extraordinary life-sustaining procedures will only postpone the otherwise imminent death of the patient.

7188. Any adult person may execute a declaration directing the withholding or withdrawal of extraordinary life-sustaining procedures in the event he or she should become a qualified patient by reason of a terminal condition. The declaration shall be signed by the declarant in the presence of two witnesses not related to the declarant by blood or marriage and who would not be entitled to any portion of the estate of the declarant upon his decease under any will of the declarant or codicil thereto then existing or, at the time of the declaration, by operation of law then existing. The declaration shall be in the following form:

Declaration made this_____day of_____(month, year)
I_____, being of sound mind, and voluntarily wishing to make known my desire that my life shall not be artificially prolonged under the circumstances set forth below, do hereby declare:
1. If at any time I should have a serious injury, disease, or illness certified to be terminal by two physicians, and which, except for the application of extraordinary life-sustaining procedures, would cause my imminent death, I desire that such procedures be withheld or withdrawn, and I be permitted to die naturally.
2. In the absence of my ability to give directions regarding the use of such extraordinary life-sustaining procedures, it is my intention that this declaration shall be honored by my family and physician(s) as the

final expression of my legal right to refuse medical or surgical treatment and accept the consequences from such refusal.

Signed_____

City, County and State of Residence_____

The declarant has been personally known to me and I believe him/her to be of sound mind.

Witness_____

Witness_____

7189. A declaration shall not become effective for 72 hours from execution thereof and may be revoked at any time by the declarant, without regard to his mental state or competency, by either of the following methods:

(a) By being canceled, defaced, obliterated, or burnt, torn, or otherwise destroyed by the declarant or by some person in his presence and by his direction.

(b) By an oral expression of the declarant of his intent to revoke made in the presence of two witnesses, only one of whom may be the attending physician or a person related to the declarant by blood or marriage. Such revocation shall become effective only upon communication to the attending physician.

7190. No physician or health facility which, acting in good faith and in accordance with the requirements of this chapter, causes the withholding or withdrawal of extraordinary life-sustaining procedures from a qualified patient, shall be subject to civil liability therefrom. No physician who participates in the withholding or withdrawal of extraordinary life-sustaining procedures in accordance with the provisions of this chapter shall be guilty of any criminal act or of unprofessional conduct.

7191. (a) Prior to effecting a withholding or withdrawal of extraordinary life-sustaining procedures from a mentally competent qualified patient pursuant to the qualified patient's declaration, the physician in charge of the qualified patient's care shall determine that the declaration complies with Section 7188, and that the declaration and all steps proposed by the physician to be undertaken are in accord with the desires of the qualified patient.

(b) Prior to effecting a withholding or withdrawal of extraordinary life-sustaining procedures, pursuant to a declaration, from a qualified patient who is mentally incompetent or incapable of communication, the physician in charge of the qualified patient's care shall determine that the declaration complies with Section 7188 and shall verify with reasonably reliable evidence that the qualified patient was of sound mind at the time of making the declaration.

7192. (a) The withholding or withdrawal of extraordinary life-sustaining procedures from a qualified patient in accordance with the provisions of this chapter shall not, for any purpose, constitute a suicide.

(b) The making of a declaration pursuant to Section 7188 shall not restrict, inhibit, or impair in any manner the sale, procurement, or issuance of any policy of life insurance, nor shall it be deemed to modify the terms of an existing policy of life insurance. No policy of life insurance shall be legally impaired or invalidated in any manner by the withholding or withdrawal of extraordinary life-sustaining procedures from an insured qualified patient, notwithstanding any term of the policy to the contrary.

7193. No physician shall be criminally or civilly liable for failing to effectuate the declaration of the qualified patient that extraordinary life-sustaining procedures be withheld or withdrawn, unless the physician refuses to make necessary arrangements, or fails to take the necessary steps, to effect the transfer of the qualified patient to the care of another physician who will effectuate the declaration of the qualified patient. Such refusal or failure shall constitute unprofessional conduct.

7194. Nothing in this chapter shall impair or supersede any right which any person may have to effect the withholding or withdrawal of extraordinary life-sustaining procedures in any lawful manner. In such respect the provisions of this chapter are cumulative.

7195. Any person who wilfully conceals, cancels, defaces, obliterates, damages, falsifies, or forges the declaration of another, or who wilfully conceals or withholds personal knowledge of an oral revocation made before him as provided in subdivision (b) of Section 7189 with intent to cause a withholding or withdrawal of extraordinary life-sustaining procedures contrary to the declarant's wishes, shall be guilty of a misdemeanor.

SECTION 2. No appropriation is made by this act, nor is any obligation created thereby under Section 2231 of the Revenue and Taxation Code, for the reimbursement of any local agency for any costs that may be incurred by it in carrying on any program or performing any service required to be carried on or performed by it by this act.

🌿 Appendix C
The Living Will

TO MY FAMILY, MY PHYSICIAN, MY LAWYER, MY CLERGYMAN
TO ANY MEDICAL FACILITY IN WHOSE CARE I HAPPEN TO BE
TO ANY INDIVIDUAL WHO MAY BECOME RESPONSIBLE FOR MY
HEALTH, WELFARE OR AFFAIRS

Death is as much a reality as birth, growth, maturity and old age—it is the one certainty of life. If the time comes when I, _____ can no longer take part in decisions for my own future, let this statement stand as an expression of my wishes, while I am still of sound mind.

If the situation should arise in which there is no reasonable expectation of my recovery from physical or mental disability, I request that I be allowed to die and not be kept alive by artificial means or "heroic measures." I do not fear death itself as much as the indignities of deterioration, dependence and hopeless pain. I, therefore, ask that medication be mercifully administered to me to alleviate suffering even though this may hasten the moment of death.

This request is made after careful consideration. I hope you who care for me will feel morally bound to follow its mandate. I recognize that this appears to place a heavy responsibility upon you, but it is with the intention of relieving you of such responsibility and of placing it upon myself in accordance with my strong convictions, that this statement is made.

Signed _____

Date _____
Witness _____
Witness _____

Copies of this request have been given to _____
_____
_____
_____

Appendix D

Confidential Financial Checklist for the Terminally Ill

Edwin Nadel and John Parker

Confidential Checklist

Date _____

Name _____ Company _____

Residence Address _____ Business Address _____

Phone _____ Years there _____ Phone _____ Years there _____

Date of Marriage _____ Nature of Business   Title _____

FAMILY DATA

Name	Relation-ship	Birth Date	Birth Place	M or S	Health*	Height Weight
___	___	___	___	__	___	___
___	___	___	___	__	___	___
___	___	___	___	__	___	___
___	___	___	___	__	___	___

Family Information _____ Stepchildren—Adopted _____

Earning Ability _____

Other Dependents—Parents, In—Laws, etc. _____ Extent of Support _____

Previous Marriage Divorce _____ Separation Agreement Date _____

*Physician   A.P.S. _____ Seen Dr. last 5 yrs. _____

                                                         Why   When

HOME OWNERSHIP

1. Mortgage—Date_____Amount_____Interest_____% Term_____

   Monthly charges_____Unpaid balance_____Prepayment privilege_____

2. Do you wish home free and clear?_____Or extra monthly payments?_____

3. Have you applied for Veterans Exemption for reduction of Assessed

   Valuation?_____

   Mustering out pay _____ Past Div. _____ G.I. Mortgage _____

52–20 Club _____ Future Div. _____ G.I. Bill_____

N.Y. State Bonus _____ C.V. Refunds _____

Should your Veterans insurance be used for this purpose at death? _____

FAMILY CASH AND INCOME REQUIREMENTS

A. Monthly Income

1. Dependency period $_____

2. Readjustment for
   _____ yrs.   _____

3. Life income   _____

   (Outside income $_____)
   Source

B. Special Cash Needs

1. Mortgage $_____

2. Emergency fund   _____

3. Educational fund   _____

4. Any litigation?   _____

5. Any special bequest?   _____

6. Charity   _____

7. _____   _____

C. Settlement Funds

1. Current expenses $_____

2. Obligations   _____

3. Final expenses   _____

4. Taxes: a) Income $\frac{1}{4}$ est.   _____

   b) Property   _____

   c) Death   _____

5. Administration

   (Assets executor must
   pay from estate within
   9 months of your death.)
   Is there enough
   liquidity? _____

D. Special Income Needs

1. Parents? _____ _____

2. _____ _____

3. _____ _____

FAMILY BUDGET CALCULATION——MONTHLY INCOME

1. Shelter
   Taxes $_____

   Mortgage   _____

   Maintenance
   Repairs
   Gardener   _____

   Rent   _____ $_____

4. Clothing $_____

5. Personal
   Auto   _____

   Recreational   _____

   Medical–
   Dental   _____

   Insurance   _____

2. House Operation
   Heating $_____   Contributions   _____

   Gas & Elec.   _____   Educational   _____ $_____

   Telephone   _____   6. Previous
                                      Subtotal   _____ _____
   Laundry   _____   10-15% Contin-
                                      gencies and
   House Help   _____ $_____   incidentals $_____ $_____

3. Food   _____ $_____   GRAND TOTAL   _____ $_____

   Subtotal   _____ $_____

DISABILITY INCOME

1. Total Income required during disability $_____

2. Professional Overhead Expense

   Rent $_____   Equip. Depreciation $_____

   Property Taxes   _____   Liability Ins. Prems.   _____

   Property Ins. Prem.   _____   Elec., Oil, Gas, etc.   _____

   Property Mtge. Int.   _____   Dues   _____

   Employees' Salaries   _____   Telephone   _____

   Periodicals   _____   Other Fixed Expense   _____

   Maintenance Service   _____

   Subtotal $_____   Subtotal $_____

                                     TOTAL $_____

3. a) Major Medical Plan?_____ b) Hospitalization?_____

4. How long is secy./nurse working for you?_____Any benefits?_____

5. To what professional societies do you belong? _____

6. Termination clause in lease? _____

7. What will business be worth in event of serious disability?_____

8. How much shrinkage in event of disability?_____

RETIREMENT INCOME

1. Age_____ Desired $_____Minimum $ _____

2. Amount you wish guaranteed $_____

3. Company pension $_____Contribution rate_____Vested Interest $ _____

4. Hobbies_____Retirement aims if income assured_____Survivor rights __

5. Have you considered HR-10?_____Incorporation?_____

STORAGE OF IMPORTANT PAPERS

1. Wills _____ Deeds _____ Trust Instr.?_____

2. Birth Certs. _____ Tax Return _____ Bonds-Stocks _____

3. Marriage Certs._____ Discharge _____ Mutual Funds
Insured? _____

LIFE INSURANCE DETAILS

Where are ins. policies stored?_____Who owns them?_____

Are there any loans?_____Are they insured?_____

What are you doing with your dividends?_____Any with company? _____

Do you have your last premium notices?_____Do you have any group ins? _____

Is there ins. on your wife or children?_____Why?
Why not?_____

Is your life ins. bene. the same as your will?_____Has this been checked? _

What are your insurance objectives? _____

INVESTMENT PLANS

1. Investment Plans_____Surplus for Investment _____

2. Special program for children? _____

3. Investment ability of wife_____

ESTATE OBJECTIVES

1. Appreciation?

2. Conservation?

3. Dissipation?

TAXES

Income Tax paid last year - State $_____Federal $_____City $_____

Please furnish copies of last years tax returns.

ASSETS AT DEATH

	Date Acq.	Cost Value	Situs State	Gross Values Husb.	Gross Values Wife	Gross Values Joint*	Loans**	Income	Probate	Liquid
Real Estate										
Savings Acct's										
Checking Acct's										
Gov't Bonds										
Mutual Funds										
Stocks										
Bonds										
Personal Effects										
Special Equip.										
Notes										
Mortgages										
Patents & Royalties										
Life Ins.**** Face Amount										
Ins. Cash Values Other Lives										

Pension/Profit Sharing						
Interest in Trusts						
Deferred Compensation Stock Option						
Vested Interests						
Business Int.***						
Power of Appointments						
Children's Assets (owned by H. or W.)						
Total						
Any Loans Separate H.W. Joint						
Net Assets at Death						

* Percentage of gift
** Indicate husband, wife or joint
*** If any, complete confidential business information
**** For value, see analysis folder

DISTRIBUTION CONSIDERATIONS

1. Special Family needs:

2. Charitable bequests:

3. Trusts (Describe): Past:

   Contemplated:

4. Should current assets of children be used for education or living expenses?

5. Disposition of Business Interests (Retention or Sale):

				Present or Future Value	Return Submitted	Total Exemption Used
6. Gifts:	Past:	To Whom	When			

   Contemplated:

MATURING TRUSTS, ANTICIPATED INHERITANCES, LEGACIES

1. Self

2. Other Family Members

PERTINENT DATA

1. Social Security Coverage?_____No._____Since _____

2. Veteran?_____Entered_____Discharged_____GI# _____

   Service Connected Disability?_____Reason_____%C# _____

3. Reserve Status?_____Flying Time _____

4. Will?_____Date_____State_____Executor_____

   Your Estate Distribution: to whom, what amount, how _____

   _____

5. Spouse's Will?_____Date_____State_____Executor_____

6. Guardian _____

7. Advisers: Attorneys: Insurance Adviser:

                Accountant: Trust Officer

                Investments:

8. Banks: Checking   Safe Deposit

                 Savings   Credit

9. Final Decisions:

    Do you make them?_____Or will you consult your wife?_____

10. Income: Current $_____Other Family Members $_____

     Expectations in 5 yrs. $_____10 yrs. $_____

     Peak?_____Continue?_____

11. Any other information which may be important to analysis?

Receipt issued_____For_____Pick up policies_____
              date   No. Pols.   date   time

Appointment for next

    interview_____,_____Mail to res. or off. _____

DOCUMENTS REQUIRED FOR ANALYSIS

ASSETS:

_____ 1. Business Agreements and/or Employment Agreements

_____ 2. Stock option and/or Stock Bonus Agreements

_____ 3. Pension and/or Profit Sharing trust instrument

_____ 4. Deferred Compensation and/or Split–Dollar Agreements

_____ 5. Royalty, Patent, Leasehold Agreement

_____ 6. Owner of record of:
        _____A. Bank Accounts
        _____B. Real Estate
        _____C. Investments (Stocks, Bonds, Mutual Funds)

_____ 7. Wills and/or Trusts
        _____A. Revocable Trusts
        _____B. Irrevocable Trusts
        _____C. Short Term Trusts

_____ 8. Social Security Number and/or Government Pension

_____ 9. Insurance Policies:
        _____A. Life – Personal (Self, Wife, Children, Others)
        _____B. Life – Business, Group, Pension, Profit Sharing
        _____C. Accident – Sickness Disability, D.B.L.–N.Y., T.D.B.–N.Y.
        _____D. Professional Overhead Expense Disability
        _____E. Business Overhead Expense Disability

_____F. Hospitalization and/or Major Medical
_____G. Liability:
       _____1. Personal
       _____2. Professional
       _____3. Office
       _____4. Automobile
       _____5. Excess

_____10. Amount of last premium and period paid for all policies

_____11. Amount of last dividend and dividend option for all policies

_____12. Most recent Federal and State Tax Returns

LIABILITIES:

_____1. Taxes – Income and/or Real Estate

_____2. Amount of Loans – Mortgages, Notes or other Debts

_____3. Litigation

_____4. Leases

_____5. Other

General Bibliography

Benjamin B. 1971. "Bereavement and Heart Disease," *Journal of Biosocial Science* (January), 3:61–67.

Blacher, Richard S. and S. H. Basch. 1970. "Psychological Aspects of Pacemaker Implantation," *Archives of General Psychiatry* (April), 22:319–23.

Dlin, B. M., H. K. Fischer, and B. Huddell. 1968. "Psychologic Adaptation to Pacemaker and Open Heart Surgery," *Archives of General Psychiatry* (November), 19:599–610.

Drugg, R. and D. Kornfeld. 1967. "Survivors of Cardiac Arrest," *Journal of the American Medical Association* (July 31), 201:291–96.

Dudley, D. et al. 1969. "Long-Term Adjustment, Prognosis and Death in Irreversible Diffuse Obstructive Pulmonary Syndromes," *Psychosomatic Medicine* (July–August), 4:310–25.

Eastwood, R. T. et al., 1969. *Cardiac Replacement: Medical, Ethical, Psychological and Economic Implications.* A Report by the Ad Hoc Task Force on Cardiac Replacement, National Heart Institute, National Institutes of Health, Public Health Service, U.S. department of Health, Education, and Welfare. Washington, D.C.: Superintendent of Documents, U.S. government Printing Office.

Franulis, M. F. 1972. "Loss: A Factor Affecting the Welfare of the Coronary Patient," *Nursing Clinics of North America* (September), 7:445–55.

Hackett, Thomas P., and Ned H. Cassem. 1972. "Patients Facing Sudden Cardiac Death." In Schoenberg, B., A. C. Carr, D. Peretz, and A. H. Kutscher, eds., *Psychosocial Aspects of Terminal Care*. New York: Columbia University Press.

Hackett, Thomas P., Ned H. Cassem, and H. A. Wishnie. 1968. "The Coronary Care Unit: An Appraisal of Its Psychological Hazards," *New England Journal of Medicine* (December 19), 279:1365–70.

* From Martin L. Kutscher, Daniel J. Cherico, Austin H. Kutscher, Amy E. Hanninen, Steven Johnson, and David Peretz. 1975. *A Comprehensive Bibliography of the Thanatology Literature.* New York: Arno Press. Reprinted by permission of Arno Press, Inc.

James, T. N. 1969. "QT Prolongation and Sudden Death," *Modern Concepts in Cardiovascular Disease* (July), 38:34.

Hackett, Thomas P. and Avery D. Weisman. 1969. "Denial as a Factor in Patients with Heart Disease and Cancer," *Annals of the New York Academy of Science* (December 19), 164:802–17.

Jokl, E. 1971. "Exercise and Cardiac Death," *Journal of the American Medical Association* (December), 218:1707.

Kubler-Ross, Elisabeth. 1971. "On Learning from the Dying," *American Journal of Nursing* (January), 71:56–60.

Moore, F. D. et al. 1968. "Bethesda Conference Report: Cardiac and Other Organ Transplantation in the Setting of Transplant Science as a National Effort," *Journal of the American Medical Association* (December 9), 206:489–500.

Page, Irving R. 1969. "The Ethics of Heart Transplantation," *Journal of the American Medical Association* (January 6), 207:109–13.

Solitaire, G. B. 1970. "Sudden Unexpected Death," *Lancet* (March).

Index

❧ List of Contributors

James Reiffel, M.D., Assistant Professor of Clinical Medicine, College of Physicians and Surgeons, Columbia University, New York, New York

Robert DeBellis, M.D., Assistant Professor of Clinical Medicine, College of Physicians and Surgeons, Columbia University, New York, New York

Lester C. Mark, M.D., Professor of Anesthesiology, College of Physicians and Surgeons, Columbia University, New York, New York

Austin H. Kutscher, D.D.S., Associate Professor (in Dentistry), Department of Psychiatry, College of Physicians and Surgeons; Associate Professor of Stomatology, School of Dental and Oral Surgery, Columbia University; President, The Foundation of Thanatology, New York, New York

Paul R. Patterson, M.D., Professor of Pediatrics, Albany Medical College of Union University, Albany, New York

Bernard Schoenberg, M.D., Professor of Clinical Psychiatry and Associate Dean, College of Physicians and Surgeons, Columbia University, New York, New York (deceased)

Adrienne Baranowitz, Medical Student, Downstate Medical Center, Brooklyn, New York

Michael D. Bieri, M.D., Washington University School of Medicine, St. Louis, Missouri

Donal M. Billig, M.D., Professor of Surgery, Hahnemann Medical College, Philadelphia, Pennsylvania; Attending Thoracic and Cardiovascular Surgeon, Monmouth Medical Center, Long Branch, New Jersey

Richard S. Blacher, M.D., Clinical Professor of Psychiatry; Lecturer in Surgery, Tufts University School of Medicine, Boston, Massachusetts

James A. Blumenthal, Ph.D., Clinical Assistant Professor, Department of Psychiatry, Duke University Medical Center, Durham, North Carolina

John G. Bruhn, Ph.D., Professor of Preventive Medicine and Community Health; Associate Dean for Community Affairs, The University of Texas Medical Branch, Galveston, Texas

John C. M. Brust, M.D., Director, Department of Neurology, Harlem Hospital Center, College of Physicians and Surgeons, Columbia University, New York, New York

George E. Burch, M.D., Professor of Medicine, Tulane University School of Medicine, New Orleans, Louisiana

Arthur C. Carr, Ph.D., Professor of Clinical Psychology in Psychiatry, Cornell University Medical College; Attending Psychologist, New York Hospital (Westchester Division), White Plains, New York

Joan Chan, M.S.W., Director, Child Life Program; Clinical Assistant Professor, Department of Pediatrics, Downstate Medical Center, Brooklyn, New York

Rita K. Chow, Ed.D., F.A.A.N., Nurse Director in the United States Public Health Service; Chief, Quality Assurance Branch, Division of Long-Term Care, Office of Standards and Certification, Health Standards and Quality Bureau, Health Care Financing Administration, Department of Health, Education and Welfare, Baltimore, Maryland

Paula J. Clayton, M.D., Professor of Psychiatry, Washington University School of Medicine, St. Louis, Missouri

R. K. Coombs, R.N., B.Sc.N., M.N., Director of Cardiac Nursing, Ottawa Civic Hospital, Ontario, Canada

Franklin H. Epstein, M.D., Herrman L. Blumgart Professor of Medicine, Harvard Medical School; Physician-in-Chief, Beth Israel Hospital, Boston, Massachusetts

Morris E. Eson, Ph.D., Professor, Department of Psychology, State University of New York at Albany; Adjunct Associate Professor (Neurosurgery), Albany Medical College of Union University, Albany, New York

A. Formo, M.A., Former Research Scientist, Social and Community Psychiatry Section, Clarke Institute of Psychiatry, Toronto, Ottawa, Canada

Robert W. M. Frater, M.B., Ch.B., Professor and Chief of Cardiothoracic Surgery, Albert Einstein College of Medicine, Montefiore Hospital and Medical Center, Bronx, New York

K. Freedman, Former Research Assistant, "Bereavement Project"; Director of Survivor Support Program, Clarke Institute of Psychiatry, Toronto, Ottawa, Canada

S. J. J. Freeman, M.D., D. Psych., Psychiatrist-in-Charge, Social and Community Psychiatry Section, Clarke Institute of Psychiatry; Professor, Department of Psychiatry, University of Toronto, Ottawa, Canada

W. Doyle Gentry, Ph.D., Professor of Psychiatry and Behavioral Sciences, University of Texas Medical Branch, Galveston, Texas

Frank Glenn, M.D., Professor of Surgery Emeritus, Cornell University Medical College; Attending Surgeon, The New York Hospital, New York, New York

Gerald Glick, M.D., Director, Cardiovascular Institute, Michael Reese Hospital and Medical Center, Chicago, Illinois

Maurice H. Greenhill, M.D., Professor Emeritus and Director, Department of Psychiatry, The Hospital of the Albert Einstein College of Medicine, Bronx, New York

Raymond Harris, M.D., Clinical Associate Professor of Medicine, Albany Medical College of Union University, Albany, New York; President, Center for the Study of Aging; Chief, Subdepartment of Medicine, St. Peter's Hospital, Albany, New York

George H. Humphreys II, M.D., Emeritus Professor of Surgery, College of Physicians and Surgeons, Columbia University, New York, New York

Arnold A. Hutschnecker, M.D., Fellow, American Association of Psychoanalytic Physicians; (former) Consultant, President's Special Action Office of Drug Abuse Prevention

W. J. Keon, M.D., F.R.C.S. (C), Professor and Chairman, University of Ottawa Department of Surgery and Director, University of Ottawa Cardiac Unit, Ontario, Canada

Nathan Lefkowitz, Ph.D., Assistant Professor (Sociology), School of Public Health of the Faculty of Medicine, College of Physicians and Surgeons, Columbia University, New York, New York (deceased)

W. A. L. Lyall, M.D., D. Psych., Staff Psychiatrist, Social and Community Psychiatry Section, Clarke Institute of Psychiatry; Associate Professor, Department of Psychiatry, University of Toronto, Ottawa, Canada

Marvin Moser, M.D., Clinical Professor of Medicine, New York Medical College, Valhalla, New York; Emeritus Chief of Cardiology, White

Plains (New York) Hospital Medical Center; Senior Medical Consultant, National High Blood Pressure Education Program, National Heart, Lung and Blood Institute, Bethesda, Maryland

Rabbi Steven A. Moss, Coordinator, Jewish Chaplaincy Services, Memorial Sloan-Kettering Cancer Center; Chaplaincy Supervisor, New York Board of Rabbis; Spiritual Leader, B'nai Israel Reform Temple, Oakdale, New York

Irvine H. Page, M.D., Cleveland Clinic, Cleveland, Ohio

Ramon H. Parilla, Jr., M.D., Washington University School of Medicine, St. Louis, Missouri

Yvonne M. Parnes, R.N.C., B.S., Nurse-Practitioner, Community Health Program of Queens-Nassau, Inc., New Hyde Park, New York

Boris J. Paul, M.D., Clinical Professor (Rehabilitation Medicine and Family Practice), Albany Medical College of Union University; Chief Medical Consultant, Office of Vocational Rehabilitation, New York State Department of Education, Albany, New York

J. Rogers, R.N., Mental Health Consultant, Social and Community Psychiatry Section, Clarke Institute of Psychiatry, Toronto, Ottawa, Canada

Ray H. Rosenman, M.D., Associate Chief, Department of Medicine, Mt. Zion Hospital and Medical Center; Senior Research Physician, Stanford Research Institute, Menlo Park, California; formerly, Associate Director, Harold Brunn Institute, Mt. Zion Hospital, San Francisco, California

Jack B. Rostoker, P.M.I., F.R., F.I., D.O.N.,* Securities Broker, Toronto, Ontario, Canada

H. D. Ruskin, M.D., F.A.C.P., Professor of Clinical Medicine, State University of New York at Stony Brook; Director, Cardiac Work Evaluation Unit, South Nassau Communities Hospital, Oceanside, New York; Director, Coronary Care Unit, Lydia E. Hall Hospital, Freeport, New York

Aaron B. Shaffer, M.D., Clinical Associate Professor of Medicine, Abraham Lincoln School of Medicine, University of Illinois, Chicago, Illinois

Lillie M. Shortridge, R.N., Ed.D., Assistant Professor, Department of Family Health Care Nursing, University of California, San Francisco, California

*Past Myocardial Infarct, Fully Rehabilitated, Fully Involved, Dependent on No One

M. L. S. Vachon, R.N., Ph.D., Research Scientist, Social and Community Psychiatry Section, Clarke Institute of Psychiatry; Assistant Professor, Department of Psychiatry, University of Toronto, Ottawa, Canada

Jan van Eys, Ph.D., M.D., The Mosbacher Professor of Pediatrics, The University of Texas System Cancer Center, M.D. Anderson Hospital and Tumor Institute, Houston, Texas

Roger R. Williams, M.D., Assistant Professor of Internal Medicine, Cardiology Division, University of Utah Medical Center, Salt Lake City, Utah

Raphael L. Wittstein, Heart Club Founder, Long Island, New York

Stewart G. Wolf, Jr., M.D., Professor of Medicine, Temple University School of Medicine, Philadelphia, Pennsylvania; Vice President for Medical Affairs, St. Luke's Hospital, Bethlehem, Pennsylvania

Irving S. Wright, M.D., M.A.C.P., F.R.C.P. (London), Emeritus Clinical Professor of Medicine, Cornell University Medical College, New York, New York; Past President, American College of Physicians; Past President, American Heart Association; Past President, American Geriatrics Society

Columbia University Press / Foundation of Thanatology Series

Teaching Psychosocial Aspects of Patient Care
Bernard Schoenberg, Helen F. Pettit, and Arthur C. Carr, editors

Loss and Grief: Psychological Management in Medical Practice
Bernard Schoenberg, Arthur C. Carr, David Peretz, and Austin H. Kutscher, editors

Psychosocial Aspects of Terminal Care
Bernard Schoenberg, Arthur C. Carr, David Peretz, and Austin H. Kutscher, editors

Psychosocial Aspects of Cystic Fibrosis: A Model for Chronic Lung Disease
Paul R. Patterson, Carolyn R. Denning, and Austin H. Kutscher, editors

The Terminal Patient: Oral Care
Austin H. Kutscher, Bernard Schoenberg, and Arthur C. Carr, editors

Psychopharmacologic Agents for the Terminally Ill and Bereaved
Ivan K. Goldberg, Sidney Malitz, and Austin H. Kutscher, editors

Anticipatory Grief
Bernard Schoenberg, Arthur C. Carr, Austin H. Kutscher, David Peretz, and Ivan K. Goldberg, editors

Bereavement: Its Psychosocial Aspects
Bernard Schoenberg, Irwin Gerber, Alfred Wiener, Austin H. Kutscher, David Peretz, and Arthur C. Carr, editors

The Nurse as Caregiver for the Terminal Patient and His Family
Ann M. Earle, Nina T. Argondizzo, and Austin H. Kutscher, editors

Social Work with the Dying Patient and the Family
Elizabeth R. Prichard, Jean Collard, Ben A. Orcutt, Austin H. Kutscher, Irene Seeland, and Nathan Lefkowitz, editors

Home Care: Living with Dying
Elizabeth R. Prichard, Jean Collard, Janet Starr, Josephine A. Lockwood, Austin H. Kutscher, and Irene B. Seeland, editors

Psychosocial Aspects of Cardiovascular Disease: The Life-Threatened Patient, the Family, and the Staff
James Reiffel, Robert DeBellis, Lester C. Mark, Austin H. Kutscher, and Bernard Schoenberg, editors

DATE DUE